Unusual Conditions That Every Orthopaedic Surgeon Should Know

Wilhelm A. Zuelzer • Sreenivasulu Metikala
Editors

Unusual Conditions That Every Orthopaedic Surgeon Should Know

A Case-Based Guide

Springer

Editors
Wilhelm A. Zuelzer
Orthopaedic Surgery
Virginia Commonwealth University
Medical School
Richmond, VA, USA

Sreenivasulu Metikala
Orthopaedic Surgery
Virginia Commonwealth University
Medical School
Richmond, VA, USA

ISBN 978-3-031-58945-4 ISBN 978-3-031-58946-1 (eBook)
https://doi.org/10.1007/978-3-031-58946-1

This Springer imprint is published by the registered company Springer Nature Switzerland AG
The registered company address is: Gewerbestrasse 11, 6330 Cham, Switzerland

This book is dedicated to Willhelm Zuelzer, MD, my father, who I have tried to honor all my life.

—Willhelm Zuelzer, Jr MD

Dedicated to my wife, Reddy Prathyusha Soma - my best friend and honest critic.

—Sreenivasulu Metikala, MD

Foreword

With great pleasure, I write this foreword to *Unusual Conditions that Every Orthopaedic Surgeon should Know*. The editors have made a comprehensive study of unusual, rare, odd, and frequently missed conditions over the course of their career. With great passion, they have taught residents and colleagues about these "Zebra" conditions that we all seem to encounter in practice. It is essential to know about the unusual and odd presentations of conditions that we encounter so that we can provide the finest quality of care in a timely manner to our patients. Recognition of the unusual condition and appropriate treatment is essential and helps to differentiate the good surgeon from a great one.

This text covers many unusual conditions that most of us will see once or twice during a career. Some are little bit more frequent such as allergic reactions to commonly used drugs and antiseptics, whereas others are much rarer in the typical orthopaedic surgeon's practice. Recognition of problems such as necrotizing fasciitis, epidural hematoma, adrenal insufficiency, or popliteal entrapment syndrome are essential to prevent severe harm or death to our patients. Other problems such as Ogilvie syndrome and hyponatremia are more common in the postop period. Some of the chapters offer an opportunity to save the patient's life during the care and need to be kept in mind when assessing a patient in an emergent situation pre- or postoperatively.

Reading and learning more about these unusual conditions will make the owner of this book a better orthopaedic surgeon. When you see these unusual conditions, remember their presentation and management, and make a positive intervention in your patient's life at that moment. I enthusiastically recommend reading, learning, and retaining this information for the benefit of your patients. The editors have done a tremendous service to the orthopaedic profession by producing this fine book and are to be commended on an excellent job writing their individual chapters. A tremendous amount of work goes into producing a text such as this, and I hope that the reader enjoys and appreciates the effort that has gone into it.

Department of Orthopaedic Surgery
Virginia Commonwealth University
Richmond, VA, USA

Stephen Kates

Preface: "Little Things"

I remember, many years ago, arranging for an orthopaedic surgeon, who was retiring, to talk to the residents about lessons learned during his 40 years of practicing medicine. Virtually no one paid attention to his talk. No one asked questions. Maybe it could have been better organized, but my sense is that the audience did not engage. The audience did not want to look backwards, or even look forward, but was more interested in what was happening "now." Dealing with "now" is hard enough, and reflecting takes energy and may divert focus. Energy conservation is a priority, because the residents and faculty are often overwhelmed. They often have poor sleep and exercise habits. They have critical relationships to satisfy, including their significant others, children, leaders, patients, and family of patients. They also need to be kind to themselves.

We live in a world where errors will occur, including the ones we make, and we typically use weak defense mechanisms, such as denial. Orthopaedists often talk about the stress of constantly have to be on guard for another disaster, another failure, and another angry patient or leader. I wished I had reflected early in my career, rather than sailing through the stresses. It would have been much better if I actually organized myself proactively. Reflection is not a little thing. It is in this spirit that I am asking for your attention.

We freely admit to being imperfect. And we have the burden of having a patient allow us to inflict hopefully temporary pain and disability, at great expense, on them. What an incredible honor! To justify this honor, we must deal with our imperfections. It took me many years to conclude that to justify this honor we must commit ourselves to being a relentless improvement machine. We will never be perfect, but in order to look in the mirror and answer the question whether we are good enough for this honor, we must honestly reflect on what we do, reflect on what others do with empathy, and again, for emphasis, be thoroughly honest. Agree that to err is human, but to improve is divine. It allows us to be kinder to ourselves. Kinder to others. Transparency and mutually addressing opportunities for improvement is a much better way to enjoy this profession. Be part of a system that relentlessly learns and improves. Do not hide your learning. Have everyone else participate in an honest, appropriately kind, review of events that should not be repeated, and outcomes that should not be. Learning from each other ultimately increases the return exponentially.

We have participated in marvelous changes in patient care. We have refined our technology and can accomplish surgical tasks that are truly amazing. Placing patient in traction is now rare. We have a large variety of tools in our shed to stabilize fractured bones and soft tissue injuries. The changes in surgical care are truly amazing. Learning techniques and selecting appropriate implants have their own set of challenges. The surgical options dominate our meetings. And how to bill. And more recently how to avoid and deal with burnout.

In the spirit of the relentless improvement machine, we need to address the issue of knowing the patient—not just the fracture or the arthritic joint or nerve injury which needs to be addressed. To minimize risks and reduce preventable complications, we must know the patient and the high-risk issues associated with the patient. We must pay attention to details. Many years ago, I heard an attending state that we need to only teach the residents the common things—the things they will most likely see in private practice. I disagree. The National Organization for Rare Disorders (NORD) estimated that, in the United States, there are more than 7000 rare diseases (defined as less than 200,000 people in the United States) affecting more than 30 million Americans—roughly 10% of the population [1]. In this NORD rare disease database, there are listed necrotizing fasciitis, syphilis, polymyalgia rheumatica, Addison (adrenal insufficiency) disease, and Ogilvie's syndrome. The patients with these conditions will be seeing the Orthopaedic Surgeon. Maybe only once or twice a year. Delay in diagnosis may have a major impact on management of these potentially life-shortening conditions. Cumulatively, the rare diseases and conditions likely cost the United States more than 1 trillion dollars annually [2]. We need to balance the technical skills required for our profession, with engagement of our profession with the entire patient. We should strive to be a musculoskeletal expert, but with roots in being still a physician. Unfortunately, it requires energy and focus. A history and physical examination will need to be more thorough to identify these conditions. Diagnosing these conditions requires re-education. This text must be thorough enough, that if you get through it, you have a good chance of placing the important clues on your long-term memory banks and will try to identify and manage them early. I argue this is much more enjoyable than being blindsided. This is the goal of this book.

You will have a hard time seeing what you do not know. The most cost-effective management of patient is to use technology to confirm your clinical impression [3]. We have seen each of the listed conditions repeatedly, with a variety of outcomes. If you come across a patient with resistant hypotension, without obvious cause, do you think of Addison's disease? You should. Should you worry about hyponatremia preoperatively? Few patients really have a true penicillin allergy, but, potentially, if you change prophylactic antibiotics, infection rates increase with surgical joint replacement. A patient is given a steroid injection in the clinic and has an obvious allergic reaction, and no one really knows what to do. How much epinephrine? Where? This must be hardwired. It will occur in your practice 5 years, 2 months, 3 hours from now. Patients are being sent home the same day or the next day after joint replacement. Do we warn total joint and spine patients about abdominal distension and make sure we minimize anticholinergic medications preoperatively in elderly patient? Do we make sure Ogilvie’s syndrome is appropriately addressed since patients are discharged so soon after surgery? A patient needs anticoagulation prophylaxis for joint replacement and is on antiseizure medication? What anticoagulant should we use? A young woman receives a gunshot and has retained lead. Should she be warned and followed? Methyl methacrylate is increasingly recommended for fixation of joint replacement for geriatric patients with a hip fracture. What complication is associated with usage and how do we minimize the occurrence? A patient presents to hand clinic with wrist synovitis and ataxia and even has personality changes per family. Do we consider syphilis? Do we realize that this terrible plague is on the rise? A New York Times article notes that alpha gal allergy is identified by meat allergy—do we need to change our protocols for surgery if we identify a meat allergy history?

This book should be considered the beginning of a journey. We need many more chapters. We hope other books and articles and educational effort are made to address other unusual conditions that are important. If you engage early in your career with this topic, return on your investment will be staggering. May this text be the beginning of a journey both for the reader and other writers/editors. It hopefully will provide a basis for AI systems to aid our memory banks. The key is to hardwire your vigilance and perform a thorough history and physical; acknowledge the concept that it is hard to see what you do not know. Technology must be a servant to your mind. There is no substitute.

1. National Organization for Rare Disorders at https://rarediseases.org/
2. Garrison S, Kennedy A, et al. The economic burden of rare diseases: quantifying the sizeable collective burden and offering solutions health affairs (Feb 1 2022). doi: 10.1377/forefront.20220128.987667
3. Zuelzer WA. Magnetic imaging and musculoskeletal assessments (A surgeon’s prospective). Top Magn Reson Imaging. 1996;8(1):68–77

Richmond, VA, USA W. Zuelzer
Richmond, VA, USA S. Metikala

Contents

Contributors

Eric Appelbaum, MD Marietta, GA, USA

J. Christian Barrett, MD Division of Hematology/Oncology, Department of Internal Medicine, Virginia Commonwealth University, Richmond, VA, USA

Jaime Bohl, MD Department of Surgery, Virginia Commonwealth University, Richmond, VA, USA

John Butterworth, MD Department of Anesthesiology, Virginia Commonwealth University, Richmond, VA, USA

Laura Carucci, MD Department of Radiology, Virginia Commonwealth University, Richmond, VA, USA

Jaharris Collier, MD Phoenix, AZ, USA

Shaunette Davey, DO Department of Orthopaedic Surgery, Virginia Commonwealth University, Richmond, VA, USA

Departments of Orthopaedic Surgery and Pediatrics, Children's Hospital of Richmond, Virginia Commonwealth University, Richmond, VA, USA

Monika Debkowska, MD Ocean Township, NJ, USA

Nidhi Desai, MD Department of Anesthesiology, Virginia Commonwealth University, Richmond, VA, USA

Neel Dixit, MD Department of Neurology, Virginia Commonwealth University, Richmond, VA, USA

Christopher Doern, PhD, D(ABMM) Department of Pathology, Virginia Commonwealth University, Richmond, VA, USA

Evan Dombrosky, MD Division of Rheumatology, Allergy, and Immunology, Department of Internal Medicine, Virginia Commonwealth University, Richmond, VA, USA

Catherine Dong, MD Department of Emergency Medicine, Virginia Commonwealth University, Richmond, VA, USA

Brady Ernst, MD Department of Orthopaedic Surgery, Virginia Commonwealth University, Richmond, VA, USA

Syeda Farooq, MD Division of Vascular Surgery, Virginia Commonwealth University, Richmond, VA, USA

Jacob Farrar, MD Department of Orthopaedic Surgery, Virginia Commonwealth University, Richmond, VA, USA

Gregory Golladay, MD Department of Orthopaedic Surgery, Virginia Commonwealth University, Richmond, VA, USA

R. Scott Graham, MD Department of Neurosurgery, Virginia Commonwealth University, Richmond, VA, USA

Dallas Hampton, Medical Student Eastern Virginia Medical School, Norfolk, VA, USA

Khalid Hasan, MD Department of Orthopaedic Surgery, Virginia Commonwealth University, Richmond, VA, USA

Callie Herman, Medical Student Campbell University School of Osteopathic Medicine, Lillington, NC, USA

Soobin Kang, MD Morganville, NJ, USA

Emily Kershner, MD Division of Toxicology, Department of Emergency Medicine, Virginia Commonwealth University, Richmond, VA, USA

Victoria Kuester, MD Departments of Orthopaedic Surgery and Pediatrics, Children's Hospital of Richmond, Virginia Commonwealth University, Richmond, VA, USA

Department of Orthopaedic Surgery, Virginia Commonwealth University, Richmond, VA, USA

Daniel Layon, MD Department of Orthopaedic Surgery, Virginia Commonwealth University, Richmond, VA, USA

Wesley Lemons, MD Department of Orthopaedic Surgery, Virginia Commonwealth University, Richmond, VA, USA

Mark Maas, PharmD, BCPS Department of Pharmacy Services, VCU Health System, Richmond, VA, USA

Ritu Madan, MD Division of Endocrinology, Diabetes and Metabolism, Department of Medicine, Virginia Commonwealth University, Richmond, VA, USA

Priyanka Majety, MD Division of Endocrinology, Diabetes and Metabolism, Department of Medicine, Virginia Commonwealth University, Richmond, VA, USA

Meric Mericliler, MD Division of Hematology/Oncology, Virginia Commonwealth University, Richmond, VA, USA

Sreenivasulu Metikala, MD Department of Orthopaedic Surgery, Virginia Commonwealth University School of Medicine, Richmond, VA, USA

Jaime Moore, MD Department of Otolaryngology, Virginia Commonwealth University, Richmond, VA, USA

Sergio Navarrete, MD Department of Anesthesiology, Virginia Commonwealth University, Richmond, VA, USA

Daniel H. Newton, MD Division of Vascular Surgery, Virginia Commonwealth University, Richmond, VA, USA

William Obremskey, MD, MPH, MMHC Department of Orthopaedic Surgery, Vanderbilt University, Nashville, TN, USA

Milan Patel, MD Division of Gastroenterology, Hepatology and Nutrition, Department of Medicine, Virginia Commonwealth University, Richmond, VA, USA

Grace Prince, MD Division of Endocrinology, Department of Medicine, Virginia Commonwealth University, Richmond, VA, USA

Ezoza Rajabaliev, MD Department of Anesthesiology, Virginia Commonwealth University, Richmond, VA, USA

Megan Rajagopal, MD Department of Neurosurgery, Virginia Commonwealth University, Richmond, VA, USA

Julie Reznicek, DO Division of Infectious Disease, Department of Internal Medicine, Virginia Commonwealth University, Richmond, VA, USA

William Rothstein, MD Division of Vascular Surgery and Endovascular Therapy, University of Pennsylvania, Philadelphia, PA, USA

Hannah Ruggles, MD Department of Internal Medicine, Virginia Commonwealth University, Richmond, VA, USA

Jibanananda Satpathy, MD Department of Orthopaedic Surgery, Virginia Commonwealth University, Richmond, VA, USA

Lawrence Schwartz, MD Department of Internal Medicine, Virginia Commonwealth University, Richmond, VA, USA

Shalin Shah, DO Department of Orthopaedic Surgery, Virginia Commonwealth University, Richmond, VA, USA

Matthew S. Smith, MD Department of Orthopaedic Surgery, Virginia Commonwealth University, Richmond, VA, USA

Jacqueline Szilagyi, MD Department of Anesthesia, Virginia Commonwealth University, Richmond, VA, USA

Shilen Thakrar, MD Department of Anesthesiology, Virginia Commonwealth University, Richmond, VA, USA

Madana Mohana Vallem, MD Department of Orthopaedic Surgery, Virginia Commonwealth University, Richmond, VA, USA

Jennifer L. Vanderbeck, MD Department of Orthopaedic Surgery, Virginia Commonwealth University School of Medicine, Richmond, VA, USA

Dirk W. Verheul, MD Department of Orthopaedic Surgery, Virginia Commonwealth University School of Medicine, Richmond, VA, USA

Christopher Wise, MD Division of Rheumatology, Allergy, and Immunology, Department of Internal Medicine, Virginia Commonwealth University, Richmond, VA, USA

Wei Zhao, MD Division of Allergy and Immunology, Department of Pediatrics, Virginia Commonwealth University, Richmond, VA, USA

Wilhelm A. Zuelzer, MD Orthopaedic Surgery, Virginia Commonwealth University Medical School, Richmond, VA, USA

Department of Orthopaedic Surgery, VCUHS, Richmond, VA, USA

Chapter 1
Necrotizing Fasciitis

Victoria Kuester, Julie Reznicek, William Obremskey, and Jacqueline Szilagyi

Clinical Vignettes

Case 1

A 69-year-old male, with no previous medical history, presented to a large academic tertiary care center in 2021 with worsening left thumb pain, swelling and purulent drainage (Fig. 1.1) after a human bite which occurred 2 weeks prior. The bite occurred when another person attempted to bite the thumb off. Within 24 h of the initial incident, the left thumb became erythematous, with clear drainage from the bite wounds. Over the next 48–72 h, the drainage changed color and consistency turning yellow/green and thick. He did not report any fevers or chills. He presented to a community walk-in clinic 1 week after the initial injury, but he was not given any antibiotics at that time. The patient stated that he delayed seeking care because he believed that only "animal bites got infected".

V. Kuester (✉)
Departments of Orthopaedic Surgery and Pediatrics, Children's Hospital of Richmond, Virginia Commonwealth University, Richmond, VA, USA
e-mail: victoria.kuester@vcuhealth.org

J. Reznicek
Division of Infectious Disease, Department of Internal Medicine, Virginia Commonwealth University, Richmond, VA, USA
e-mail: julie.reznicek@vcuhealth.org

W. Obremskey
Department of Orthopaedic Surgery, Vanderbilt University, Nashville, TN, USA
e-mail: william.obremskey@vumc.org

J. Szilagyi
Department of Anesthesia, Virginia Commonwealth University, Richmond, VA, USA
e-mail: jacqueline.szilagyi@vcuhealth.org

W. A. Zuelzer, S. Metikala (eds.), *Unusual Conditions That Every Orthopaedic Surgeon Should Know*, https://doi.org/10.1007/978-3-031-58946-1_1

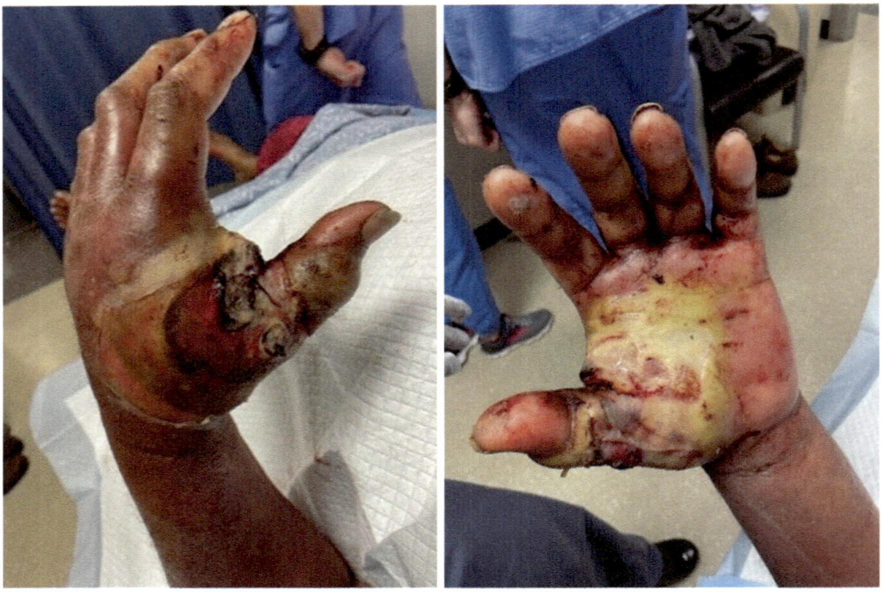

Fig. 1.1 Skin lesions of a patient presenting with NF

He denied illicit drug or tobacco use but did consume one bottle of wine per day. No pets in the home or other animal exposures. He denied any family history of recurrent infections or diabetes mellitus.

On presentation to our Emergency Department at 06:30, he was afebrile and normotensive. His labs were significant for a white blood cell count (WBC) of 13.6 cells/mm^3, erythrocyte sedimentation rate (ESR) of 91 mm/h, C-reactive protein (CRP) of 18.4 mg/dL, lactate of 1.7 mmol/L, and a hemoglobin A1C (HgbA1C) of 8.9%. Radiographs of the left hand showed extensive soft tissue hematoma and laceration and a chronic fracture of the base of the first metacarpal.

Initially, the patient was scheduled for an operative irrigation and debridement (I&D), but throughout the first hospital day, there was rapid progression of this necrotizing infection, as evidenced by increasing pain, swelling and erythema. This prompted emergent operative left upper extremity disarticulation at the wrist joint. Per the operative note, "dishwater pus" was encountered in the carpal tunnel. The tendons of the carpal tunnel were fibrotic and dehydrated in appearance, and the skin and fascia around the wrist and overlying the metacarpal bones were completely necrotic. The amputation site was initially covered with a wound vacuum-assisted closure (VAC). He returned to the operating room 48 h later for a repeat I&D and VAC change, and then required one final surgery on hospital day #8 for revision of the left wrist trans-radial amputation and surgical wound closure.

Two months after the amputation, the patient has recovered very well. He is not experiencing any phantom limb pain and wears a prosthesis daily, allowing him to garden, prepare meals, and perform all of his activities of daily living.

Case 2: Type 2

A 5-year-old female with no other past medical history presented to clinic with a 2-day history of ankle pain and difficulty ambulating after jumping in a puddle. There was no break in the skin, but her father reported a temperature of 100 °F accompanied by worsening pain at home. Upon arrival in clinic, her temperature was found to be 103.1 °F, and she appeared lethargic. On exam, she had no obvious wounds, but displayed exquisite tenderness along the lateral aspect of the distal fibula and mild erythema. Her labs were as follows: WBC of 40.6 × 10^9/L, HGB of 11.7 g/dL, CRP of 5.9 mg/dL H, Na of 131 mmol/L. An initial ultrasound did not show any drainable fluid collection, but raised concern for possible cellulitis, therefore she was started on clindamycin.

Overnight, she began to experience high fevers and worsening redness of her leg up to her knee. Blood cultures drawn that evening came back positive for MRSA. An emergent MRI was then performed (see Fig. 1.2 below), which showed fluid tracking up most of the fascial planes all the way to the knee circumferentially. She was taken emergently to the OR for debridement along both sides of the leg up to the knee with all fascial compartments being opened. Purulence was found around the fibula and murky fluid tracked all along the tissue planes medially and laterally from

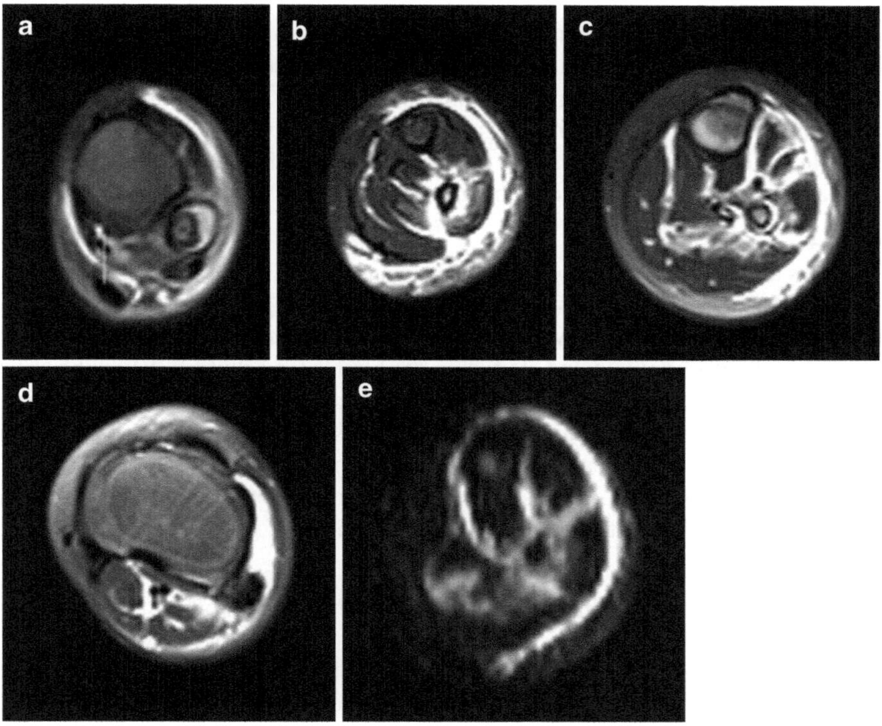

Fig. 1.2 MRI axial views. (**a**) T2 FS distally, (**b**) T2 FS distal third, (**c**) T2 FS proximal third, (**d**) T2 FS proximally, (**e**) post contrast middle of leg

the ankle to knee joint with partially devitalized peroneal musculature. Incisions were made from the foot to the knee both medially and laterally and all compartments opened. She was placed on Vancomycin and Clindamycin for 1 week and then remained on Vancomycin for 14 days from negative blood cultures. She took oral clindamycin for another week.

Following surgery, she was initially placed on the floor, however, she was brought to the PICU for closer monitoring due to her tachycardia and low oxygen saturation. She was supported in the PICU with fluids but did not need intubation. At her second debridement, she had some more debridment of devitalized tissue over the gastric and soleus muscle bellies, and after four debridements, her skin was closed. Fortunately, she recovered with permanent residuals in the involved leg.

Case 3: Type 2

A 55-year-old male patient with type 2 diabetes presented with worsening bilateral leg pain, malaise, and fevers 4 days after bricks fell on him. Initially, he was alert, but tachypneic and his vitals were T 97.4, HR 126, BP 109/65, R 22 and oxygen saturation at 90%. His left thigh had ecchymosis with one bullous lesion and the right leg had a smaller area of ecchymosis, but rapidly got worse. (See Image 5). His initial labs were WBC 17,000, HCT 54, CO_2 9, Cr 2.73, and glucose 265. He deteriorated clinically with altered mental status, hypotension requiring Levophed and respiratory failure requiring intubation. He was placed on Zosyn and Vancomycin and General Surgery was consulted. He was brought to the OR emergently after consultation within 1 h of intubation to excise all of the deep tissue affected by necrotizing fasciitis but the entire extremity was necrotic. As the surgeon performed a hip disarticulation in an attempt to save his life he was stuck with the electrocautery. He removed his gloves, washed the wound and scrubbed back in. In the following days the patient succumbed to the infection.

Case 4

Ten days afterward, the surgeon for case 3 began to feel ill and fatigued. He noticed some increasing redness on his foot and right thigh (see Fig. 1.3). The redness began to progress quickly while he was getting his total hip checked for a possible site of infection. He was admitted and started on antibiotics for cellulitis or lymphangitis and became critically ill. The surgeon was then taken to the OR where necrotizing fasciitis was found spreading from his foot to his groin and he developed toxic shock syndrome with renal and liver failure. He went to the operating room multiple times over the next week. He also received high dose steroids. He then began to improve and later was extubated on day 8. He survived.

Case 5—Type 2

A 21 y/o male, with a past medical history of a splenic vein thrombosis, was admitted to a large academic tertiary care center with a 5-day history of worsening left ankle pain. The pain began after he "twisted" his ankle while playing basketball. One day after the injury, he presented to a local hospital where he was diagnosed with an ankle sprain and given crutches. He returned to this same hospital 48 h later because of worsening left ankle pain, new right wrist pain and bilateral shoulder

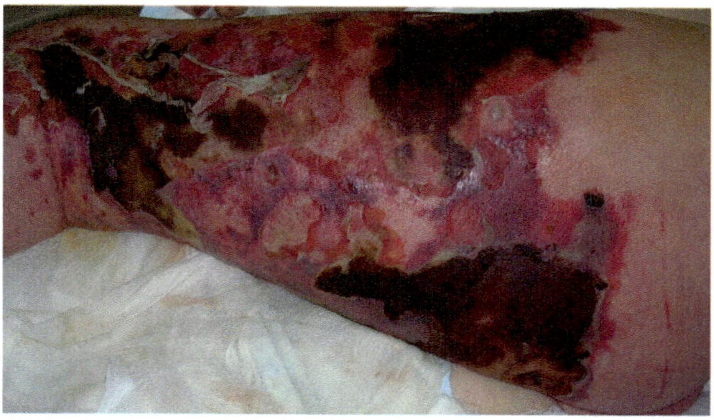

Fig. 1.3 Lower extremity of 55 year old (permission from Dr. Obremskey)

pain. These new symptoms were attributed to the use of crutches. Over the next 48 h, he developed fevers, severe diarrhea, and peeling of his lips. He sought out care at an Urgent Care center and another Emergency Room; both sent him home with supportive treatment.

On admission, he was afebrile (37.3 °C), tachycardic (heart rate 115) and hypotensive (blood pressure 92/55). Laboratory evaluation revealed an elevated white blood cell (WBC) count of 19.2 cells//mm^3, erythrocyte sedimentation rate (ESR) of 37 mm/h, C-reactive protein (CRP) of 25.6 mg/dL, lactate of 3.8 mmol/L, and a creatinine kinase (CPK) of 1289. On examination, he had a very large vesicle on the lateral aspect of the left ankle and evolving vesicles on the posterior ankle (see Fig. 1.4 below). There was also extensive erythema from the left ankle to the knee. This area was exquisitely tender to palpation. He also had swelling of both deltoid areas with fluctuance palpated over the right deltoid muscle. His right forearm (dorsal) felt tense as well.

Given the concern for necrotizing fasciitis, he was emergently taken to the operating room for irrigation and debridement with fasciotomies of the left lower extremity, right forearm, right lateral shoulder, and left lateral shoulder. Murky fluid was encountered in the right forearm and left lower leg. Purpura was seen along the posterior compartment fascia of the left lower leg. The surgical team also noted progressive vesicles of the lateral left lower leg in comparison to the examination that was performed 1 h prior. He returned to the operating room for six additional debridements. Blood cultures from admission as well as intraoperative cultures from the left lower extremity and right forearm were all positive for Group A Streptococcus.

The patient initially required pressor support and intubation. He was started on broad spectrum antibiotics which were eventually de-escalated to clindamycin and cefazolin after culture results returned. He was also given 3 days of intravenous immunoglobulin (IVIG).

After this 19-day hospitalization, he went to a rehabilitation center for 1 week and subsequently recovered.

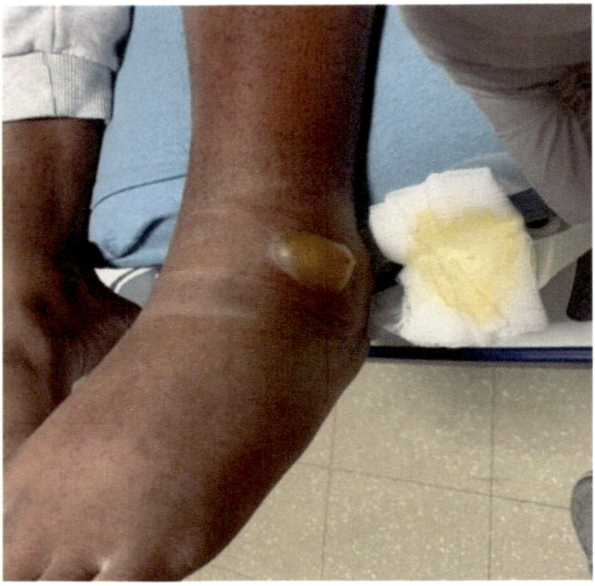

Fig. 1.4 Image of Case 5 at presentation

Questions

1. What role do imaging modalities have in the diagnosis of necrotizing fasciitis?
2. Which laboratory values are included in the LRINEC score?
3. What are some common risk factors for the development of necrotizing fasciitis?
4. Is Fournier's Gangrene classified as a Type 1 or 2 necrotizing fasciitis?

Introduction

Necrotizing Fasciitis (NF) is a potentially life-threatening soft tissue infection characterized by rapid disease progression and extensive necrosis of the fascia and subcutaneous tissue [1]. NF is one of the most challenging infections faced by surgeons, because it is rare and lacks early, pathognomonic signs. Most often, patients with NF present with symptoms of sepsis, systemic toxicity, or evidence of skin inflammation with pain that is disproportionate to the degree of swelling [2]. Because clinical manifestations range from a fulminant presentation to a subtle and insidious development, it can be extremely difficult to diagnose. Diagnosis of NF is further impeded because infection progresses below the surface and cutaneous manifestations are late and accordingly disguise the severity of the disease. Without treatment, NF can lead to systemic toxicity, amputation of the affected extremity, and loss of life [2, 3]. As a result, patient survival requires a high index of suspicion, early detection, and immediate, aggressive treatment by physicians.

Standard treatment of NF infection involves broad-spectrum antibiotics, surgical debridement, and supportive care. Frequently, multiple surgical debridements are required [4]. Even with optimal treatment, NF infections result in significant morbidity and also a mortality rate of up to 35% [3].

This chapter discusses the epidemiology, etiology, causative organisms, and pathophysiology of NF. It then outlines the clinical presentation, diagnosis, and treatment of the disease, placing particular emphasis on achieving better patient outcomes through early diagnosis and treatment.

Epidemiology

NF is relatively rare with an incidence of approximately 1000 new cases per year reported in the United States [5]. The incidence of NF has increased in recent years, perhaps due to better disease reporting, increased population morbidity with obesity and diabetes or increased microbial virulence and resistance as a result of increased antibiotic use [6, 7]. Mortality rates from NF infections are estimated to be between 12–35% and are largely dependent upon timing and adequacy of debridement, with a significant increase in mortality when surgery is delayed for greater than 24 h [8]. Approximately 20% of NF cases result in amputations and 30% result in permanent functional limitations [9].

NF also occurs in children and is frequently misdiagnosed. Several features differ from those of NF in adults. Risk factors for NF in the pediatric population include malnutrition and skin infections, such as varicella. In addition, immunosuppression is the most significant risk factor associated with a fatal outcome [2, 5, 10]. It is important to emphasize that physicians should not rule out NF in normal healthy patients including children with minor dermatologic trauma.

Etiology

NF infection can present in any area of the body and requires proliferation with a causal bacteria in the subcutaneous tissue. Causal bacteria can come from hematogenous or inoculation via a break in the epithelial or mucosal. In many cases, the initiating factor may be as minor as an insect bite or scratch, which the patient may fail to mention [11]. Examples of reported precipitating events are listed in Table 1.1 [2, 11]. Inoculation with causative microbes may also occur via hematogenous spread to sites of nonpenetrating trauma (e.g. muscle strain), as suggested in the case of patients with streptococcal NF [12]. In many cases, NF has been reported without any known trauma [13].

Table 1.1 Precipitating events leading to necrotizing fasciitis

Surgery
Minor invasive procedures such as joint aspirations
Acupuncture
Use of intravenous drugs
Penetrating injuries such as insect or animal bites
Soft tissue infection
Contusions
Closed or open fractures
Hematomas
Burns

Puvanendran, R., Huey, J. C., & Pasupathy, S. (2009). Necrotizing fasciitis. *Canadian family physician Medecin de famille canadien*, *55* (10), 981–987

Microbiology and Risk Factors

Necrotizing skin infections can be classified into four groups based on the type of bacteria present in the infection. In addition to different microbial etiologies, each class has differences in presentation, patient demographics, and risk factors. Known risk factors for all types of NF are listed in Table 1.2 [11].

Type I Infections

Type I NF, also known as synergistic, or subacute NF is responsible for 80% of all NF cases [9]. These infections are polymicrobial and caused by a combination of gram-positive cocci, gram-negative rods, and typically at least one anaerobic species. Commonly isolated pathogens include: non-group A *Streptococcus species*, *Klebsiella* species, *Escherichia coli* and *Bacteroides* species [6]. In addition, Pseudomonas has been isolated in approximately one-fourth of microbiologically confirmed cases [14].

Type I infections commonly affect the perineum and trunk or a chronic diabetic foot wound and tend to run an initial indolent course. It may take several days for symptoms to appear fully, but may begin to rapidly progress or cause the patient to become septic. Patients who present with these infections tend to be older and have multiple medical comorbidities such as diabetes mellitus and peripheral vascular disease [2].

An example of a type I infection is NF of the perineum, which is more commonly referred to as Fournier's Gangrene. This infection originates from bacteria of the skin, colon, anus, and rectum and frequently involve anaerobes and species such as *E. coli, Klebsiella,* and *Enterococci* [2]. Diabetes is a major risk factor for Fournier's gangrene, but NF can also occur after vasectomy in adults or in neonates with

Table 1.2 Risk factors for the development of necrotizing fasciitis

Cirrhosis
Diabetes
Immunosuppression
Advanced age (>60)
Steroid use
Renal failure
Peripheral vascular disease
Underlying malignancy Pregnancy
Childbirth
IV Drug abuse
Malnutrition
Obesity

Davoudian, P. & Flint, N. J. (2012). Necrotizing fasciitis. *Continuing Education in Anaesthesia Critical Care & Pain*, *12*(5), 245–250.

omphalitis or following circumcision [15, 16]. Fournier's gangrene affects men overwhelming more than women [17].

Type II Infections

Type II infections account for approximately 15% of cases and are usually monomicrobial and caused by gram-positive organisms [8]. Compared to type I infections, type II infections are initially more insidious, but progress far more rapidly [18]. The most common type II NF is usually caused by group A beta-hemolytic Streptococcus (GAS) alone or infrequently with *Staphylococcus aureus* [2]. Type II infections tend to occur on the extremities, but also can arise on the trunk [3]. Patients who present with type II infections are typically young, previously healthy, and immunocompetent. These patients may have a history of recent trauma, laceration, burn, surgery, or IV drug use [19–21]. However, in many cases, the disease may appear to have arisen spontaneously. In these cases, the infection is usually perpetuated via hematogenous spread from foci such as the throat, ascending vaginitis, primary peritonitis, or necrotizing proctitis. Initial symptoms in these cases are typically ascribed to influenza, gastroenteritis, muscle strain, or a minor sporting injury in athletes, thus delaying the diagnosis of NF [18]. In approximately 50% of cases, necrotizing infections caused by GAS can also be associated with toxic shock syndrome [22].

Although previously an uncommon cause of NF, community-acquired methicillin-resistant *S. aureus* (MRSA) is an emerging pathogen in type II infections [23]. Within the past five years there has been an increasing incidence of MRSA in IV drug users, athletes, and institutionalized patients. MRSA is now cultured in up to 40% of NF infections [6].

Type III Infections

Type III infections account for less than 5% of NF cases and are caused by gram-negative estuarine or marine organisms [9]. These infections are predominantly acquired through an open wound or break in the skin and the causative pathogen can vary based on what type of water (e.g. fresh, brackish, salt) the individual was exposed to. They can also be acquired by consuming or handling raw or undercooked seafood or injury by fish fins or fish hooks [24]. Instances of type III NF are typically reported along warm water coastal regions in the US, Central and South America, and Asia [3]. The major microorganism associated with saltwater infections is *Vibrio vulnificus*. Mono-microbial gram-negative non-vibrio NF is rare, but does happen with *Pasteurella multocida, Haemophilus influenzae, Shewanella* spp.*, and Aeromonas hydrophila.* Infections caused by freshwater exposure are usually caused by *Aeromonas hydrophila* [25]. The biggest risk factors for type III NF are advanced age, chronic hepatitis B, alcoholism, and liver cirrhosis [26].

It is important to note that type III NF, while rare, presents with a fulminant course which leads to septicemia and multisystem organ failure within 24 h of infection. If not detected early and treated aggressively, the mortality rate is 100% [5].

Type IV Infections

Although rare, Type IV NF can be seen in severe burn, trauma, or immune-compromised patients. This type of NF is caused by fungal infections including: *aspergillus, zygomycetes*, and in rare cases *candida* spp. [5]

Pathology

The underlying pathophysiology of NF is similar among all types. However, the clinical features and speed of disease progression differ depending upon the causal organism. The primary site of pathology for NF infections is the superficial fascia. Typically, NF infections begin innocuously after minor trauma to the skin or spread from the colon, rectum, anus, or another perforated visceral surface [27]. Bacteria then invade subcutaneous tissue, producing endotoxins, exotoxins, and enzymes such as hyaluronidase, which cause the infection to spread rapidly and lead to tissue ischemia, liquefactive necrosis, and systemic illness. Underlying infections may progress as rapidly as one inch per hour with innocuous changes to the outer layers of skin [6].

In NF infections, some organisms such as *Staphylococcus aureus* and *Streptococcus Group A* develop M-1 and M-3 proteins, which serve to improve the pathogens' ability to adhere to tissue and evade phagocytosis. In addition, bacterial pathogens frequently produce exotoxins A, B, C, Streptolysin O, and superantigens. Production of exotoxins can make pathogens more virulent and increase the rate of infection. Exotoxins A and B damage endothelium, compromise microvascular integrity, and exit blood vessels, causing tissue edema and reduced capillary blood flow. Toxins A, B, and streptolysin O, trigger the production of cytokines by CD4 cells and macrophages. Production of the Th1 cytokine leads to the formation of TNF alpha and can eventually aid in the development of myonecrosis. In addition, massive cytokine release produces a systemic inflammatory response syndrome (SIRS) which may progress to septic shock, multisystem organ failure, and loss of life [18].

The key feature of the pathophysiology of NF is thrombosis of perforating vessels of the skin and subcutaneous tissue. An inexperienced surgeon might not recognize the seriousness or extent of infection based on examination of the skin alone. The extent of infection is usually much larger than what is evidenced by skin findings alone because thrombosis of large numbers of vast dermal capillary beds must occur before skin changes reflecting necrosis arise. Thrombosis in NF patients is the result of the local hypercoagulable state, platelet-neutrophil plugging of vessels, and increased interstitial pressure. These three factors combined contribute to decreased capillary blood flow to end tissues and result in tissue ischemia [6]. Superantigens stimulate T cells directly, activating the complement system, the bradykinin-kallikrein system, and the coagulation cascade, thereby worsening small vessel thrombosis and tissue ischemia [18].

Tissue ischemia prevents oxidative destruction of bacteria by polymorphonuclear cells, which eventually become lysed producing a classic 'dishwater fluid.' Further, tissue ischemia prevents adequate delivery of antibiotics, therefore, antibiotic therapy alone does not provide much value. Surgical debridement is crucial for the treatment of NF infections [18].

Pathology of NF Disease Progression

Migration of infection results from rapid bacterial multiplication within viable tissue. Fibrous attachments between subcutaneous tissues and fasciae limit spread to areas like the hands, feet, and scalp. However, a lack of fibrous attachments in the trunk and limbs, leaves the potential for widespread infection and tissue damage. NF can also spread to venous and lymphatic channels, resulting in edema [28]. As mentioned previously, the spread of bacteria results in thrombosis of blood vessels in dermal papilla, resulting in ischemia and gangrene of subcutaneous fat and dermis. As more blood vessels become occluded and nerves become infarcted, patients typically experience progressive skin ischemia and a worsening, "crescendo" pain, which is similar to pain from compartment syndrome of an extremity. The skin is essentially becoming ischemic [18]. If the infection reaches the muscle, myositis occurs. Gas-producing organisms can lead to the formation of gas within the tissues but is not required or present in the majority of infections [2].

As NF infections progress, an increasing number of nutrient vessels become occluded, resulting in worsening ischemia and producing more visible manifestations. Without treatment, infections continue to spread beneath apparently healthy skin in a horizontal manner, progressively leading to bullae formation, ulceration, and finally, skin necrosis [27, 29]. The following pathway in Fig. 1.5 shows the pathogenesis and clinical findings of necrotizing fasciitis.

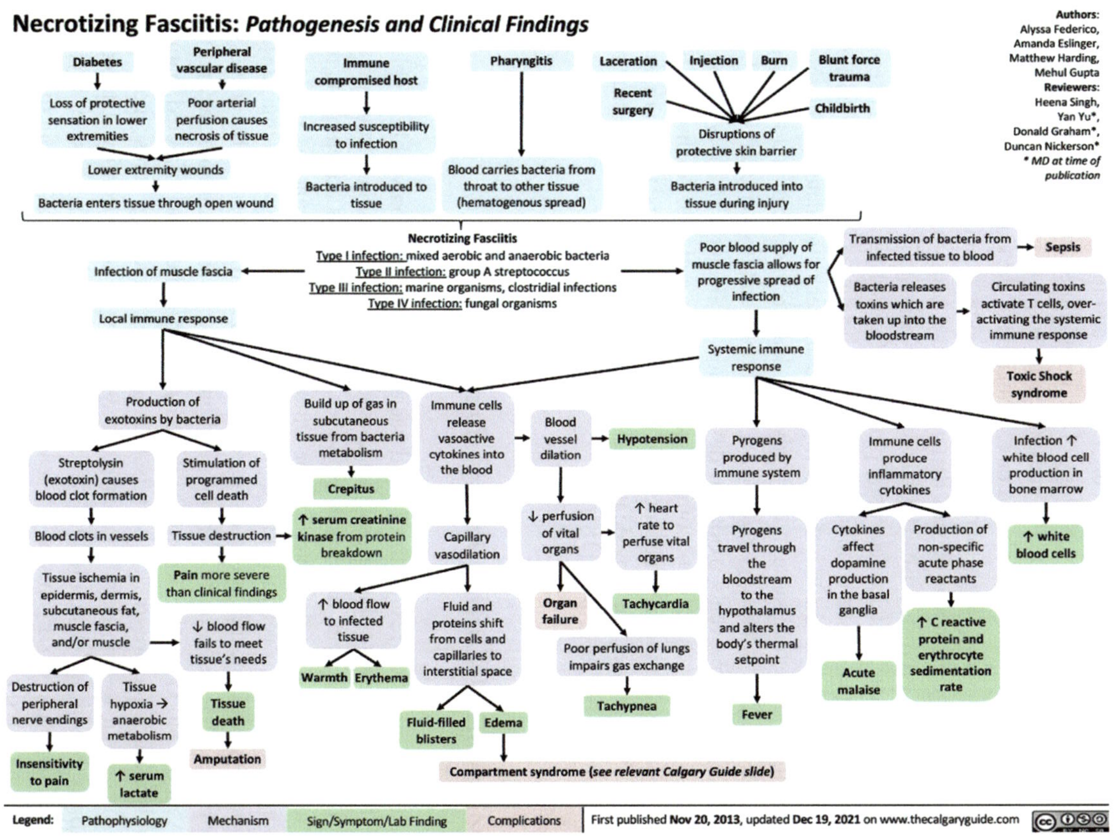

Fig. 1.5 Pathogenesis and clinical findings of necrotizing fasciitis. [Reproduced with permission from The Calgary Guide to Understanding Disease, a collaborative student/faculty project of the University of Calgary. For this, and other materials which illuminate the connection between pathophysiology and clinical manifestation of disease, visit www.thecalgaryguide.com]

Clinical Manifestations

NF manifests in a variety of ways making it extremely difficult to recognize and diagnose. It has been shown that only 10–40% of patients present with a 'classic' history of rapidly worsening pain related to trauma or a break in the skin within 48 h of symptom onset [6]. Although it can affect any region or part of the body, NF is most often seen in the extremities (lower extremities more commonly than upper extremities), perineum, and genitalia. These infections typically present acutely over the course of a few hours, but have also been known to present sub-acutely, taking several days to develop [3]. Due to the potential for extensive tissue destruction, systemic toxicity, amputation, and death, early recognition of NF is crucial.

Although some patients present with little or no pain, the most critical early distinctive symptom of NF is a disproportionate level of pain as compared to physical findings. These patients will be in severe pain, but they occasionally display only mild erythema or swelling over the affected area. Further, because NF initially affects the subcutaneous tissue, these patients experience tenderness and pain that commonly extends far beyond the apparent site of infection [6]. Pain assessment may be more difficult in the post-operative patient, further complicating the diagnosis.

Unlike cellulitis, where the infection begins at the junction between the dermis and superficial fascia, in NF, the infection starts at the level of subcutaneous fat and deep fascia. As a result, the subcutaneous tissue in patients infected with NF can be firm and indurated, such that the underlying muscle groups cannot be palpated distinctly [29]. Because the epidermal and dermal layers are spared in the early stages of infection, erythema and edema of skin are not obvious, making it difficult to discern the extent of infection clinically.

Subcutaneous gas is often present in the polymicrobial (type I) form of necrotizing fasciitis, particularly in patients with diabetes. See Fig. 1.6 for an example seen on plain film. Although crepitus or skin necrosis is often taught to be a hallmark symptom of NF infection, a study by Sarani and colleagues showed that it was present in only 13–31% of patients [6].

In addition to pain that is out of proportion to physical exam findings, the other most common signs of NF include local erythema (72%), swelling (75%), and fever (60%) [30]. In some cases, marked edema may become so severe that it leads to compartment syndrome with complicating myonecrosis requiring fasciotomy. Table 1.3 lists other clinical manifestations frequently observed in cases of NF [2].

In some patients a Group A Strep infection may present solely with systemic symptoms such as fever (102–105 °F), tachycardia, and systemic toxicity. They may also present with hypotension initially or develop hypotension as the infection progresses [5]. Some other common, generalized symptoms that these patients have been reported to experience include: malaise, myalgias, diarrhea, and anorexia (Table 1.3) [2, 30, 31]. These patients require a thorough physical exam to try and elicit a localizing area, especially in cases of non-penetrating trauma.

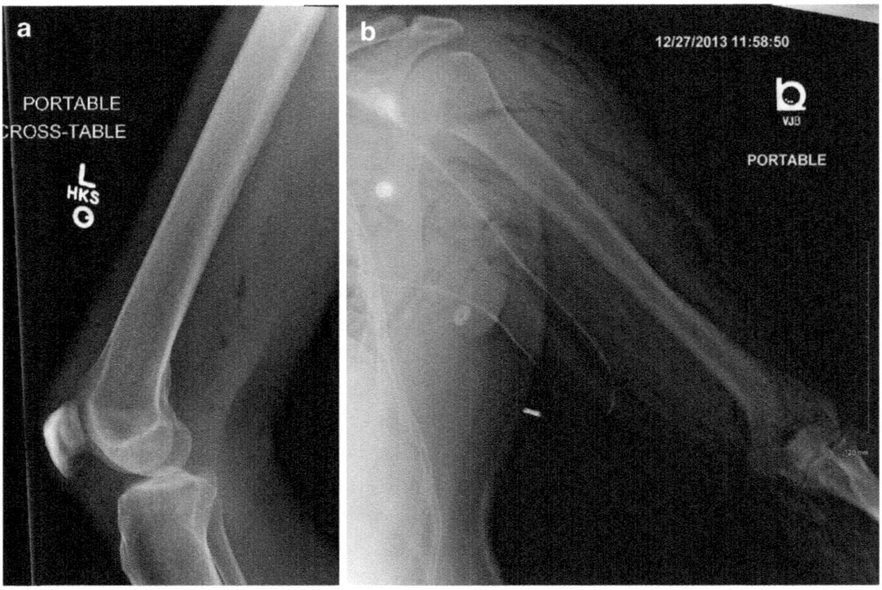

Fig. 1.6 (**a**) X-ray of the left lateral thigh from an adult with NF shows evidence of mild fascial air-tracking. (**b**) X-ray of the left upper extremity from an adult with NF showing extensive subcutaneous and fascial tracking air in a severe case of NF

Table 1.3 Clinical features commonly seen with necrotizing fasciitis

Skin findings	Pain symptoms	General findings	
Erythema	Extends past apparent area of infection	Fever	Anorexia
Edema with gray or brown discharge	Disproportionate to physical findings	Altered mental state	Diarrhea
Vesicles/bullae (may be hemorrhagic)		Tachycardia	Tachypnea
Necrosis		Hypotension	
Crepitus		Myalgia/malaise	
Absence of lymphadenopathy		Presentation with diabetic ketoacidosis or sepsis	

Puvanendran, R., Huey, J. C., & Pasupathy, S. (2009). Necrotizing fasciitis. *Canadian family physician Medecin de famille canadien*, *55* (10), 981–987

The infective process of NF progresses rapidly over several hours or days. Skin color typically changes from reddish-purple to patches of blue-gray. Within 3–5 days of onset, the skin begins to break down and bullae (containing thick pink or purple fluid) can be seen [32]. Blister and bulla formation is a late feature indicating that ischemia of the skin is occurring, resulting in thrombosis of penetrating vessels (see Figs. 1.1 and 1.3 above).

As noted previously, the skin might have a normal appearance in the early stages of disease because the infection tracks subcutaneously. Lymphatics frequently become obstructed; therefore, lymphangitis and lymphadenitis are rare. Patients can develop diminished sensations to pain in the affected area as thrombosis of small blood vessels and destruction of superficial nerves occurs. This may precede the appearance of skin necrosis and provide a clue to the presence of necrotizing fasciitis [32].

The rate of progression of NF can vary. Patients with NF in the later stages of the disease often show symptoms and signs of septic shock, toxic shock syndrome, and multiorgan failure. The following may occur: tachycardia, tachypnoea, fever or hypothermia, hypotension, cardiac arrhythmias, confusion, metabolic acidosis, abnormal renal and liver function, coagulopathy, and thrombocytopenia. These patients carry a high rate of mortality [11].

Staging

In tracking cases of suspected NF, a staging system that correlates with disease progression can be useful. One such staging system, put forth by Wang and colleagues in a retrospective analysis of cutaneous manifestations, is based on the principle that progressive skin ischemia is responsible for development of many clinical features. This system is divided into the following three main stages: [33]

Stage 1 (Early stage) Defined by nonspecific signs such as erythema, tenderness beyond the erythema, swelling, pain beyond the confines of erythema, and hot skin. In this stage, diagnosis is particularly difficult because symptoms often mimic those of cellulitis or erysipelas.

Stage 2 (Intermediate Stage) Defined by the formation of skin bullae, blister, and skin fluctuation. See Fig. 1.4 in Case 5 above.

Stage 3 (Late Stage) Manifests with hemorrhagic bullae, crepitus, skin necrosis/discoloration, skin anesthesia, and gangrene. Patients in late stage may be apathetic and unaware of their surroundings [11, 33].

Laboratory Findings

Laboratory findings in NF patients are generally nonspecific. Abnormalities may include leukocytosis with a left shift, coagulopathy, thrombocytopenia, elevated inflammatory markers [C-reactive protein (CRP) and/or erythrocyte sedimentation rate (ESR)], and elevations in serum creatinine, lactate, creatine kinase (CK), and aspartate aminotransferase (AST) concentrations. Raised serum CK or AST concentrations suggest deep infection involving muscle or fascia (myositis or myonecrosis as opposed to cellulitis). Hypocalcemia is a sign of fat necrosis and calcium deposit in necrotic tissues. Bacterial infection, inflammation, and necrosis cause raised CRP. As in severe sepsis, abnormal renal function, hypoalbuminemia, hyponatremia, abnormal liver function, and metabolic acidosis may occur. It is also possible to see anemia in these patients either from fluid resuscitation or hemolysis [30, 34–36]. As in any severe case of sepsis, disseminated intravascular coagulation may also be seen [37].

Blood cultures are positive in approximately 60% of patients with monomicrobial (type II) NF and are routinely positive in patients with necrotizing myositis [38]. However, the blood culture yield is much lower (as low as 20%) in patients with polymicrobial (type I) NF [8, 20]. In addition, cultures may not reflect all of the organisms involved in polymicrobial infections. Although percutaneous needle aspiration of the advancing edge can be useful, tissue biopsy is preferred. Both tissues and aspirates should be Gram stained and cultured. Fungal culture is recommended in high-risk immunocompromised patients [6, 39].

Diagnosis and Decision for Surgical Exploration

Early recognition of necrotizing infection is critical. Rapid progression to extensive destruction can occur, leading to systemic toxicity, limb loss, and/or death [34, 40, 41]. Due to a wide variety of clinical manifestations, diagnosis is frequently very difficult and incorrect diagnoses or delayed diagnoses can have serious implications. In a large systemic review of over 1400 patients, the rate of misdiagnosis of NF ranged from 41 to 96% (mean 71.4), with most patients being misdiagnosed with cellulitis or abscess [24].

NF should be suspected in patients with soft tissue infection (erythema, edema, warmth) and signs of systemic illness (fever, hemodynamic instability) in association with crepitus, rapid progression of clinical manifestations, and/or severe pain (out of proportion to skin findings in some cases) [5].

Although history and physical examination are important clues that can aid in increasing suspicion of NF, diagnosis of NF is essentially clinical. The gold standard is surgical exploration, during which infected tissue is debrided [3]. When there is clinical suspicion of a NF infection, surgical exploration should not be delayed while awaiting results of radiographic imaging, tissue culture, or other diagnostic information. Tissue biopsy may be obtained during surgery, but it is not required to establish the diagnosis of NF [42].

The diagnosis of necrotizing infection is confirmed upon operative findings that include: dull-gray, swollen, necrotic fascia, easy separation of normally adherent superficial fascia during blunt dissection accompanied by a lack of bleeding, and presence of foul smelling "dishwater" pus [43]. The presence of fascial necrosis and myonecrosis or loss of fascial integrity along tissue planes and evidence of muscle involvement are also diagnostic. In addition to histology, intraoperative specimens should be sent for Gram stain and culture [11].

Blood Culture

Before beginning antimicrobial therapy, two sets of blood cultures should be obtained. Appropriate serum lab testing includes complete blood count with differential, chemistries, liver function tests, creatinine concentration, coagulation studies, creatine kinase concentration, lactate concentration, and inflammatory markers such as C-reactive protein and/or erythrocyte sedimentation rate [30, 34–36, 44, 45].

Finger Test

The finger tissue test can also be used to diagnose NF. This test can be performed by making a 2 cm incision down to the deep fascia of the affected area while the patient is under local anesthesia. The superficial fascia can then be probed and observed for any signs that may be indicative of NF, such as lack of bleeding, presence of dishwater pus, and minimal tissue resistance to finger dissection. If these three things are present, this is considered sufficient to be diagnostic of NF [2, 5].

Frozen Section Biopsy

There is some evidence of improved survival by using frozen section biopsy for early NF detection. Studies by Stamenkovic recommend excision of a 1 cm [3] piece of tissue from an affected site under local anesthesia and immediate frozen section, culture and Gram stain. If the sample comes back positive, the patient should be sent to undergo immediate surgical debridement [46]. An additional study by Majeski and Majeski successfully utilized this procedure to confirm 28% of the NF cases they reviewed, further supporting the use of frozen section biopsy as an effective diagnostic tool [39]. It is important to note that, while effective, this technique would require strong collaboration from pathologists. Also, if patient is septic or in extremis, a biopsy may only delay definitive surgical debridement. Surgeons should err on early surgical exploration over a biopsy if concerned of about NF.

Histology

As mentioned above, deep incisional biopsies and frozen sections with Gram staining of tissues can be diagnostic of NF. When samples are taken, physicians should be sure to include the advancing edge and central necrotic areas. These areas allow for the detection of underlying thrombi, necrosis, polymorphonuclear infiltrates, microorganisms, and vasculitis [11]. Histologic criteria have also been proposed by Majeski and Majeski and include: necrosis of superficial fascia, fibrinous thrombi of arteries and veins coursing through fascia, angiitis and fibrinoid necrosis of arteries and veins, presence of microorganisms within the destroyed fascia and dermis and absence of muscle involvement [39, 47].

Imaging

Radiographic imaging studies can be useful to help determine whether a NF infection is present. However, it is important to realize that imaging is not a definitive diagnostic procedure and therefore it should never delay surgery. Plain films may show gas in the soft tissues which is concerning for necrotizing fasciitis (see Fig. 1.6 below).

Computed tomography (CT) scan, ultrasound, and magnetic resonance imaging (MRI) have all been used to image cases of NF [48]. CT scans are capable of revealing deep fascial thickening and the presence of fluid and gas within soft tissue planes in and around the superficial fascia. Ultrasound identifies features suggestive of thickening, distortion, and fluid collections along the deep fascia. MRI with gadolinium differentiates necrotic and inflamed or edematous tissue. T2-weighted images on MRI are probably the best radiological adjunctive investigation for NF (see Fig. 1.2 in Case 2 above). The best initial radiographic imaging exam is a CT scan [49]. CT scans have a sensitivity of 88.5% and specificity of 93.3% when looking for fascial gas, which is more commonly seen in patients with clostridial infection or polymicrobial (type I) NF [50]. This finding is highly specific for NF and should result in immediate surgical intervention. Other radiographic findings may include fluid collections, absence or heterogeneity of tissue enhancement with intravenous contrast, and inflammatory changes beneath the fascia. MRI is not as useful as CT for detection of gas in soft tissues because it can be overly sensitive, and it has the potential to overestimate deep tissue involvement. Therefore, this imaging technique should not be used to reliably distinguish between necrotizing cellulitis and deeper infection. Ultrasound may be used for detection of localized abscesses and gas in tissues but has not been well studied in necrotizing fasciitis. Frequently, imaging studies demonstrate soft tissue swelling; this finding is not specific since it is not possible to distinguish between swelling caused by infection, trauma, surgery, or inflammation. Therefore, in such cases, the diagnosis of necrotizing infection can be established only by surgical exploration and surgical exploration should not be delayed if patient is deteriorating [51].

Laboratory Scoring Systems for the Prediction of Necrotizing Fasciitis

It is widely known that early operative debridement is a major determinant of patient outcome in NF. However, early recognition and diagnosis is clinically very difficult. In 2004, Wong and colleagues recognized this critical problem and developed the LRINEC (Laboratory Risk Indicator for Necrotizing Fasciitis) scoring system, which is a clinical tool that is designed to distinguish NF from other soft tissue infections. The tool is based on laboratory indicators, including the following six values; white cell count, hemoglobin, sodium, serum glucose, creatinine, and C-reactive protein [52]. Each variable is awarded a certain number of points based upon its independent predictive value for positive diagnosis. The overall LRINEC score is calculated by adding up each of the six predictive factors. A diagram of the LRINEC scoring system is shown in Table 1.4 [11].

Patients with scores of 6 or more, have a positive predictive value of 92% and a negative predictive value of 96%. A score of 8 or more is strongly predictive of NF (positive predictive value of 93.4%) [53]. All these tests are routinely available, and it is easy to enumerate them even in the emergency department. Su et al.

Table 1.4 Laboratory risk indicator for necrotizing fasciitis

Variable	Score
C-reactive protein (mg/L)	
<150	0
≥150	4
WBC (cells/mm^3)	
<15	0
15–25	1
>25	2
Hemoglobin (g/dL)	
>13.5	0
11–13.5	1
<11	2
Sodium (mmol/L)	
≥135	0
<135	2
Creatinine (μg/L)	
≤141	0
>141	2
Glucose (mmol/L)	
≤10	0
>10	1

Davoudian, P. & Flint, N. J. (2012). Necrotizing fasciitis. *Continuing Education in Anaesthesia Critical Care & Pain*, *12*(5), 245–250.

demonstrated that LRINEC score may also indicate outcomes as mortality and amputation rates are higher when the score is >6 [54].

Although the LRINEC was initially noted to have high specificity and negative predictive value, subsequent studies have demonstrated limited sensitivity [29]. Patients who have a score of <6 are considered low risk, but this lower LRINEC value should never completely dismiss the possibility of NF, especially in patients where the clinical presentation is rapidly evolving. In the pioneering study conducted by Wong, 10% of patients with NF had a LRINEC score <6 [20, 52]. Further, the LRINEC remains not validated in larger prospective studies [6]. Therefore, this tool should not be used to rule out NF. It is important to note that if suspicion is high for NF based upon clinical history and physical exam, a LRINEC score should not be calculated or further imaging attained, and surgical care should be initiated immediately.

Clinical factors that may make diagnosis of NSTI difficult include: [30]

- Absence of fever—In some cases, use of NSAIDs can mask the presence of a fever [55].
- Absence of cutaneous manifestations and/or portal of entry—Patients may present with no obvious lesions or superficial signs of infection. In some cases, superficial signs of infection may not appear until later in disease.
- Attribution of pain to alternative causes—Pain may be mistakenly attributed to recent known conditions, such as a previous surgery.
- Nonspecific imaging tests—Imaging may show edema with no gas in the deep tissue, which may confound diagnosis.
- Systemic manifestations may be attributed to other causes—Non-specific symptoms such as nausea, vomiting, and diarrhea may be early manifestations of systemic toxicity due to GAS infection, but may be wrongly attributed to other conditions, such as a nonspecific viral illness.

Differential Diagnosis

Many patients with NF are initially misdiagnosed. Initial misdiagnosis leads to delayed and inappropriate disease management and frequently results in increased morbidity and mortality. Some common differential diagnoses for NF infections are discussed below.

- **Cellulitis**—Cellulitis presents with skin erythema, edema, and warmth. Fever may be present, but cellulitis is generally not associated with hemodynamic instability or exquisite tenderness. Unlike cellulitis, where the infection begins at the junction between the dermis and superficial fascia, in NF, the infection starts at the level of subcutaneous fat and deep fascia. It is because of this sparing of the epidermal and dermal layers in the early stages of the disease that erythema and edema of the skin are not obvious, and so the extent of infection clinically is not clear. Further, lymphadenopathy and lymphangitis are rare in NF, but are often present in cellulitis [56, 57]. Blister or bulla formation is an important, late-occurring feature of NF. In contrast, blistering and bullae are rare findings in cellulitis (see Fig. 1.3). Elevations in serum CK or AST concentrations are also suggestive of deep infection involving muscle or fascia [30, 34–36].

- **Pyoderma gangrenosum**—Pyoderma gangrenosum, an ulcerative, non-infectious skin disorder, may be difficult to distinguish from necrotizing fasciitis. It is important to distinguish between these two diseases because inappropriate surgical debridement of pyoderma gangrenosum can cause extension of the lesion and potential disfigurement. Inappropriate administration of immunosuppressive therapy may worsen necrotizing fasciitis. Typically, pyoderma gangrenosum will have a slower progression and a poor response to antibiotics, but a rapid response to corticosteroids. Distinguishing features are summarized in the Table 1.5 [58–62].
- **Gas gangrene (clostridial myonecrosis)**—Gas gangrene is an invasion of healthy tissue that can arise either spontaneously or after traumatic injury. Like gas gangrene, polymicrobial NF can be associated with gas in the tissues. Gram stain is often used to differentiate between these two diseases. In gas gangrene, the Gram stain typically displays anaerobic gram-positive rods, whereas in necrotizing fasciitis, the Gram stain will be polymicrobial with a mix of both aerobes and anaerobes [63].
- **Pyomyositis**—Pyomyositis can sometimes be confused with necrotizing myositis. However, pyomyositis is generally associated with abscess formation in skeletal muscle, whereas necrotizing myositis is characterized by gangrenous necrosis. In addition, pyomyositis tends to result in less systemic toxicity than necrotizing myositis [64].

Table 1.5 NF vs pyoderma gangrenosum-distinguishing features

NF	Pyoderma gangrenosum
No link to inflammatory bowel disease	Associated with inflammatory bowel disease
Progression is rapid	Progression is slow
May resemble cellulitis	Not similar to cellulitis
Violaceous ulcer edge is not characteristic	Characteristic violaceous edge is often present
Likely to develop sepsis	Sepsis unlikely to occur
Responsive to surgery	Worsens with surgery
Fascial planes are easily dissected	Fascial planes have normal resistance to dissection
Immunosuppressive therapy is detrimental	Immunosuppressive therapy is effective
Responsive to antibiotics (in conjunction with surgery)	Not responsive to antibiotics
Blood and tissue cultures are typically positive	Blood and tissue cultures are typically negative

Bisarya, K., Azzopardi, S., Lye, G., & Drew, P. J. (2011). Necrotizing fasciitis versus pyoderma gangrenosum: securing the correct diagnosis! A case report and literature review. *Eplasty*, *11*, e24.

- **Deep venous thrombosis**—Like NF, deep venous thrombosis (DVT) is characterized by swelling, pain, and warmth around the affected area, typically the extremities. However, the pain in patients with DVT is far less extreme than the pain that patients feel when battling a necrotizing infection. Although fever may be present with a DVT, it is more commonly seen as a manifestation of a contiguous soft tissue infection [65].

Treatment

Treatment of NF requires a combination of aggressive surgical debridement, broad-spectrum antibiotics, and hemodynamic support. It is important to emphasize that NF is a surgical emergency, therefore early debridement is critical. Studies have shown that administration of antibiotic therapy alone, without surgical debridement, is associated with a mortality rate near 100% [66]. The goal of surgical treatment is to aggressively debride all necrotic tissue until healthy, bleeding tissue is present. Debridement should be continued every 24–48 h until no necrotic tissue remains [67]. For severe cases of NF, amputation may be necessary to achieve source control. Empiric treatment of NF should also include broad-spectrum antibiotic therapy with coverage of both aerobes, including MRSA, and anaerobes [66]. Antibiotics should be administered immediately after obtaining blood cultures and should be continued until no further debridement is needed and the patient's hemodynamic status has normalized [68]. NF can be complicated by other infections, such as endocarditis or osteomyelitis. In these cases, the antibiotic duration may be extended for treatment of the non-NF diagnosis.

The recommended empiric antibiotic regimen is a carbapenem (imipenem, meropenem, or ertapenem) or beta-lactam-beta-lactamase inhibitor (piperacillin-tazobactam, ampicillin-sulbactam, or ticarcillin-clavulanate) along with an agent that covers methicillin-resistant S. aureus (MRSA), such as vancomycin or daptomycin. In cases where patients have a hypersensitivity to the preceding beta-lactam-beta-lactamase inhibitors, an aminoglycoside or a fluoroquinolone plus metronidazole may be used. If there is clinical concern for Group A Strep NF, clindamycin should be added for suppression of the streptococcal toxin and cytokine production [69].

In infants and children, the most frequently used empiric antibiotic for MRSA is vancomycin (15 mg/kg/dose every 6–8 h) along with clindamycin for its antitoxin effects (40 mg/kg per day divided every 8 h) The recommended carbapenem for children and infants older than 7 days is meropenem (20 mg/kg per dose every 8 h).

Empiric therapy for patients who experienced trauma in freshwater or seawater and may have been exposed to *Aeromonas* or *V. vulnificus* should include antibiotics with activity against those causative organisms [40, 51, 70–74].

Hemodynamic support—Patients with hemodynamic instability may need supportive care with fluids and vasopressors. In certain cases, especially in cases associated with streptococcal toxic shock syndrome, Intravenous fluids and albumin replacement may be required [30].

Intravenous immune globulin—It is recommended that patients with NF and streptococcal toxic shock syndrome (STSS) be given intravenous immune globulin (IVIG). This recommendation is supported by a recent meta-analysis conducted by Parks et al. that showed that use of IVIG in treating STSS was correlated with nearly 50% decline in mortality at 30 days as compared to the use of clindamycin alone [75, 76].

Surgical Exploration

Indications for/timing and location of initial debridement—Patients with NF may appear well in the early stages of infection. However, because they often deteriorate within hours of presentation, a high index of suspicion of NF is sufficient to initiate surgical exploration [51, 66, 77]. Studies show that failure to recognize the severity of infection and delays in initial debridement, especially those greater than 24 h, are associated with high morbidity and mortality [52, 78, 79].

Because time is critical, whenever possible, initial debridement by an experienced surgeon should take place at the facility where the diagnosis is first suspected. Although immediate transfer to a facility with expertise in managing advanced soft tissue infections may seem appropriate, a comprehensive study conducted by Holena et al. showed that patients debrided at the hospital to which they initially presented had a significantly lower mortality rate (8.7%) than those who were transferred without debridement (15.5%) [80]. After initial debridement, it is recommended that patients be transferred to a tertiary center or similar facility accustomed to caring for infections of this nature [3, 81–84].

Patient optimization—Prior to surgery, without causing a delay in initial debridement, the patient's physiological condition should be optimized in an intensive care setting, where aggressive fluid resuscitation and vasoactive support are available [85].

Antibiotics—If not already started, broad-spectrum antibiotics should be administered and continued intraoperatively and postoperatively until the causative organism(s) are identified from surgical specimens. Empiric antimicrobial therapy should cover both gram-negative and gram-positive microbes, including methicillin-resistant *Staphylococcus aureus*, in conjunction with an anti-ribosomal agent, such as clindamycin, to target potential toxin production by gram-positive organisms. Once the causative organism(s) have been identified, treatment should be tailored accordingly [86].

Informed consent—If possible, informed consent should be obtained from the patient. Given the significant mortality associated with NF, advance care directives may need to be initiated. The urgency and purpose of the initial surgical debridement and the possibility for adjunctive procedures, including amputation and the creation of a stoma, should be discussed with the patient and family.

Debridement procedure

1. Make an initial long extensile incision to include all overtly necrotic skin and extend beyond the apparently involved tissue. If no necrotic skin is evident, make the incision over the area presumed to be the center of the infection.
2. Debride aggressively in a circular pattern beginning with the most severely affected anatomical area and working progressively outward until healthy, bleeding tissue is reached [3]. Because capillary thrombosis precedes skin necrosis, incision through affected areas will not bleed normally. Often the necrotic region is much larger than what is initially expected based upon general physical exam. If diagnosis is early, then no skin may need debridement and incision is extended to fascia and proximally and distally beyond the affected area into more normal tissue. A fasciectomy is not necessary.
3. For the most rapid and effective debridement of large areas, use a #10 scalpel blade and large curved Mayo scissors. For more specialized areas including the face and hands, use a #15 blade and Metzenbaum scissors.
4. Do not consider the subsequent reconstruction. Doing so may result in an incomplete initial debridement, which correlates with an increase in the incidence of septic shock, renal failure, and death.
5. To ensure that debridement is comprehensive, explore the margin and depth of the wound thoroughly. It may be necessary to probe between muscle planes below the fascia. Assess viability of muscles with a cautery to assess if muscle is reactive and viable. Remove all non-viable tissue (skin, fascia and muscle).
6. Early on in debridement, obtain tissue biopsies and cultures from multiple sites and perform histologic tests to identify causative organism(s) and guide antimicrobial treatment. Samples at the margins of the wound should also be taken to ensure that all infected tissue has been removed.
7. Subcutaneous necrosis, polymorphonuclear cell infiltration, fibrinous vascular thrombosis, and the presence of microbes within the destroyed tissue are histologic findings commonly seen in NF patients.
8. Use a broad-spectrum antiseptic solution, such as 0.025% sodium hypochlorite, to thoroughly clean the wound.
9. Debris can be removed by gravity flow or via a water jet debridement system set on low to prevent tissue damage [3, 87].
10. Hemostasis should be achieved via electrocautery. Avoid the use of epinephrine injections in this context because it may compromise the procedure by allowing the infection to spread. If needed, use dilute epinephrine applied topically [88].
11. Upon conclusion of debridement, apply an antiseptic dressing, such as 0.025% sodium hypochlorite or a negative pressure dressing if feasible, to the affected area.

12. Return the patient to the intensive care unit for continued treatment.

Fecal diversion—As many NF infections affect the perineal region, it is sometimes beneficial for patients to undergo a diverting colostomy early on in their course of treatment to decrease the risk of secondary infection from enteric bacteria. Another strategy that is effective for NF cases occurring near the anal verge is the insertion of a rectal diversion device, such as a silicone catheter with a balloon and irrigation port. These devices are less invasive than a diverting colostomy, however, possible complications include rectal erosion and bleeding [89, 90].

Amputation—Approximately 10–20% of NF patients, especially those with comorbidities such as diabetes and peripheral artery disease, may require an amputation [91]. All decisions for amputation should involve a second opinion from another healthcare expert. Amputation should be considered in life threatening cases, if repeated debridements are unlikely to achieve source control, or when no good reconstructive options exist [7, 92–94]. In emergency situations, a guillotine amputation should be performed at a healthy site proximal to the infection. In such cases, it is not necessary to consider creating bone flaps, as the bone is usually shortened to allow for closure.

Need for Additional Debridement—Upon completion of the initial debridement, a subsequent debridement surgery should be scheduled and performed within 24 h. However, if the patient's condition begins to decline, an earlier procedure may be warranted. Lab results can be monitored and may signal the need for earlier or repeat debridement. Multiple debridements may be necessary prior to beginning reconstruction [3, 84, 95]. Two C-reactive protein (CRP), lactate, or procalcitonin (PCT) levels should be obtained and compared to baseline values every 6–8 h. These biomarkers may indicate the severity of infection. PCT most closely correlates with infection severity and aids in determining the course of antibiotic treatment [36, 96].

Wound Care

Dressings—It is important to avoid wound dressings that inhibit mobility, especially in cases that involve the head, neck, and extremities. Negative pressure wound therapy (NPWT) has proven to be effective and allows for patient mobility. See Table 1.6 below for the possible type of dressings.

Topical antimicrobial dressings—Available topical antimicrobials for treating NF include:

Negative pressure wound therapy (NPWT)—NPWT has been shown to be useful in treating patients with NF and is typically used when dressing changes occur more than 48 h apart. This type of therapy involves the continuous or intermittent application of sub-atmospheric pressure to either foam or gauze placed on the wound surface. The use of NPWT in the treatment of NF has many benefits. In addition to protecting the wound in a moist, closed environment, NPWT allows for excess exudate to be controlled. It also stimulates the formation of

Table 1.6 Topical antimicrobials and therapies used in the treatment of NF [97, 98]

Timing	Antimicrobials/therapies	Notes
Early (before formation of granulation tissue, when dressing changes are frequent)	[a]0.025% Sodium hypochlorite (1:20 Dakin solution[b]) *alternating with* polyhexamethylene biguanide (PHMB)/ betaine	• Potent, broad-spectrum • Low host-cell cytotoxicity[b] • Ability to perforate biofilms • Resistance is rare
	Acetic acid	• Bactericidal against most gram (+) and gram (−) organisms, including Pseudomonas • Inhibits epithelialization/can be cytotoxic • Limited activity against biofilms
	Mafenide acetate	• Potent carbonic anhydrase inhibitor • Covers pseudomonas • Inhibits epithelialization/can be cytotoxic • Used as an alternative to silver sulfadiazine
	Povidone iodine	• Broad-spectrum • Limited use due to cytotoxicity • Causes stinging and erythema • Resistance is rare
Late (after formation of granulation tissue, when dressing changes are less frequent)	[a]Silver-containing dressings (e.g.: Acticoat)	• Broad-spectrum coverage • Useful to prepare wounds for skin grafting • Can result in silver toxicity • Minimal resistance to pathogens • Permits dressing change intervals up to 72 h
	[a]Negative Pressure Wound Therapy (NPWT)	• Used for dressing changes >48 h apart • Allows for control of excess exudate • Stimulates granulation tissue formation • Useful in preparation for skin grafts or flaps

[a]Indicates favored treatment regimens
[b]Sodium hypochlorite solution becomes significantly more cytotoxic at concentrations >0.025%

granulation tissue, which aids in the preparation of a wound bed for skin grafts or tissue flaps [98–104]. Another benefit of NPWT is that it allows for easy, automatic irrigation of the wound. This system enables preset volumes of fluid to be delivered through the tubing to soak the wound for a given amount of time. The system also allows for drainage of the fluid and any exudates by applying negative pressure when desired [99–105]. The cycle of irrigation and drainage is automatic and specific settings, including duration of therapy, can be adjusted based upon clinical need.

Hyperbaric Oxygen (HBO)—Current evidence for treating NF with hyperbaric oxygen therapy is contradictory. Although some studies suggest that there may be benefits when it comes to limb salvage for patients following the initial debridement, other studies have shown that transfer to another facility for HBO negatively impacts patient outcomes during the perioperative period [106–108].

Reconstructive Surgery

Wound coverage and closure become important when surgical debridement is no longer required. This stage of the treatment process should not be considered until the patient is stable and all necrotic or infected areas have been completely debrided. At this stage, healthy granulation tissue can often be seen in the wound bed.

In order to reduce heat and fluid loss and protect the wound from exposure to inflammatory stimuli, temporary deceased donor allografts may be used. Use of this form of skin coverage allows the patient time to further recover and allows the surgical team time to develop a reconstruction plan that is best for the patient. If the temporary allograft adheres, it is likely that an autograft will also be effective [109, 110].

Split-thickness autografting can be used for definitive reconstruction in the majority of NF cases. Some patients may need additional forms of coverage such as fasciocutaneous or muscle flaps if they have exposed bones, tendons, or neurovascular structures. Benefits of muscle flaps include their predictable blood supply pattern and their ability to conform to defects and thus these are often favored. However, fasciocutaneous flaps should be utilized when covering pressure areas such as the elbow, sacrum, or ischial tuberosity because of their increased durability [111].

Use of dermal substitutes, such as Matriderm or Integra may be beneficial in some NF patients. Although such substances are avoided during the acute stages because infection can complicate their application, they have been correlated with increased skin durability and laxity and in some cases may replace the need for flap surgery [112–114].

Morbidity and Mortality

Recent data shows that with surgical intervention and intravenous antibiotics, the mortality rate for community-acquired NF is 16.4%, while the mortality rate for postprocedural NF is 36.3%. Without surgery, the mortality rate nears 100% [66]. Mortality rates are significantly higher for patients with streptococcal toxic shock syndrome, for patients who are diabetic, and in cases where surgery is delayed more than 24 h [91, 115, 116]. Postoperative morbidity is considerable. Many patients experience muscle loss as a result of extensive debridement and require rehabilitation. Substantial scarring and disfigurement may occur [2].

Pearls and Pitfalls

- Early detection of NF is imperative because without intervention, mortality rates approach 100%.
- NF cannot be ruled out based on the absence of severe pain, fever, or crepitus.
- Despite its association with risk factors like diabetes, NF can occur in otherwise healthy patients with or without minor traumatic injury, or at the site of a non-penetrating trauma.

- Suspicion for NF should be increased upon imaging that reveals gas in the tissues and symptoms that include pain that is out of proportion to cutaneous findings.
- If there is any suspicion for NF, broad-spectrum antibiotic use should be immediately considered, and surgical debridement should not be delayed. Surgical intervention is necessary to definitively diagnose NF.
- A diagnostic finger test intraoperatively can be used to confirm NF. A small incision is made, and fingers are inserted into the deep fascia. If the fascial planes dissect easily with the fingers, NF can be confirmed.
- Debridement should be performed aggressively with a long extensile incision and then, in a circular pattern, beginning with the most severely affected area and working outward until healthy, bleeding tissue is reached.
- Early on in debridement, tissue biopsies and cultures from multiple sites should be obtained to identify causative organism(s) and guide antimicrobial treatment.
- Multiple debridements are necessary to ensure that all infected tissue has been removed.

Questions with answers

1. What role do imaging modalities have in the diagnosis of necrotizing fasciitis?
   This is a clinical diagnosis for the most part; however, if air is found on plain films or CTs, it likely points to NF. This can also be true of fluid tracking around fascial planes seen on T2 weighted images of an MRI, however MRIs may take too much time to help determine if a patient has NF.
2. Which laboratory values are included in the LRINEC score?
   CRP, WBC, HGB, Na, Cr, Glucose.
3. What are some common risk factors for the development of necrotizing fasciitis?
   Cirrhosis, diabetes, immunosuppression, advanced age >60yo, steroid use, renal failure, peripheral vascular disease, malignancy, pregnancy, childbirth, IV drug use, malnutrition and obesity.
4. Is Fournier's Gangrene classified as a Type 1 or 2 necrotizing fasciitis?
   Type 1

References

1. Schuster L, Nuñez DE. Using clinical pathways to aid in the diagnosis of necrotizing soft tissue infections synthesis of evidence. Worldviews Evid Based Nurs. 2012;9(2):88–99. https://doi.org/10.1111/j.1741-6787.2011.00235.x.
2. Puvanendran R, Huey JC, Pasupathy S. Necrotizing fasciitis. Can Fam Physician. 2009;55(10):981–7.
3. Hakkarainen TW, Kopari NM, Pham TN, Evans HL. Necrotizing soft tissue infections: review and current concepts in treatment, systems of care, and outcomes. Curr Probl Surg. 2014;51(8):344–62. https://doi.org/10.1067/j.cpsurg.2014.06.001.
4. Leong HN, Kurup A, Tan MY, Kwa ALH, Liau KH, Wilcox MH. Management of complicated skin and soft tissue infections with a special focus on the role of newer antibiotics. Infect Drug Resist. 2018;11:1959–74. https://doi.org/10.2147/IDR.S172366.
5. Misiakos EP, Bagias G, Patapis P, Sotiropoulos D, Kanavidis P, Machairas A. Current concepts in the management of necrotizing fasciitis. Front Surg. 2014;1:36. https://doi.org/10.3389/fsurg.2014.00036.

6. Sarani B, Strong M, Pascual J, Schwab CW. Necrotizing fasciitis: current concepts and review of the literature. J Am Coll Surg. 2009;208(2):279–88. https://doi.org/10.1016/j.jamcollsurg.2008.10.032.
7. Angoules AG, Kontakis G, Drakoulakis E, Vrentzos G, Granick MS, Giannoudis PV. Necrotising fasciitis of upper and lower limb: a systematic review. Injury. 2007;38(Suppl 5):S19–26. https://doi.org/10.1016/j.injury.2007.10.030.
8. Wong CH, Chang HC, Pasupathy S, Khin LW, Tan JL, Low CO. Necrotizing fasciitis: clinical presentation, microbiology, and determinants of mortality. J Bone Jt Surg Am. 2003;85(8):1454–60.
9. Yahav D, Duskin-Bitan H, Eliakim-Raz N, Ben-Zvi H, Shaked H, Goldberg E, Bishara J. Monomicrobial necrotizing fasciitis in a single center: the emergence of gram-negative bacteria as a common pathogen D. Int J Infect Dis. 2014;28:13–6. https://core.ac.uk/download/pdf/82468655.pdf
10. Fustes-Morales A, Gutierrez-Castrellon P, Duran-Mckinster C, Orozco-Covarrubias L, Tamayo-Sanchez L, Ruiz-Maldonado R. Necrotizing fasciitis: report of 39 pediatric cases. Arch Dermatol. 2002;138(7):893–9. https://doi.org/10.1001/archderm.138.7.893.
11. Davoudian P, Flint NJ. Necrotizing fasciitis. Contin Educ Anaesth Crit Care Pain. 2012;12(5):245–50.
12. Wong CJ, Stevens DL. Serious group a streptococcal infections. Med Clin N Am. 2013;97(4):721–12. https://doi.org/10.1016/j.mcna.2013.03.003.
13. Childers BJ, Potyondy LD, Nachreiner R, Rogers FR, Childers ER, Oberg KC, Hendricks DL, Hardesty RA. Necrotizing fasciitis: a 14-year retrospective study of 163 consecutive patients. Am Surg. 2002;68(2):109–16.
14. Reisman JS, Weinberg A, Ponte C, Kradin R. Monomicrobial pseudomonas necrotizing fasciitis: a case of infection by two strains and a review of 37 cases in the literature. Scand J Infect Dis. 2012;44(3):216–21. https://doi.org/10.3109/00365548.2011.626441.
15. Brook I, Frazier EH. Clinical and microbiological features of necrotizing fasciitis. J Clin Microbiol. 1995;33(9):2382–7.
16. Hsieh WS, Yang PH, Chao HC, Lai JY. Neonatal necrotizing fasciitis: a report of three cases and review of the literature. Pediatrics. 1999;103(4):e53. https://doi.org/10.1542/peds.103.4.e53.
17. Voelzke BB, Hagedorn JC. Presentation and diagnosis of Fournier gangrene. Urology. 2018;114:8–13. https://doi.org/10.1016/j.urology.2017.10.031.
18. Morgan MS. Diagnosis and management of necrotising fasciitis: a multiparametric approach. J Hosp Infect. 2010;75(4):249–57. https://doi.org/10.1016/j.jhin.2010.01.028.
19. Hasham S, Matteucci P, Stanley PR, Hart NB. Necrotising fasciitis. BMJ (Clinical research ed). 2005;330(7495):830–3. https://doi.org/10.1136/bmj.330.7495.830.
20. Wong CH, Wang YS. The diagnosis of necrotizing fasciitis. Curr Opin Infect Dis. 2005;18(2):101–6. https://doi.org/10.1097/01.qco.0000160896.74492.ea.
21. Eneli I, Davies HD. Epidemiology and outcome of necrotizing fasciitis in children: an active surveillance study of the Canadian Paediatric surveillance program. J Pediatr. 2007;151(1):79–84.e1. https://doi.org/10.1016/j.jpeds.2007.02.019.
22. Ross A, Shoff HW. Toxic shock syndrome. In: StatPearls. Treasure Island (FL): StatPearls Publishing; 2020. https://www.ncbi.nlm.nih.gov/books/NBK459345/.
23. Miller LG, Perdreau-Remington F, Rieg G, Mehdi S, Perlroth J, Bayer AS, Tang AW, Phung TO, Spellberg B. Necrotizing fasciitis caused by community-associated methicillin-resistant *Staphylococcus aureus* in Los Angeles. N Engl J Med. 2005;352(14):1445–53. https://doi.org/10.1056/NEJMoa042683.
24. Goh T, Goh LG, Ang CH, Wong CH. Early diagnosis of necrotizing fasciitis. Br J Surg. 2014;101(1):e119–25. https://doi.org/10.1002/bjs.9371.
25. Tsai YH, Huang KC, Huang TJ, Hsu RW. Case reports: fatal necrotizing fasciitis caused by *Aeromonas sobria* in two diabetic patients. Clin Orthop Relat Res. 2009;467(3):846–9. https://doi.org/10.1007/s11999-008-0504-0.
26. Shaikh N. Necrotizing fasciitis: facts and figures. Scientific Research Publishing, Incorporated; 2016.

27. Roje Z, Roje Z, Matić D, Librenjak D, Dokuzović S, Varvodić J. Necrotizing fasciitis: literature review of contemporary strategies for diagnosing and management with three case reports: torso, abdominal wall, upper and lower limbs. World J Emerg Surg WJES. 2011;6(1):46. https://doi.org/10.1186/1749-7922-6-46.
28. Navinan MR, Yudhishdran J, Kandeepan T, Kulatunga A. Necrotizing fasciitis—a diagnostic dilemma: two case reports. J Med Case Rep. 2014;8:229. https://doi.org/10.1186/1752-1947-8-229.
29. Kiat HJ, En Natalie YH, Fatimah L. Necrotizing fasciitis: how reliable are the cutaneous signs? J Emerg Trauma Shock. 2017;10(4):205–10. https://doi.org/10.4103/JETS.JETS_42_17.
30. Stevens DL, Bryant AE. Necrotizing soft tissue infections. N Engl J Med. 2017;377:23. http://www.egradu.fmed.edu.uy/sites/www.dbc.fmed.edu.uy/files/Residentes/Archivospar/d)%20Necrotizing%20Soft-Tissue%20Infections.pdf.
31. Elliott DC, Kufera JA, Myers RA. Necrotizing soft tissue infections. Risk factors for mortality and strategies for management. Ann Surg. 1996;224:672–83.
32. Lakhani NA, Narsinghani U, Kumar R. Necrotizing fasciitis of the abdominal wall caused by *Serratia marcescens*. Infect Dis Rep. 2015;7(2):5774. https://doi.org/10.4081/idr.2015.5774.
33. Wang YS, Wong CH, Tay YK. Staging of necrotizing fasciitis based on the evolving cutaneous features. Int J Dermatol. 2007;46(10):1036–41. https://doi.org/10.1111/j.1365-4632.2007.03201.x.
34. Stevens DL, Tanner MH, Winship J, Swarts R, Ries KM, Schlievert PM, Kaplan E. Severe group A streptococcal infections associated with a toxic shock-like syndrome and scarlet fever toxin A. N Engl J Med. 1989;321(1):1–7. https://doi.org/10.1056/NEJM198907063210101.
35. Simonart T, Simonart JM, Derdelinckx I, De Dobbeleer G, Verleysen A, Verraes S, de Maubeuge J, Van Vooren JP, Naeyaert JM, de la Brassine M, Peetermans WE, Heenen M. Value of standard laboratory tests for the early recognition of group A beta-hemolytic streptococcal necrotizing fasciitis. Clin Infect Dis. 2001;32(1):E9–E12. https://doi.org/10.1086/317525.
36. Yaghoubian A, de Virgilio C, Dauphine C, Lewis RJ, Lin M. Use of admission serum lactate and sodium levels to predict mortality in necrotizing soft-tissue infections. Arch Surg (Chicago, Ill.: 1960). 2007;142(9):840–6. https://doi.org/10.1001/archsurg.142.9.840.
37. van Sambeek CHL, van Stigt SF, Brouwers L, Bemelman M. Necrotising fasciitis: a ticking time bomb? BMJ Case Rep. 2017;2017:bcr2017221770. https://doi.org/10.1136/bcr-2017-221770.
38. Yoder EL, Mendez J, Khatib R. Spontaneous gangrenous myositis induced by *Streptococcus pyogenes*: case report and review of the literature. Rev Infect Dis. 1987;9(2):382–5. https://doi.org/10.1093/clinids/9.2.382.
39. Majeski J, Majeski E. Necrotizing fasciitis: improved survival with early recognition by tissue biopsy and aggressive debridement. South Med J. 1997;90(11):1065–8.
40. Stevens DL. Streptococcal toxic-shock syndrome: spectrum of disease, pathogenesis, and new concepts in treatment. Emerg Infect Dis. 1995;1:69.
41. Chelsom J, Halstensen A, Haga T, Høiby EA. Necrotising fasciitis due to Group A Streptococci in western Norway: incidence and clinical features. Lancet (London, England). 1994;344(8930):1111–5. https://doi.org/10.1016/s0140-6736(94)90629-7.
42. Bakleh M, Wold LE, Mandrekar JN, Harmsen WS, Dimashkieh HH, Baddour LM. Correlation of histopathologic findings with clinical outcome in necrotizing fasciitis. Clin Infect Dis. 2005;40(3):410–4. https://doi.org/10.1086/427286.
43. Parikh RP, Pappas-Politis E. Soft tissue infection of the upper extremity. Eplasty. 2011;11:ic6.
44. Butterworth SA, Murphy JJ. Necrotizing soft tissue infections—are they different in healthy vs immunocompromised children? J Pediatr Surg. 2006;41(5):935–9. https://doi.org/10.1016/j.jpedsurg.2006.01.012.
45. Wall DB, Klein SR, Black S, de Virgilio C. A simple model to help distinguish necrotizing fasciitis from non-necrotizing soft tissue infection. J Am Coll Surg. 2000;191(3):227–31. https://doi.org/10.1016/s1072-7515(00)00318-5.
46. Stamenkovic I, Lew PD. Early recognition of potentially fatal necrotizing fasciitis. The use of frozen-section biopsy. N Engl J Med. 1984;310(26):1689–93. https://doi.org/10.1056/NEJM198406283102601.

47. Brumann M, Bogner V, Völkl A, Sotlar K, Euler E, Mutschler W. Necrotizing fasciitis in a young patient with acute myeloid leukemia—a diagnostic challenge. Patient Saf Surg. 2014;8:28. https://doi.org/10.1186/1754-9493-8-28.
48. Tso DK, Singh AK. Necrotizing fasciitis of the lower extremity: imaging pearls and pitfalls. Br J Radiol. 2018;91(1088):20180093. https://doi.org/10.1259/bjr.20180093.
49. Wysoki MG, Santora TA, Shah RM, Friedman AC. Necrotizing fasciitis: CT characteristics. Radiology. 1997;203(3):859–63. https://doi.org/10.1148/radiology.203.3.9169717.
50. Fernando SM, Tran A, Cheng W, Rochwerg B, Kyeremanteng K, Seely AJE, Inaba K, Perry JJ. Necrotizing soft tissue infection: diagnostic accuracy of physical examination, imaging, and LRINEC score: a systematic review and meta-analysis. Ann Surg. 2019;269(1):58–65. https://doi.org/10.1097/SLA.0000000000002774.
51. Stevens DL, Bisno AL, Chambers HF, Dellinger EP, Goldstein EJ, Gorbach SL, Hirschmann JV, Kaplan SL, Montoya JG, Wade JC, Infectious Diseases Society of America. Practice guidelines for the diagnosis and management of skin and soft tissue infections: 2014 update by the Infectious Diseases Society of America. Clin Infect Dis. 2014;59(2):e10–52. https://doi.org/10.1093/cid/ciu444.
52. Wong CH, Khin LW, Heng KS, Tan KC, Low CO. The LRINEC (laboratory risk indicator for necrotizing fasciitis) score: a tool for distinguishing necrotizing fasciitis from other soft tissue infections. Crit Care Med. 2004;32(7):1535–41. https://doi.org/10.1097/01.ccm.0000129486.35458.7d.
53. van Stigt SF, de Vries J, Bijker JB, Mollen RM, Hekma EJ, Lemson SM, Tan EC. Review of 58 patients with necrotizing fasciitis in The Netherlands. World J Emerg Surg WJES. 2016;11:21. https://doi.org/10.1186/s13017-016-0080-7.
54. Su Y-C, Chen H-W, Hong Y-C, Chen C-T, Hsiao C-T, Chen I-C. Laboratory risk indicator for necrotizing fasciitis score and the outcomes. ANZ J Surg. 2008;78:968–72. https://doi.org/10.1111/j.1445-2197.2008.04713.x.
55. Holder EP, Moore PT, Browne BA. Nonsteroidal anti-inflammatory drugs and necrotising fasciitis. An update. Drug Saf. 1997;17(6):369–73. https://doi.org/10.2165/00002018-199717060-00003.
56. Seal DV. Necrotizing fasciitis. Curr Opin Infect Dis. 2001;14(2):127–32. https://doi.org/10.1097/00001432-200104000-00003.
57. Green RJ, Dafoe DC, Raffin TA. Necrotizing fasciitis. Chest. 1996;110(1):219–29. https://doi.org/10.1378/chest.110.1.219.
58. Bisarya K, Azzopardi S, Lye G, Drew PJ. Necrotizing fasciitis versus pyoderma gangrenosum: securing the correct diagnosis! A case report and literature review. Eplasty. 2011;11:e24.
59. Berger N, Ebenhoch M, Salzmann M. Postoperative pyoderma gangrenosum in children: the case report of a 13-year-old boy with pyoderma gangrenosum after hip reconstruction surgery and a review of the literature. J Pediatr Orthop. 2017;37(6):e379–83. https://doi.org/10.1097/BPO.0000000000000952.
60. Touil LL, Gurusinghe DA, Sadri A, El-Gawad A, Fahmy FS. Postsurgical pyoderma gangrenosum versus necrotizing fasciitis: can we spot the difference? Ann Plast Surg. 2017;78(5):582–6. https://doi.org/10.1097/SAP.0000000000001070.
61. Hradil E, Jeppsson C, Hamnerius N, Svensson Å. The diagnosis you wish you had never operated on: pyoderma gangrenosum misdiagnosed as necrotizing fasciitis—a case report. Acta Orthop. 2017;88(2):231–3. https://doi.org/10.1080/17453674.2016.1260403.
62. Karimi K, Odhav A, Kollipara R, Fike J, Stanford C, Hall JC. Acute cutaneous necrosis: a guide to early diagnosis and treatment. J Cutan Med Surg. 2017;21(5):425–37. https://doi.org/10.1177/1203475417708164.
63. Buboltz JB, Murphy-Lavoie HM. Gas gangrene. In: StatPearls. Treasure Island (FL): StatPearls Publishing; 2020. https://www.ncbi.nlm.nih.gov/books/NBK537030/.
64. Seok JH, Jee WH, Chun KA, Kim JY, Jung CK, Kim YR, Eo WK, Kim YS, Chung YG. Necrotizing fasciitis versus pyomyositis: discrimination with using MR imaging. Korean J Radiol. 2009;10(2):121–8. https://doi.org/10.3348/kjr.2009.10.2.121.
65. Rahman A, Abou-Foul AK, Yusaf A, Holton J, Cogswell L. Necrotising myositis, the deadly impersonator. Case Rep Surg. 2014;2014:485651. https://doi.org/10.1155/2014/485651.

66. Anaya DA, Dellinger EP. Necrotizing soft-tissue infection: diagnosis and management. Clin Infect Dis. 2007;44(5):705–10. https://doi.org/10.1086/511638.
67. Sudarsky LA, Laschinger JC, Coppa GF, Spencer FC. Improved results from a standardized approach in treating patients with necrotizing fasciitis. Ann Surg. 1987;206(5):661–5. https://doi.org/10.1097/00000658-198711000-00018.
68. Lauerman MH, Kolesnik O, Sethuraman K, Rabinowitz R, Joshi M, Clark E, Stein D, Scalea T, Henry S. Less is more? Antibiotic duration and outcomes in Fournier's gangrene. J Trauma Acute Care Surg. 2017;83(3):443–8. https://doi.org/10.1097/TA.0000000000001562.
69. Stevens DL, Bryant AE, Hackett SP. Antibiotic effects on bacterial viability, toxin production, and host response. Clin Infect Dis. 1995;20(Suppl 2):S154–7. https://doi.org/10.1093/clinids/20.supplement_2.s154.
70. Stevens DL, Gibbons AE, Bergstrom R, Winn V. The Eagle effect revisited: efficacy of clindamycin, erythromycin, and penicillin in the treatment of streptococcal myositis. J Infect Dis. 1988;158(1):23–8. https://doi.org/10.1093/infdis/158.1.23.
71. Eagle H. Experimental approach to the problem of treatment failure with penicillin. I. Group A streptococcal infection in mice. Am J Med. 1952;13(4):389–99. https://doi.org/10.1016/0002-9343(52)90293-3.
72. Stevens DL, Yan S, Bryant AE. Penicillin-binding protein expression at different growth stages determines penicillin efficacy in vitro and in vivo: an explanation for the inoculum effect. J Infect Dis. 1993;167(6):1401–5. https://doi.org/10.1093/infdis/167.6.1401.
73. Stevens DL, Bryant AE, Yan S. Invasive group A Streptococcal infection: new concepts in antibiotic treatment. Int J Antimicrob Agents. 1994;4(4):297–301. https://doi.org/10.1016/0924-8579(94)90029-9.
74. Zimbelman J, Palmer A, Todd J. Improved outcome of clindamycin compared with beta-lactam antibiotic treatment for invasive streptococcus pyogenes infection. Pediatr Infect Dis J. 1999;18(12):1096–100. https://doi.org/10.1097/00006454-199912000-00014.
75. Parks T, Wilson C, Curtis N, Norrby-Teglund A, Sriskandan S. Polyspecific intravenous immunoglobulin in clindamycin-treated patients with streptococcal toxic shock syndrome: a systematic review and meta-analysis. Clin Infect Dis. 2018;67(9):1434–6. https://doi.org/10.1093/cid/ciy401.
76. Laho D, Blumental S, Botteaux A, Smeesters PR. Invasive Group A Streptococcal infections: benefit of clindamycin, intravenous immunoglobulins and secondary prophylaxis. Front Pediatr. 2021;9:697938. https://doi.org/10.3389/fped.2021.697938.
77. Sartelli M, Malangoni MA, May AK, Viale P, Kao LS, Catena F, Ansaloni L, Moore EE, Moore FA, Peitzman AB, Coimbra R, Leppaniemi A, Kluger Y, Biffl W, Koike K, Girardis M, Ordonez CA, Tavola M, Cainzos M, Di Saverio S, Yuan KC. World Society of Emergency Surgery (WSES) guidelines for management of skin and soft tissue infections. World J Emerg Surg WJES. 2014;9(1):57. https://doi.org/10.1186/1749-7922-9-57.
78. Kalaivani V, Hiremath BV. Necrotising soft tissue infection-risk factors for mortality. J Clin Diagn Res. 2013;7(8):1662–5. https://doi.org/10.7860/JCDR/2013/5535.3240.
79. Gelbard RB, Ferrada P, Yeh DD, Williams BH, Loor M, Yon J, Mentzer C, Khwaja K, Khan MA, Kohli A, Bulger EM, Robinson B. Optimal timing of initial debridement for necrotizing soft tissue infection: a practice management guideline from the Eastern Association for the Surgery of trauma. J Trauma Acute Care Surg. 2018;85(1):208–14. https://doi.org/10.1097/TA.0000000000001857.
80. Holena DN, Mills AM, Carr BG, Wirtalla C, Sarani B, Kim PK, Braslow BM, Kelz RR. Transfer status: a risk factor for mortality in patients with necrotizing fasciitis. Surgery. 2011;150(3):363–70. https://doi.org/10.1016/j.surg.2011.06.005.
81. Endorf FW, Supple KG, Gamelli RL. The evolving characteristics and care of necrotizing soft-tissue infections. Burns. 2005;31(3):269–73. https://doi.org/10.1016/j.burns.2004.11.008.
82. Faucher LD, Morris SE, Edelman LS, Saffle JR. Burn center management of necrotizing soft-tissue surgical infections in unburned patients. Am J Surg. 2001;182(6):563–9. https://doi.org/10.1016/s0002-9610(01)00785-1.
83. Bernal NP, Latenser BA, Born JM, Liao J. Trends in 393 necrotizing acute soft tissue infection patients 2000–2008. Burns J Int Soc Burn Inj. 2012;38(2):252–60. https://doi.org/10.1016/j.burns.2011.07.008.

84. Shah AK, Kumar NB, Gambhir RP, Chaudhry R. Integrated clinical care pathway for managing necrotising soft tissue infections. Indian J Surg. 2009;71(5):254–7. https://doi.org/10.1007/s12262-009-0076-6.
85. Weiss A, Sandler B. Lower extremity necrotizing fasciitis: a unique initial presentation of Crohn's disease. Ann Med Surg (2012). 2015;4(3):215–6. https://doi.org/10.1016/j.amsu.2015.05.007.
86. Leekha S, Terrell CL, Edson RS. General principles of antimicrobial therapy. Mayo Clin Proc. 2011;86(2):156–67. https://doi.org/10.4065/mcp.2010.0639.
87. Rennekampff HO, Schaller HE, Wisser D, Tenenhaus M. Debridement of burn wounds with a water jet surgical tool. Burns J Int Soc Burn Inj. 2006;32(1):64–9. https://doi.org/10.1016/j.burns.2005.07.010.
88. Nicks BA, Ayello EA, Woo K, Nitzki-George D, Sibbald RG. Acute wound management: revisiting the approach to assessment, irrigation, and closure considerations. Int J Emerg Med. 2010;3(4):399–407. https://doi.org/10.1007/s12245-010-0217-5.
89. Eray IC, Alabaz O, Akcam AT, Ulku A, Parsak CK, Sakman G, Seydaoglu G. Comparison of diverting colostomy and bowel management catheter applications in Fournier gangrene cases requiring fecal diversion. Indian J Surg. 2015;77(Suppl 2):438–41. https://doi.org/10.1007/s12262-013-0868-6.
90. Merchant N, Boudana D, Willoughby L, Lin J, Rehou S, Shahrokhi S, Jeschke MG. Management of adult patients with buttock and perineal burns: the Ross Tilley burn Centre experience. J Trauma Acute Care Surg. 2014;77(4):640–8. https://doi.org/10.1097/TA.0000000000000405.
91. McHenry CR, Piotrowski JJ, Petrinic D, Malangoni MA. Determinants of mortality for necrotizing soft-tissue infections. Ann Surg. 1995;221(5):558–65. https://doi.org/10.1097/00000658-199505000-00013.
92. Busse JW, Jacobs CL, Swiontkowski MF, Bosse MJ, Bhandari M, Evidence-Based Orthopaedic Trauma Working Group. Complex limb salvage or early amputation for severe lower-limb injury: a meta-analysis of observational studies. J Orthop Trauma. 2007;21(1):70–6. https://doi.org/10.1097/BOT.0b013e31802cbc43.
93. Stineman MG, Kwong PL, Xie D, Kurichi JE, Ripley DC, Brooks DM, Bidelspach DE, Bates BE. Prognostic differences for functional recovery after major lower limb amputation: effects of the timing and type of inpatient rehabilitation services in the veterans health administration. PM R. 2010;2(4):232–43. https://doi.org/10.1016/j.pmrj.2010.01.012.
94. Uehara K, Yasunaga H, Morizaki Y, Horiguchi H, Fushimi K, Tanaka S. Necrotising soft-tissue infections of the upper limb: risk factors for amputation and death. Bone Jt J. 2014;96-B(11):1530–4. https://doi.org/10.1302/0301-620X.96B11.34888.
95. Glass GE, Sheil F, Ruston JC, Butler PE. Necrotising soft tissue infection in a UK metropolitan population. Ann R Coll Surg Engl. 2015;97(1):46–51. https://doi.org/10.1308/003588414X14055925058553.
96. Borschitz T, Schlicht S, Siegel E, Hanke E, von Stebut E. Improvement of a clinical score for necrotizing fasciitis: 'pain out of proportion' and high CRP levels aid the diagnosis. PLoS One. 2015;10(7):e0132775. https://doi.org/10.1371/journal.pone.0132775.
97. Hirsch T, Seipp HM, Jacobsen F, Goertz O, Steinau HU, Steinstraesser L. Antiseptics in surgery. Eplasty. 2010;10:e39.
98. Paddle-Ledinek JE, Nasa Z, Cleland HJ. Effect of different wound dressings on cell viability and proliferation. Plast Reconstr Surg. 2006;117(7 Suppl):110S–20S. https://doi.org/10.1097/01.prs.0000225439.39352.ce.
99. Kairinos N, Hudson DA, Solomons M. The influence of different sizes and types of wound fillers on wound contraction and tissue pressure during negative pressure wound therapy. Int Wound J. 2011;8(6):656–7. https://doi.org/10.1111/j.1742-481X.2011.00825.x.
100. Kairinos N, Hudson D, Solomons M. Depth of penetration of negative pressure wound therapy into underlying tissues. Wound Repair Regener. 2009;17(3):456. https://doi.org/10.1111/j.1524-475X.2009.00493.x.
101. Kairinos N, Voogd AM, Botha PH, Kotze T, Kahn D, Hudson DA, Solomons M. Negative-pressure wound therapy II: negative-pressure wound therapy and increased perfusion.

Just an illusion? Plast Reconstr Surg. 2009;123(2):601–12. https://doi.org/10.1097/PRS.0b013e318196b97b.
102. Kairinos N, Solomons M, Hudson DA. Negative-pressure wound therapy I: the paradox of negative-pressure wound therapy. Plast Reconstr Surg. 2009;123(2):589–600. https://doi.org/10.1097/PRS.0b013e3181956551.
103. Birke-Sorensen H, Malmsjo M, Rome P, Hudson D, Krug E, Berg L, Bruhin A, Caravaggi C, Chariker M, Depoorter M, Dowsett C, Dunn R, Duteille F, Ferreira F, Francos Martínez JM, Grudzien G, Ichioka S, Ingemansson R, Jeffery S, Lee C, Smith J. Evidence-based recommendations for negative pressure wound therapy: treatment variables (pressure levels, wound filler and contact layer)—steps towards an international consensus. J Plast Reconstr Aesthet Surg. 2011;64(Suppl):S1–S16. https://doi.org/10.1016/j.bjps.2011.06.001.
104. Malmsjö M, Gustafsson L, Lindstedt S, Gesslein B, Ingemansson R. The effects of variable, intermittent, and continuous negative pressure wound therapy, using foam or gauze, on wound contraction, granulation tissue formation, and ingrowth into the wound filler. Eplasty. 2012;12:e5.
105. Kim PJ, Attinger CE, Crist BD, Gabriel A, Galiano RD, Gupta S, Lantis Ii JC, Lavery L, Lipsky BA, Teot L. Negative pressure wound therapy with instillation: review of evidence and recommendations. Wounds. 2015;27(12):S2–S19.
106. Crew JR, Varilla R, Iii TAR, Abdul Rani S, Debabov D. Treatment of acute necrotizing fasciitis using negative pressure wound therapy and adjunctive neutrophase irrigation under the foam. Wounds Compend Clin Res Pract. 2013;25(10):272–7.
107. Willy C, Rieger H, Vogt D. Hyperbare oxygenation bei nekrotisierenden Weichteilinfektionen: Kontra [hyperbaric oxygen therapy for necrotizing soft tissue infections: contra]. Der Chirurg Zeitschrift fur alle Gebiete der operativen Medizen. 2012;83(11):960–72. https://doi.org/10.1007/s00104-012-2284-z.
108. Soh CR, Pietrobon R, Freiberger JJ, Chew ST, Rajgor D, Gandhi M, Shah J, Moon RE. Hyperbaric oxygen therapy in necrotising soft tissue infections: a study of patients in the United States Nationwide inpatient sample. Intensive Care Med. 2012;38(7):1143–51. https://doi.org/10.1007/s00134-012-2558-4.
109. Leon-Villapalos J, Eldardiri M, Dziewulski P. The use of human deceased donor skin allograft in burn care. Cell Tissue Bank. 2010;11(1):99–104. https://doi.org/10.1007/s10561-009-9152-1.
110. Rogers AD, Allorto NL, Adams S, Adams KG, Hudson DA, Rode H. Isn't it time for a cadaver skin bank in South Africa? Ann Burns Fire Disasters. 2013;26(3):142–6.
111. Chan JK, Harry L, Williams G, Nanchahal J. Soft-tissue reconstruction of open fractures of the lower limb: muscle versus fasciocutaneous flaps. Plast Reconstr Surg. 2012;130(2):284e–95e. https://doi.org/10.1097/PRS.0b013e3182589e63.
112. Ryssel H, Germann G, Czermak C, Kloeters O, Gazyakan E, Riedel K. Matriderm® in depth-adjusted reconstruction of necrotising fasciitis defects. Burns J Int Soc Burn Inj. 2010;36(7):1107–11. https://doi.org/10.1016/j.burns.2009.12.002.
113. Payne CE, Williams AM, Hart NB. Lotus petal flaps for scrotal reconstruction combined with Integra resurfacing of the penis and anterior abdominal wall following necrotising fasciitis. J Plast Reconstr Aesthet Surg JPRAS. 2009;62(3):393–7. https://doi.org/10.1016/j.bjps.2007.09.015.
114. Bache SE, Watson SB. Bedside application of integra after debridement of necrotising fasciitis. J Plast Reconstr Aesthet Surg JPRAS. 2011;64(4):559–60. https://doi.org/10.1016/j.bjps.2010.07.032.
115. Bucca K, Spencer R, Orford N, Cattigan C, Athan E, McDonald A. Early diagnosis and treatment of necrotizing fasciitis can improve survival: an observational intensive care unit cohort study. ANZ J Surg. 2013;83(5):365–70. https://doi.org/10.1111/j.1445-2197.2012.06251.x.
116. Hadeed GJ, Smith J, O'Keeffe T, Kulvatunyou N, Wynne JL, Joseph B, Friese RS, Wachtel TL, Rhee PM, El-Menyar A, Latifi R. Early surgical intervention and its impact on patients presenting with necrotizing soft tissue infections: a single academic center experience. J Emerg Trauma Shock. 2016;9(1):22–7. https://doi.org/10.4103/0974-2700.173868.

Chapter 2
Postoperative Acute Airway Obstruction Status Post Anterior Cervical Fusion

Monika Debkowska, John Butterworth, Jaime Moore, Soobin Kang, Eric Appelbaum, and Wilhelm A. Zuelzer

Clinical Vignette

A 51-year-old male was involved in a motor vehicle collision. On arrival to our medical center he complained of neck and right shoulder pain with paresthesias in the right hand and arm. His neurological examination was notable for normal sensation in the upper and lower extremities, with right triceps weakness. He had hyperreflexia in both the upper and lower extremities. Three beats of clonus and negative Babinski signs were elicited in both ankles. He underwent magnetic resonance imaging (MRI) of the cervical spine, which revealed a C3–4 central disc bulge.

M. Debkowska (✉)
Ocean Township, NJ, USA

J. Butterworth (Deceased)
Department of Anesthesiology, Virginia Commonwealth University, Richmond, VA, USA

J. Moore
Department of Otolaryngology, Virginia Commonwealth University, Richmond, VA, USA
e-mail: jaime.moore@vcuhealth.org

S. Kang
Morganville, NJ, USA
e-mail: Soobin.kang@univrraad.com

E. Appelbaum
Marietta, GA, USA
e-mail: eric.appelbaum@wellstar.org

W. A. Zuelzer
Orthopaedic Surgery, Virginia Commonwealth University Medical School, Richmond, VA, USA

Department of Orthopaedic Surgery, VCUHS, Richmond, VA, USA
e-mail: wilhelm.zuelzer@vcuhealth.org

W. A. Zuelzer, S. Metikala (eds.), *Unusual Conditions That Every Orthopaedic Surgeon Should Know*, https://doi.org/10.1007/978-3-031-58946-1_2

The patient underwent C3–4 anterior cervical discectomy and fusion 3 days after the accident. On post-operative day 1 at 23:19, the patient had dyspnea, anxiety about swallowing, and felt that the cervical collar was too tight. The symptoms resolved after the collar was removed and the patient was comfortable on 2 L/min of supplemental oxygen by nasal cannula. On post-operative day 3, patient was talking with the nurse, when he was suddenly unable to breathe, fell to the ground and had respiratory arrest. The attending anesthesiologist arrived 4 min after the arrest but was unable to perform an orotracheal intubation; 8 minutes after the arrest, the surgical resident opened the neck wound but failed to identify a retropharyngeal hematoma; 10 minutes after the respiratory arrest, the attending surgeon arrived and performed a cricothyrotomy. However, further resuscitative efforts failed, and the patient was pronounced dead.

This review will focus on the issue of respiratory arrest after anterior cervical spine surgery and place particularly emphasis on the importance of immediately reestablishing an airway in this most precarious clinical situation.

Questions

1. What is the most likely reason for respiratory arrest.
2. What would be the preferred sequence of resuscitation.
3. What should be the required skills sets.

Introduction

When pain and disability from cervical spondylosis and disc degeneration become refractory to conservative treatment, surgical interventions such as anterior cervical discectomy and fusion (ACDF) or anterior cervical corpectomy and fusion (ACCF) may be necessary to treat or prevent cervical myelopathy or radiculopathy. Surgical treatment relieves symptoms by decompressing the spinal cord and nerve roots. ACDF is a common procedure and most patients have excellent results [1–3]. A long list of complications may arise after anterior cervical spine surgery (ACSS), with dysphagia being the most common [4–11]. Post-operative adverse events related to the airway occur in up to 14% of patients after multi-level ACSS with or without fusion [7, 12, 13]. Retropharyngeal edema occurs in up to 6% of patients with the greatest risk arising in multilevel surgery [14, 15]. The post-operative hematoma occurs in up to 2.4% in ACSS [4, 5, 10, 11, 13, 15–19]. Of patients undergoing single level ACDF, 2% may require reintubation [4, 7, 19–26] and as many as 5.2% may require reintubation after multilevel surgery [21, 27]. These are uncommon complications. However, as in our clinical vignette, airway obstruction is a potentially life-threatening event for which one must be prepared with an effective management plan. Symptoms of airway compromise after ACSS requires immediate attention, as the situation may quickly proceed to respiratory arrest. Obtaining emergent control of the airway is the key to survival of such patients. Knowing how to perform emergency intubation, cricothyrotomy or tracheostomy without delay is critical. Unfortunately, these challenging situations may occur in off-hours, when available support is limited. Our objective in this review is to describe significant acute postoperative airway complications associated with ACSS and provide recommendations on how they would be best managed.

Clinical Anatomy and Surgical Approach

Effective treatment for a patient with airway compromise following ACSS requires knowledge of the neck and upper respiratory tract anatomy as well as procedural skills. The neck contains many vital structures within a small space. Important superficial landmarks include the cricoid and thyroid cartilages (Fig. 2.1). Palpating from the inferior to superior, the cricoid cartilage is the first prominence and the thyroid cartilage is the second. Typically, in males the thyroid cartilage ("Adam's apple") is more prominent. In women, the cricoid cartilage is usually more pronounced. The soft spot between these two landmarks is the cricothyroid membrane, which is incised during a cricothyrotomy.

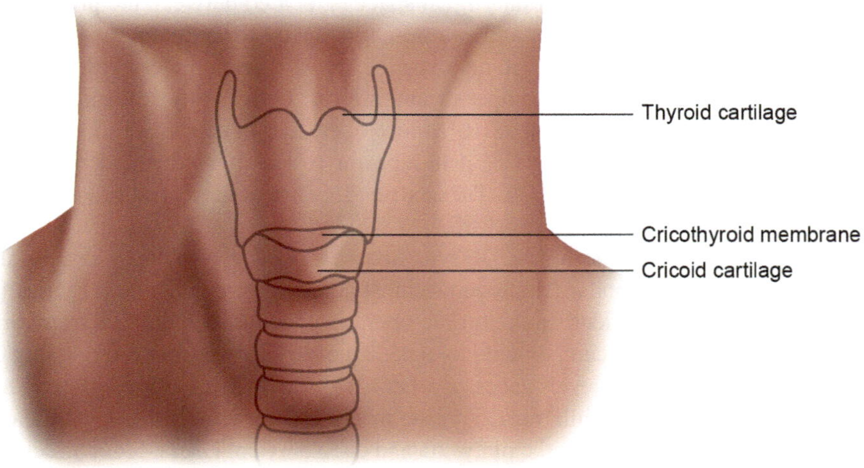

Fig. 2.1 Neck topography showing the major landmarks used for a cricothyrotomy

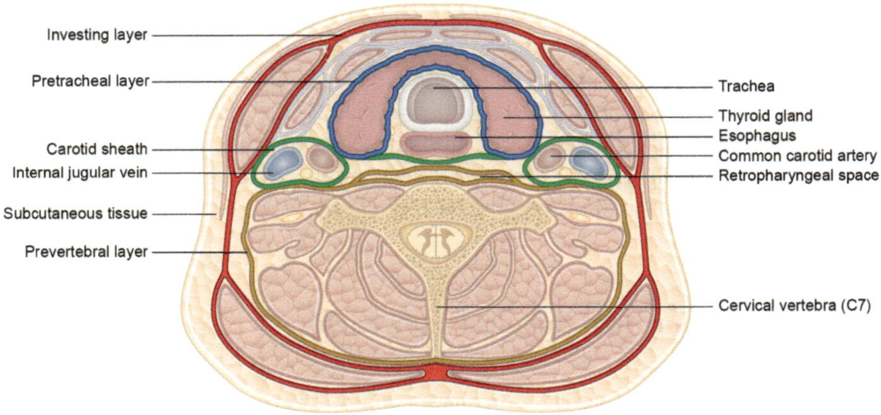

Fig. 2.2 Cross sectional drawing of the cervical spine at C7 showing the three deep cervical fascial layers: the investing layer, pretracheal layer, and prevertebral layer. The retropharyngeal space is posterior to the esophagus

Internally, the neck is divided into three deep fascial layers (Fig. 2.2). The first or investing layer is most superficial. The second or pretracheal (visceral) layer encloses the trachea, esophagus and thyroid gland. The third or prevertebral layer surrounds the cervical vertebral column. The carotid sheath is formed by contributions from all three fascial layers and encompasses the common carotid and internal carotid arteries, the internal jugular vein, the lymphatic plexus and cranial nerves IX–XII. The retropharyngeal space is located between the pretracheal and prevertebral fascial layers and is a potential space for hematomas following ACSS [15, 16]. The thyroid gland overlies the trachea and cricoid cartilage (Fig. 2.3). It is supplied by the superior and inferior thyroid arteries. Injury to the superior thyroid artery may lead to a post-operative hematoma [16, 28]. The thyroid cartilage is located at C4, just superior to the thyroid gland, while the cricoid cartilage is located at C6. These structures are at increased risk of injury during the anterior approach in ACSS.

The surgical technique for ACDF was first described by Robinson and Smith, and has become the standard approach to most anterior cervical spine surgeries [1, 2, 29, 30]. With the patient supine on the operating room table, either a transverse or longitudinal incision can be made to expose the cervical vertebrae depending on the numbers of vertebral levels necessary. For C4–5, the incision is made at the level of the thyroid cartilage while for C5–7, the incision is made at the level of the cricoid cartilage. After splitting the platysma and deep cervical fascia, blunt dissection is made medially to the carotid sheath and down through the prevertebral fascia. The trachea and larynx must be gently retracted medially.

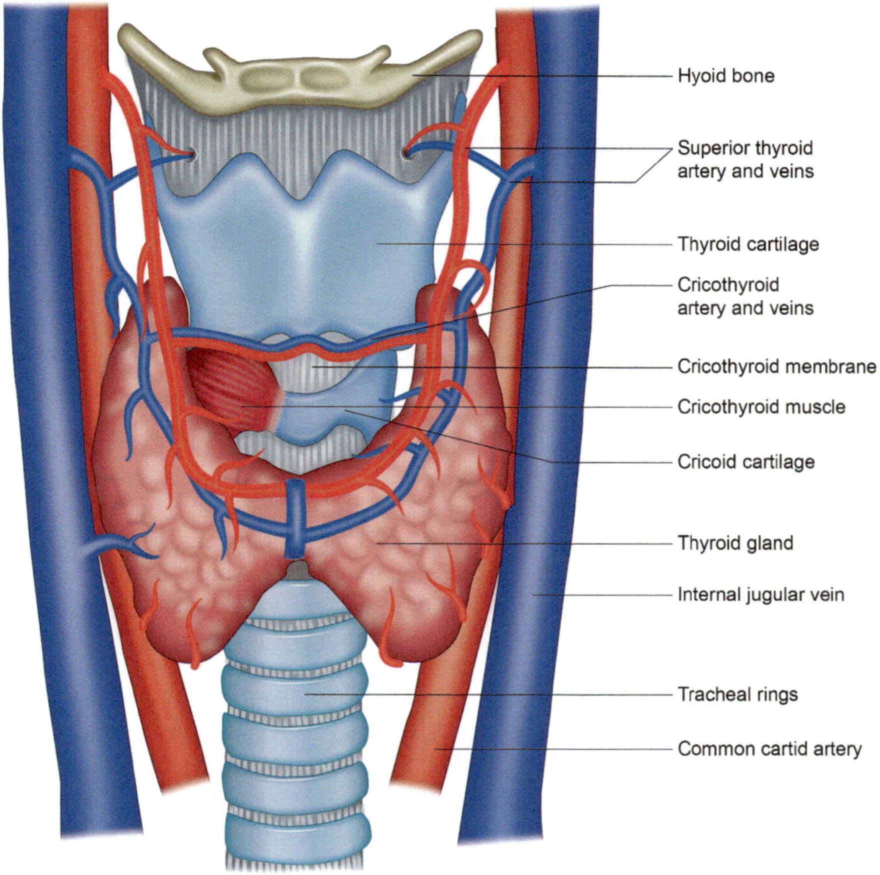

Fig. 2.3 The internal cervical neck anatomy showing the cricothyroid membrane between the thyroid and cricoid cartilage. The membrane is incised during a cricothyrotomy. The cricothyroid artery and vein are at the superior margin of the cricothyroid membrane and may be injured during cricothyrotomy

Clinical Presentation

Patients developing respiratory distress after ACSS may present in various ways. Patients may progress from being asymptomatic to having partial or complete airway obstruction in a few minutes or gradually over several days. Early on, the patient may complain of difficulty breathing, swallowing, and talking, exacerbated in the supine position [16]. Patients may complain they are suffocating or that the cervical collar is becoming too tight [31]. They may exhibit voice changes [14, 16].

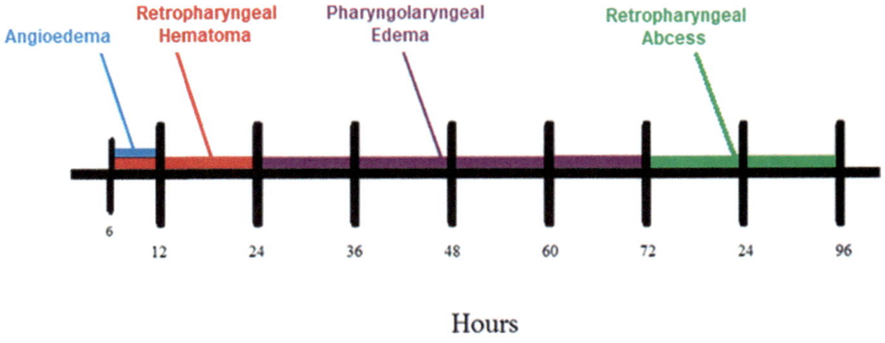

Fig. 2.4 Etiologies of post-operative airway compromise following anterior cervical surgery occur in a predictable time sequence

However, oxygen saturation will often remain normal. Therefore, a satisfactory measurement with pulse oximetry may be misleading and delay intervention. The carbon dioxide tension measured in an arterial blood gas provides a better objective assessment of the patient's respiratory status [21]. The patient may become restless and agitated as carbon dioxide levels increase; hypoxemia may or may not be present [14, 16]. They may have a look of fear or panic associated with dyspnea [16]. In later stages, the patient may use accessory respiratory muscles, or demonstrate inspiratory stridor or cyanosis [16].

Various etiologies of acute postoperative airway compromise following ACSS present in a predictable timeline (Fig. 2.4), with most adverse airway events occurring 24–48 h after surgery [7, 17, 32, 33]. Severe cases will require reintubation. Nagoshi et al. performed a retrospective multi-center cohort study of 8887 ACSS patients and found that 9 patients required reintubation, with 6 patients developing airway compromise within 24 h of surgery and the other 3 patients between 5 and 7 days [24]. Patients should be counseled on the symptoms and advised to seek immediate care as delay can result in fatality.

Angioedema

Although uncommon, angioedema may cause respiratory distress in the immediate post-operative setting, such as in the post-anesthesia care unit [34]. Patients can develop difficulty breathing with neck swelling extending into the face and oropharynx [34]. They may also have a massively swollen tongue protruding from their mouth [34]. It is essential to differentiate angioedema from a retropharyngeal hematoma to provide the patient with proper treatment. Their early findings can be very similar, however, reopening the surgical wound to evacuate a hematoma will not address the underlying cause nor relieve the symptoms of aniogedema [34]. Most cases of angioedema are idiopathic, and these cases are treated with intravenous

(IV) corticosteroids, antihistamines, and/or subcutaneous (or IV) epinephrine [34]. Hereditary angioedema represents 1–6% of cases [34], and does not respond to corticosteroids or antihistamines [35]. Instead, IV plasma-derived C1 esterase inhibitor (C1-INH) can be given prophylactically or as a lifesaving treatment. In all cases of angioedema, there should be a lower threshold for intubation as these patients can rapidly progress to respiratory failure. Endotracheal intubation may be difficult secondary to swelling and disruption of the normal cervical anatomy.

Retropharyngeal Hematoma

Clinically significant hematomas typically appear within 6–12 h of surgery [5, 14, 16]. Lied et al. found all wound hematomas presented within 6 h after surgery [5]. Song found 67% of retropharyngeal hematomas occur within 24 h and the remaining 33% within 72 h [13]. O'Neill found 65% of retropharyngeal hematomas occur within 24 h and the remaining 35% within 6 days [15]. Patients who develop a retropharyngeal hematoma typically form a tense mass under the incision, swelling of the anterior neck, and possible tracheal deviation [16, 28, 33, 36–39]. Multiple studies have investigated risk factors for post-operative retropharyngeal hematoma after cervical spine surgery (Table 2.1) [13, 15, 16, 40]. Other factors associated with hematoma formation include coagulopathies, excessive intra-operative blood loss, excessive postoperative hypertension, and prolonged excessive coughing during

Table 2.1 Risk factors reported in literature for airway compromise and reintubation following anterior cervical spine surgery

Hematoma	Pharyngolaryngeal edema	Abscess	CSF leak	Reintubation
African-American DISH OPLL Therapeutic heparin Long operative time (>5 h) Multi-level surgery (>3)	Male Older >65 years Obesity HTN OSA Mod-severe myelopathy Smoking Pulmonary disease Multiple intubation attempts/difficult intubation ACDF Multi-level surgery (>3) Exposing C2–4 Long operative time (>5 h) Prior/revision surgery EBL >300 cc Intra-operative blood transfusions (>4)	Esophageal perforation Operative contamination	OPLL Revision surgery	Male Age >60 years Obesity Smoking COPD Bleeding disorders/anemia CHF Alcohol abuse Dependent functional status ACCF ASA class >2 Multi-level surgery (>3) Exposing levels proximal to C5 Long operative time (>5 h) Greater blood loss wound class >2

extubation [16]. Inadequate intra-operative hemostasis is also a risk factor that can lead to post-operative hematomas. However, hematomas can still form despite apparently adequate intraoperative hemostasis [11, 13, 15, 16, 38]. At the time of diagnosis, a retropharyngeal hematoma should be immediately evacuated through the existing surgical incision to prevent further progression of respiratory distress. O'Neill et al. [15] found that of the 17 patients who developed a wound hematoma following ACSS, 2 required cricothyrotomy.

Pharyngolaryngeal Edema

If signs and symptoms of respiratory distress develop between 12–72 h post-operatively, pharyngolaryngeal edema should be highly suspected as the cause of respiratory failure [7, 14]. Patients can have various clinical presentations. They may progress slowly with difficulty talking and subtle changes in voice quality. Dyspnea may be exacerbated in supine position. Some patients may suddenly collapse with respiratory arrest. Multiple authors have attempted to define the risk factors leading to this complication (Table 2.1) [7, 10, 12, 21, 23, 25–27, 41–43]. Patients with multiple risk factors should have a very low threshold for maintaining post-operative intubation for 24–48 h and transferring to intensive critical care unit for observation. Patients with pharyngolaryngeal edema may pose a significant challenge for reintubation, and potential emergency cricothyrotomy should always be considered.

Cervical Abscess

Cervical abscess typically takes days to weeks to develop, and is the most likely cause of airway compromise more than 72 h after surgery [14]. A patient with a cervical abscess may complain of difficulty swallowing or choking sensation especially at night [44]. They may also notice neck swelling, fevers, and worsening leukocytosis [45]. Treatment should include irrigation and debridement as well as appropriate IV antibiotics. Specifically, a retropharyngeal abscess may develop as a result of esophageal perforation or operative contamination (Table 2.1) [45].

Cerebrospinal Fluid Leak

An intraoperative dural tear can lead to a cerebrospinal fluid (CSF) leak. This is a rare complication, which even less frequently leads to respiratory distress. CSF leaks are usually detected in the operating room. However, if the tear is missed, it can present within a variable timeframe with similar findings to a hematoma, such as swelling of the anterior neck, formation of a tense mass, and possible tracheal deviation [16, 28, 33, 36–39]. Greater risk for dural tears is associated with more complex surgeries including revisions and patients with severe ossification of the posterior longitudinal ligament (OPLL) (Table 2.1) [4, 36]. When a dural tear is observed intraoperatively it must be immediately repaired, often followed by insertion of a closed lumbar cerebrospinal fluid drain [6, 11, 36]. If a CSF leak is not treated appropriately, recurrences may prompt multiple reintubations [46].

Other Causes of Acute Postoperative Airway Complications

Other rare causes of acute postsurgical airway compromise have been described in literature. Goyal et al. reported a case of a malpositioned surgical drain that was accidentally placed through the trachea, and resting over the vocal cords, requiring intubation and mechanical ventilation [47]. A malpositioned drain should be considered if there is no significant cervical fluid collection or edema on inspection of the wound, and the drain is not functioning properly [47]. Finally, Skovrlj et al. described a case of cellulose gauze leading to post-operative respiratory compromise. The patient had no evidence of hematoma or soft tissue edema, however, on surgical exploration of the wound Surgifoam was found under high pressure obstructing the airway [48]. The authors recommended removing cellulose gauze from the surgical site after hemostasis is achieved to prevent airway compression, since it swells as it absorbs blood [48].

Imaging

Imaging is a routine part of pre- and post-operative evaluation of the cervical spine surgical patient. All radiographic studies should be reviewed in a systematic fashion so that potentially important findings are not overlooked. Plain radiographs are the mainstay of post-operative evaluation. However, computed tomography (CT) is superior for evaluation of post-operative complications, particularly soft-tissue abnormalities that could cause airway compromise. MRI is more sensitive than CT in detecting soft tissue pathology around the cervical spine [49]. However, MRI also has several disadvantages, such as increased motion artifacts, greater cost, and significantly longer acquisition time [49]. Thus, MRI is generally impractical for emergent settings such as airway compromise.

In cervical spine radiographs, the airway is best evaluated on the lateral view. Radiographic prevertebral soft tissue swelling (PSTS) is most commonly due to pharyngolaryngeal edema, which as discussed earlier is one of the most common causes of dyspnea and airway compromise after ACSS [33]. Many studies have used similar methods for quantifying PSTS after ACSS, most commonly by

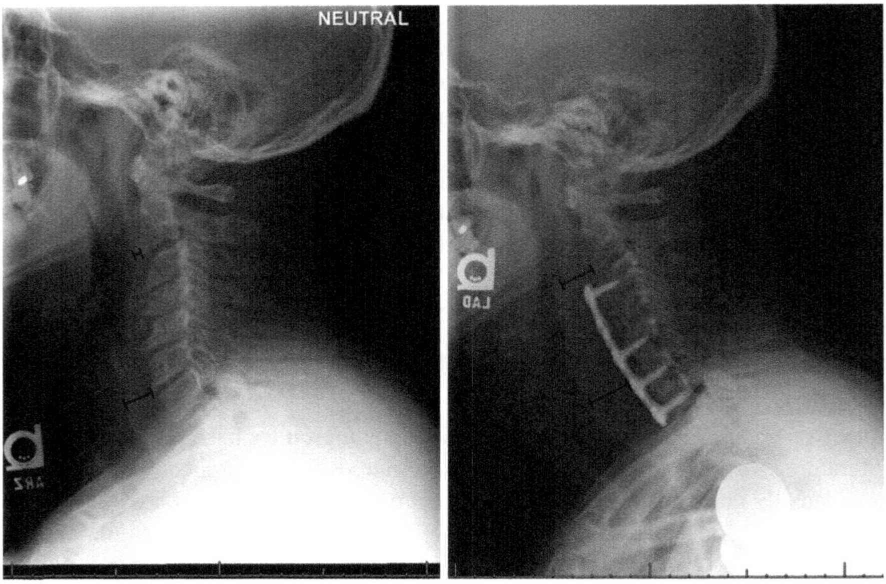

Fig. 2.5 Prevertebral soft tissue swelling (PSTS). Lateral radiographs of a 56-year-old male who underwent anterior cervical fusion of C3–C7. The pre-operative image (left) demonstrates prevertebral soft tissue thickness of 4 mm and 14 mm at the C2 and C6 levels respectively. The post-operative day 6 image (right) shows increased PSTS, measuring 27 mm and 34 mm at the C2 and C6 levels respectively, causing mild narrowing of the upper airway

measuring the distance between the anterior margin of the vertebral body to the posterior margin of the airway shadow at the same level (Fig. 2.5) [22, 32, 50, 51]. PSTS should be identified by comparing a post-operative study to a pre-operative study rather than with absolute thickness, as there is a wide range of normal prevertebral soft tissue thicknesses [50]. Most severe PSTS is found in the region of C4 [32]. PSTS is greatest on post-operative days 2 and 3, followed by a gradual decrease after day 4 [22, 51]. However, patients most frequently experienced dyspnea on post-operative days 0–2, which differs from noted maximum soft tissue swelling on post-operative days 2 or 3 [51]. Thus, degree of PSTS alone does not necessarily predict risk of dyspnea, and other contributing factors such as hematoma must also be considered.

Other common complications that can compromise the airway are hematoma, seroma, and abscess. Hematoma and seroma typically develop within the prevertebral soft tissue. On radiographs, these entities appear similar to each other and to PSTS. CT of the neck with intravenous contrast is useful for evaluating soft tissue swelling. Infected fluid collections or abscesses will have peripheral enhancement with IV contrast (Fig. 2.6) [44], whereas hematomas will typically not enhance with IV contrast, and seromas may or may not have thin peripheral enhancement. A

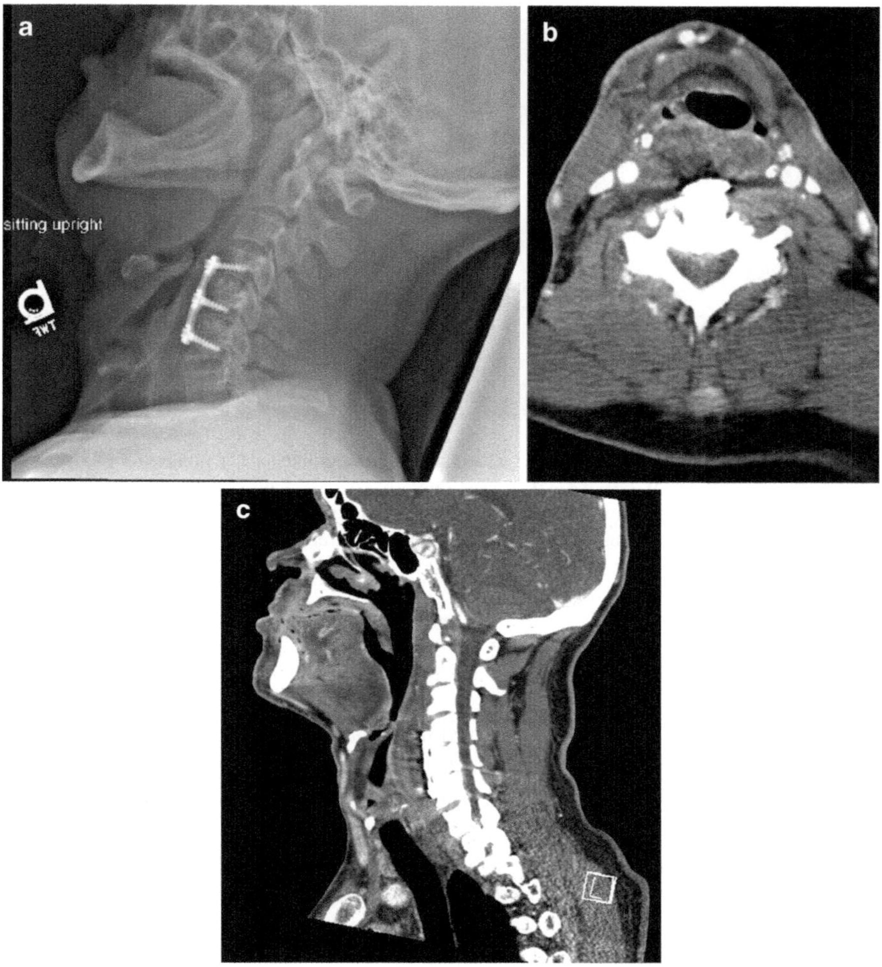

Fig. 2.6 Cervical abscess. (**a**) Immediate post-operative lateral radiograph of a 63-year-old male who underwent ACDF of C4–C6, demonstrating no significant fluid collections or edema. (**b**) Axial view of a CT with IV contrast of the same patient on post-operative day 7 demonstrating a peripherally enhancing prevertebral fluid collection found to be an abscess. (**c**) Sagittal view shows the abscess anteriorly displacing and mildly narrowing the airway

seroma will have uniform, simple-fluid density on CT, whereas an acute hematoma is generally more dense and heterogeneous (Fig. 2.7). As a hematoma ages, the density will decrease. CSF leaks, while rare, can lead to formation of a pseudomeningocele that can cause delayed airway compromise [46]. They present on CTs as a low-density fluid collection with thin peripheral enhancement [52].

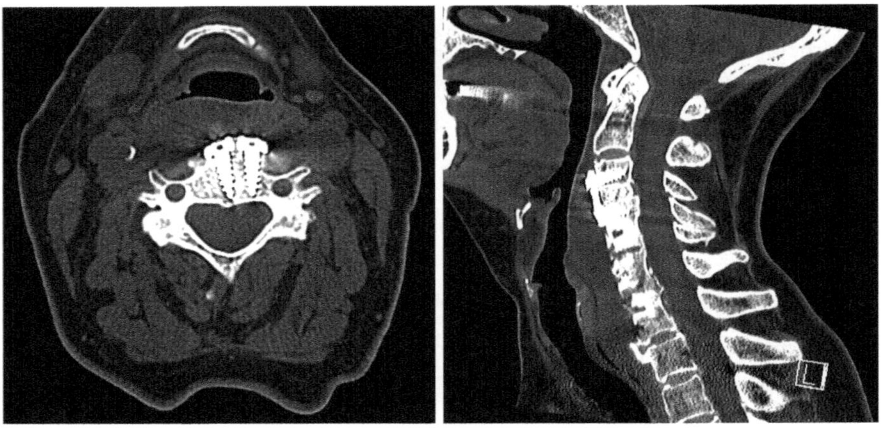

Fig. 2.7 Retropharyngeal hematoma. Axial and sagittal non-enhanced CT images of a 73-year-old female who underwent ACDF of C3–C4, post-operative day 7. A prevertebral fluid collection is seen, representing a hematoma with mild compression and narrowing of the adjacent airway. Of note, the patient had a prior fusion of C4–C6 with hardware removal

Perioperative Corticosteroids

Corticosteroids have been used in the past in the hope of decreasing laryngopharyngeal edema following prolonged tracheal intubation, and surgeries of the neck such as thyroidectomy and carotid endarterectomy [53, 54]. Nevertheless, the value of intravenous corticosteroids administered perioperatively to patients undergoing ACSS remains controversial.

Numerous studies have been conducted to investigate the effects of peri-operative corticosteroid use in ACSS, using various protocols. Multiple studies have found a reduction in PSTS on lateral radiographs or on flexible endoscopic airway examination [31, 32, 55, 56]. However, multiple studies have also found no difference in extubation timing, airway compromise, or reintubation rate following intra-operative corticosteroid treatment [20, 53, 57]. In terms of complications, corticosteroids are known to cause nonunion in bone healing. However, several studies evaluating fusion rates for patients receiving intra-operative corticosteroids for ACSS found no significant difference in bony fusion rates at 12 months [20, 57].

Side effects of systemic corticosteroids include hyperglycemia, infection, nonunion, gastritis, peptic ulcer disease, DVT, osteoporosis and avascular necrosis. Local retropharyngeal steroids have the advantage of a lower risk of systemic complications [32]. Thus, the risks and benefits of steroids should be weighed to provide the patient with the best clinical outcome.

Postoperative Intubation Protocol

There are multiple algorithms established by different national and international specialty societies as a guide for "difficult" airway placements in patients that require anesthesia. Unfortunately, there is no established standard algorithm either for postoperative airway management after ACDF or for how best to secure the airway should reintubation be required [16, 41]. We believe that it is helpful to identify patients at increased risk for postoperative airway compromise and need for reintubation. Recognizing these concerns, Epstein et al. developed a conservative protocol with for patients undergoing multi-level anterior-posterior spine surgery [26]. All patients remained intubated overnight after surgery and were extubated only after direct fiberoptic assessment confirmed that there was minimal soft tissue swelling. Most patients (40/58) could be extubated on post-operative day 1. However, a substantial number (31%) underwent delayed extubation. Only one (1.7%) patient required emergent reintubation, on post-operative day 3.

Palumbo et al. suggested an airway protection protocol following anterior cervical spine surgery based on surgical risk factors [7], stratifying the patients into low-, intermediate-, and high-risk categories [14]. Patients in the low-risk group may be safely extubated after surgery in the operating room. Patients in the high-risk group had multiple surgical risks factors, were routinely ventilated overnight, and underwent delayed extubation [14]. In the intermediate-risk group, patients had only one surgical risk factor. Palumbo et al. recommended evaluating the secondary risk factors to determine if the patient should be left intubated for overnight observation.

Kim et al. created an airway management protocol at their institution for patient undergoing anterior cervical spine surgery [41]. If patients had any one of five risk factors including: (1) exposure of greater than 3 cervical levels; (2) operative site on C3–4 or above; (3) greater than 5 h operative time; (4) blood loss greater than 300 mL and (5) significant medical comorbidity, they would remain intubated overnight [7, 41]. The cuff-leak test and lateral radiographs were repeated at 12 h intervals until the patients were extubated. If the patient passed the cuff-leak test or had no significant prevertebral soft tissue swelling on cervical lateral radiographs, they would be extubated. Kim et al. compared 275 patients in the non-protocol group to 263 patients in the protocol group and found that there was a significantly reduced postoperative airway complication rate in the protocol group [41].

Patients left intubated after surgery should have the head of the bed elevated to 30° to improve ventilation and venous drainage. Patients should be extubated only when appropriate physicians and supporting staff are available to manage a failed extubation. If a patient develops laryngeal edema and cannot be reintubated, either transtracheal jet ventilation or an emergent cricothyrotomy should be performed [16]. If there is complete airway obstruction, jet ventilation is precluded given the inability for exhaled gas to exit. Unfortunately, after ACSS, postoperative swelling and anatomical distortion may result in increased rates of failed intubations [13].

Timely restoration of ventilation and oxygenation is critical to avoid asphyxia-induced cardiac arrest and brain injury. Therefore, an emergency cricothyrotomy kit should be readily accessible near the patient's bedside, including on the floor unit. Of note, cricothyrotomy is contraindicated in patients who are under 12 years of age.

Sequence of Resuscitation After Respiratory Arrest

The sequence of resuscitation efforts is typically based on the assumption that after cardiac arrest, the brain can recover if adequate oxygen delivery resumes within 5 min [58]. However, this time limit was arrived at based on animal studies of cardiac arrest without prior asphyxia. Unfortunately, animal studies comparing cardiac arrest with or without prior asphyxia uniformly demonstrate that prior asphyxia leads to worse outcomes and reduces the potential time of cardiac arrest after which meaningful survival can be anticipated [59, 60]. We can assume that in patients who experience cardiac arrest after ACSS as a consequence of airway edema and obstruction, the cause of cardiac arrest is progressive hypoxemia and hypercarbia. Similarly, we strongly suspect that without immediate restoration of adequate oxygen delivery, such patients will likely be associated with a catastrophic brain injury following cardiac arrest [61–63].

Like all procedures, experience is a critical factor for an efficient performance of emergent cricothyrotomy. Petrosoniak et al. noted that 20 Emergency Medicine residents, in a simulation lab, had a cricothyrotomy performance time of approximately 160 s (±48 s) including assessment to technical completion of the task prior to simulation training [64]. Subsequent simulation training reduced this time to 100 s (±26 s). Many of these residents had witnessed or performed a cricothyrotomy simulation in the past, but only one resident had actually performed a cricothyrotomy on a patient. An observational study reported that experienced physicians needed a median of 73 s (range: 53–255 s), while inexperienced physicians required a median of 180 s to complete a cricothyrotomy using the standard technique in unfixed cadavers [65]. An observational study of 44 paramedic students found that an average of 46 s (range 29–63 s) were needed to complete a standard cricothyrotomy [66]. A performance time study would be beneficial using orthopaedic and neurosurgery residents. Based on this data and assuming minimal experience with cricothyrotomy, we make the following recommendations regarding emergency airway management (which can be modified based on the operator's level of experience):

1. Immediately call for help so that another physician can oversee cardiac arrest management, such as chest compressions, pharmaceutical treatments, and defibrillation. We suggest adhering to the American Heart Association/American College of Cardiology Advanced Cardiovascular Life Support (ACLS) algorithm or the relevant algorithms in other countries (e.g. Resuscitation Council in the United Kingdom).

2. Immediately upon arrival, ventilate a patient experiencing respiratory arrest with oxygen using a bag-valve mask system. Observe chest rise and level of oxygenation to assess the effectiveness of ventilation. An assistant can attach a pulse oximeter to the patient and a capnograph in line with the mask. Give particular attention to appropriate mask seal and position of mandible. The mask should have a circumferential seal over the perinasal and perioral face. The mandible should be advanced anteriorly to dilate the posterior oropharyngeal orifice.
3. If ventilation is not effective within 1 min, make 1 attempt at oral intubation using (preferably) video laryngoscopy or a conventional laryngoscope.
4. If orotracheal intubation is not successful or if more than 2 min have passed since onset of respiratory arrest, proceed directly cricothyrotomy.

Cricothyrotomy Kit

The emergency cricothyrotomy kit should only contain the essential instruments. The kit should include an antiseptic skin cleaning preparation such as ChloraPrep™, 11- or 15-blade scalpel, hemostat, a small cuffed endotracheal or tracheostomy tube, and a 10 mL syringe (Fig. 2.8). Kits are best kept on the hospital floor, in the resident room, or at the bedside of high-risk patients where they are readily accessible. Like code carts, all clinical staff should be aware of the location of emergency cricothyrotomy kits.

Steps for cricothyrotomy procedure

1. Confirm that ventilation with bag valve mask and endotracheal intubation have failed.
2. Position patient supine with the neck extended, exposing the anterior trachea.
3. Clean the skin with antiseptic solution, such as a ChloraPrep™. Double glove yourself.
4. Palpate laryngeal landmarks: thyroid cartilage notch, cricoid cartilage, and cricothyroid membrane (Fig. 2.9a).
5. Make a longitudinal midline skin incision from the thyroid notch to the cricoid cartilage and deep to the cricothyroid membrane (Fig. 2.9a).
6. Use blunt dissection to evacuate any hematomas making sure that the posterior aspect of the trachea is cleared. Having a suctioning device available may aid in exposure.
7. Make a transverse incision through the cricothyroid membrane (Fig. 2.9b). If the provider is unsure of the location of the cricothyroid membrane, a needle attached to a saline filled syringe can be inserted through the site. If there is return of air bubbles on aspiration, this will confirm location of the needle tip within the airway.
8. Insert the hemostat and dilate the opening (Fig. 2.9c).
9. Insert the cuffed endotracheal tube or tracheostomy tube into the opening (Fig. 2.9d).

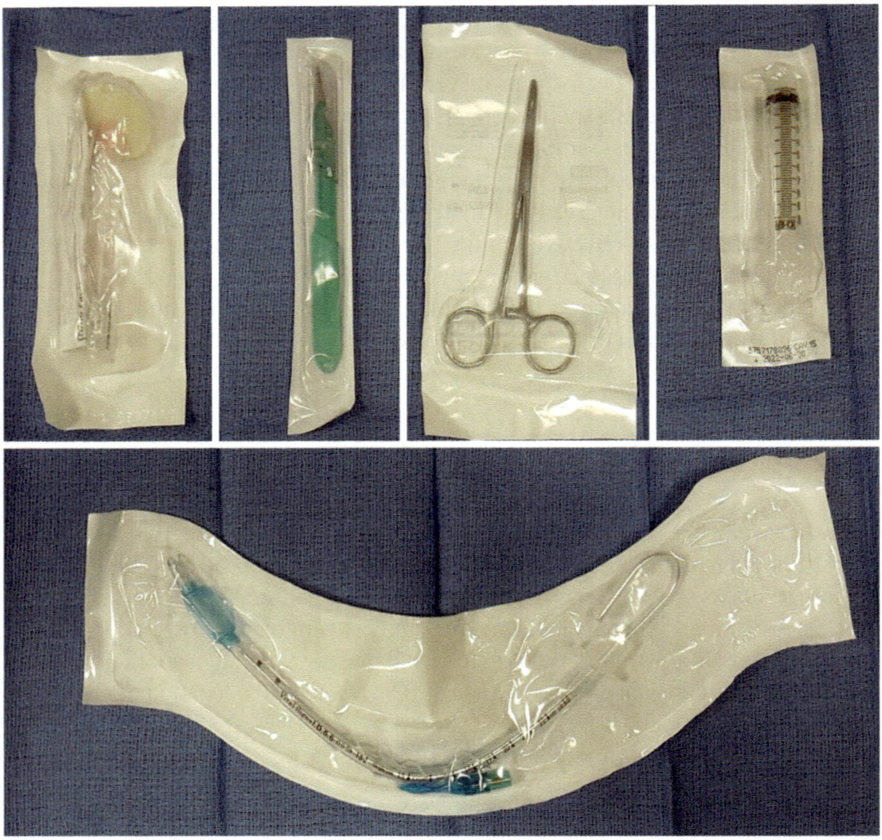

Fig. 2.8 The essential tools for a cricothyrotomy kit include antiseptic skin cleaning preparation such as ChloraPrep, scalpel, hemostat, a small cuffed endotracheal or tracheostomy tube, and a 10 mL syringe

10. Inflate the cuff to prevent an air leak.
11. Confirm endotracheal placement with return of end-tidal CO_2, increase in O_2 saturation, and chest rise.
12. Do NOT let go of the tracheal tube until it is secured with tape.
13. Take patient straight to the OR for formal wound exploration and conversion to a definitive tracheostomy (Fig. 2.10).

Pearls and Pitfalls

- Proper care of the at-risk airway begins prior to the need for a surgical airway. Patients at risk for airway compromise should be continuously monitored with pulse oximetry in an intermediate or stepdown unit with adequate nursing care. Communication between the surgical team and nursing staff regarding airway management should be part of the patient transfer process after surgery. This

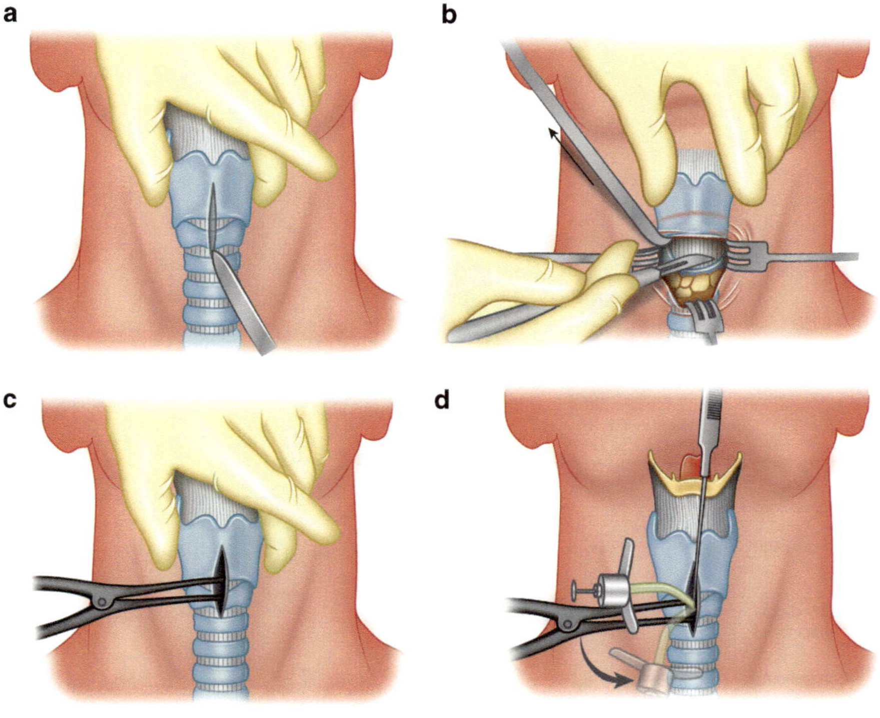

Fig. 2.9 Steps of performing a cricothyrotomy. (**a**) Position the neck extended, exposing the anterior trachea. Palpate laryngeal landmarks. Make a midline skin incision from the thyroid notch to the cricoid cartilage and deep to the cricothyroid membrane. (**b**) Make a transverse incision through the cricothyroid membrane. (**c**) Insert the hemostat and dilate the opening. (**d**) Insert the cuffed endotracheal tube or tracheostomy tube into the opening and inflate the cuff

includes instructions for elevating the head of the bed to lessen edema, aspiration precautions at re-initiation of an oral diet, and ensuring appropriate airway tools are readily available in the event of an emergency. In procedures that require extensive dissection within the neck, consideration should be given to placing a surgical drain and to administering steroids for 24 h post-operatively.

- Any changes in respiratory status should be immediately assessed. This may include bedside laryngoscopy to evaluate the airway. In the non-responsive patient with developing respiratory distress, cricothyrotomy should not be delayed by multiple intubation attempts. This is especially true in patients with evolving or changing airway anatomy such as an expanding hematoma causing laryngeal edema or angioedema.
- Airway management solutions should be initiated in parallel sequence. For example, calling for the materials for intubation should also include having the materials available to rapidly establish a surgical airway if needed.

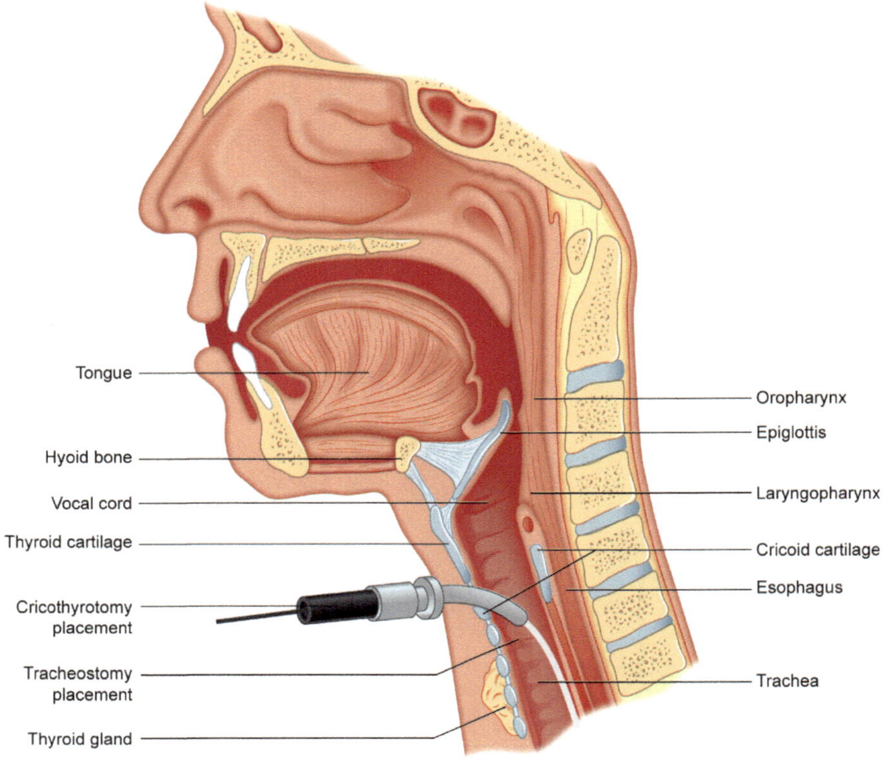

Fig. 2.10 A sagittal drawing of the upper respiratory tract showing the location of a cricothyrotomy and tracheostomy as compared to the surrounding vital structures

- There should be no delay between the time that the determination is made that a patient requires a surgical airway and performing a cricothyrotomy. Delayed placement of a surgical airway is the most common reason for adverse outcomes in cases of airway obstruction.
- All residents taking care of patients with potential need for surgical airway management (otolaryngology, orthopaedics, general surgery, neurosurgery, emergency medicine, anesthesia, etc.) should have the basic supplies to perform a cricothyrotomy in their bag or close at hand.
- The patient's neck should be positioned in extension to best show relevant laryngeal landmarks. This is an important step and may be the difference between inadequate versus good exposure of the cricothyroid membrane. Neck extension may be accomplished by placing a rolled blanket, towel, or sheet under the shoulders, and removing the pillow.
- Once the patient is adequately positioned, the surgeon should firmly grasp the larynx between their thumb and third/fourth finger of their non-dominant hand using their second finger to palpate the cricothyroid membrane. Pressure should

be applied downward (posteriorly) bilaterally to retract the vertical skin incision as it is made and facilitate exposure of the cricothyroid membrane.

- Upon piercing the cricothyroid membrane there will be a distinct popping sensation confirming entry into the larynx. The tracheostomy or endotracheal tube should be rotated from 90° to straight during insertion. If you are using an endotracheal tube with a flexible tip, be aware that the tip may flip superiorly instead of inferiorly toward the airway. Pointing the tip down and not inserting perpendicular to the skin will help direct the endotracheal tube inferiorly. If the ETT is placed superiorly, it will become evident with oxygenation failing to improve and absence of return of end-tidal CO_2 on monitoring. The tube should be removed and carefully reinserted. A rigid bougie, intubating stylet or flexible fiberoptic bronchoscope may aid with insertion.
- A cuffed, flexible tracheotomy tube such as a Shiley #4 or #6 or an endotracheal tube may be utilized. Depending on availability, either tube is an appropriate choice, but if difficultly is encountered with placement of a tracheotomy tube, the provider should switch to an endotracheal tube. A rigid tracheotomy tube can create a false passage with the pressure required for placement and the flange on the tracheotomy tube can impair visualization during placement.
- Bleeding during an emergent surgical airway is difficult to avoid as there may be several, relatively large anterior jugular veins in the area. Staying as close to midline as possible will decrease this risk. Pressure may be applied to control bleeding and the patient should be taken emergently to the OR for conversion to a formal tracheostomy and hemostasis.

Conclusion

ACSS, such as ACDF, is becoming more common as these procedures produce good outcomes with low risk for complications. Unfortunately, some perioperative complications may quickly become debilitating or fatal. The most common causes of airway compromise during recovery from ACSS are hematomas and pharyngolaryngeal edema. Certain risk factors can be used to help stratify patients into low-, intermediate- and high-risk groups for post-surgical airway compromise. Physicians must be prepared to diagnose and immediately treat these life-threatening complications to prevent cardiopulmonary arrest, anoxic brain injury, or fatality. If intubation cannot be accomplished immediately on the first attempt, physicians should not hesitate to obtain a secure, surgical airway. Although patients have had meaningful recoveries after uncomplicated cardiac arrests in which successful resuscitation required greater than 5 min, patients experiencing cardiac arrest from asphyxia differ. A brain subjected to increasing degrees of hypercarbia and hypoxemia prior to cardiac arrest has no tolerance for delayed resuscitation [61].

Questions Revisited

1. **What is the most likely reason for respiratory arrest? A combination of edema and hematoma resulting in mechanical airway obstruction.**
2. **What is the preferred sequence of resuscitation? Depending on time arrest was witnessed.**

   (a) **Call for assistance and initiate an airway alert if available, call for intubation and procedural airway supplies.**
   (b) **Attempt mask-ventilate and assess with pulse oximeter and capnograph.**
   (c) **Attempt intubation or supraglottic airway, if mask ventilation not successful with in 1 min.**
   (d) **Proceed to surgical airway, if intubation or supraglottic airway not successful within 2 min.**

3. **What should be the required skill sets to handle this condition? Ability to intubate and ability to perform a surgical airway.**

References

1. Rhee J, Voyadzis J-M. Anterior cervical diskectomy and fusion. In: Surgical anatomy and techniques to the spine; 2014. p. 131–8.
2. Helgeson MD, Albert TJ. Anterior approach to the cervical spine. In: Textbook of the cervical spine, vol. 3; 2015. p. 33–8.
3. Wilson AS, Samartzis D, Shen FH. Anterior cervical diskectomy and fusion. In: Textbook of the cervical spine; 2015. p. 285–93.
4. Daniels AH, et al. Adverse events associated with anterior cervical spine surgery. J Am Acad Orthop Surg. 2008;16(12):729–38.
5. Lied B, Sundseth J, Helseth E. Immediate (0–6 h), early (6–72 h) and late (>72 h) complications after anterior cervical discectomy with fusion for cervical disc degeneration; discharge 6 h after operation is feasible. Acta Neurochir. 2008;150:111–8.
6. Fountas KN, et al. Anterior cervical discectomy and fusion associated complications. Spine (Phila Pa 1976). 2007;32(21):2310–7.
7. Sagi HC, Beutler W, Carroll E, Connolly PJ. Airway complications associated with surgery on the anterior cervical spine. Spine (Phila Pa 1976). 2002;27(9):949–53.
8. Macdonald RL, et al. Multilevel anterior cervical corpectomy and fibular allograft fusion for cervical myelopathy. J Neurosurg. 1997;86(6):990–7.
9. Sinkiewicz A, Harat M, Furtak J. Complications after surgery of the anterior cervical spine. Neurol Neurochir Pol. 1997;31(1):135–44.
10. Boakye M, Patil CG, Ho C, Lad SP. Cervical corpectomy: complications and outcomes. Neurosurgery. 2008;63(4 SUPPL):295–302.
11. Tasiou A, et al. Anterior cervical spine surgery-associated complications in a retrospective case-control study. J Spine Surg. 2017;3(3):444–59.
12. Kwon B, Yoo JU, Furey CG, Rowbottom J, Emery SE. Risk factors for delayed extubation after single-stage, multi-level anterior cervical decompression and posterior fusion. J Spinal Disord Tech. 2006;19(6):389–93.
13. Song KJ, Choi BW, Lee DH, Lim DJ, Oh SY, Kim SS. Acute airway obstruction due to postoperative retropharyngeal hematoma after anterior cervical fusion: a retrospective analysis. J Orthop Surg Res. 2017;12(19):19.

14. Palumbo MA, Aidlen JP, Daniels AH, Bianco A, Caiati JM. Airway compromise due to laryngopharyngeal edema after anterior cervical spine surgery. J Clin Anesth. 2013;25(1):66–72.
15. O'Neill KR, Neuman B, Peters C, Riew KD. Risk factors for postoperative retropharyngeal hematoma after anterior cervical spine surgery. Spine (Phila Pa 1976). 2014;39(4):E426–252.
16. Palumbo MA, Aidlen JP, Daniels AH, Thakur NA, Caiati J. Airway compromise due to wound hematoma following anterior cervical spine surgery. Open Orthop J. 2012;6(1):108–13.
17. Bertalanffy H, Eggert HR. Complications of anterior cervical discectomy without fusion in 450 consecutive patients. Acta Neurochir. 1989;99(1–2):41–50.
18. Viejo-Fuertes D, Liguoro D, Ansari M, Rombouts JJ, Vital JM, Senegas J. Complications following anterior approaches to the cervical spine. Review of 535 surgical procedures. Eur J Orthop Surg Traumatol. 2000;10:177–81.
19. Al Maaieh M, et al. The immediate safety profile after complex anterior cervical reconstruction surgery. MOJ Orthop Rheumatol. 2015;2(1):4–9.
20. Jeyamohan SB, Kenning TJ, Petronis KA, Feustel PJ, Drazin D, Dirisio DJ. Effect of steroid use in anterior cervical discectomy and fusion: a randomized controlled trial. J Neurosurg Spine. 2015;23:137–43.
21. Li H, Huang Y, Shen B, Ba Z, Wu D. Multivariate analysis of airway obstruction and reintubation after anterior cervical surgery: a retrospective cohort study of 774 patients. Int J Surg. 2017;41:28–33.
22. Suk K-S, Kim K-T, Lee S-H, Park S-W. Prevertebral soft tissue swelling after anterior cervical discectomy and fusion with plate fixation. Int Orthop. 2006;30:290–4.
23. Marquez-Lara A, Nandyala SV, Fineberg SJ, Singh K. Incidence, outcomes, and mortality of reintubation after anterior cervical fusion. Spine (Phila Pa 1976). 2014;39(2):134–9.
24. Nagoshi N, et al. Prevalence and outcomes in patients undergoing reintubation after anterior cervical spine surgery: results from the AOSpine North America multicenter study on 8887 patients. Glob Spine J. 2017;7(1S):96S–102S.
25. Lim S, Kesavabhotla K, Cybulski GR, Dahdaleh NS, Smith ZA. Predictors for airway complications following single- and multilevel anterior cervical discectomy and fusion. Spine (Phila Pa 1976). 2017;42(6):379–84.
26. Epstein NE, Hollingsworth R, Nardi D, Singer J. Can airway complications following multilevel anterior cervical surgery be avoided? J Neurosurg. 2001;94(2 Suppl):185–8.
27. Emery SE, Smith MD, Bohlman HH. Upper-airway obstruction after multilevel cervical corpectomy for myelopathy. J Bone Jt Surg Am. 1991;73(4):544–51.
28. Yu NH, Jahng TA, Kim CH, Chung CK. Life-threatening late hemorrhage due to superior thyroid artery dissection after anterior cervical discectomy and fusion. Spine (Phila Pa 1976). 2010;35(15):E739–42.
29. Smith GW, Robinson RA. The treatment of certain cervical spine disorders by anterior removal of the intervertebral disc and interbody fusion. J Bone Jt Surg Am. 1958;40(3):607–24.
30. Cheung KMC, Mak KC, Luk KDK. Anterior approach to cervical spine. Spine (Phila Pa 1976). 2012;37(5):297–302.
31. Pedram M, Castagnera L, Carat X, Macouillard G, Vital J-M. Pharyngolaryngeal lesions in patients undergoing cervical spine surgery through the anterior approach: contribution of methylprednisolone. Eur Spine J. 2003;12:84–90.
32. Lee SH, Kim KT, Suk KS, Park KJ, Il Oh K. Effect of retropharyngeal steroid on prevertebral soft tissue swelling following anterior cervical discectomy and fusion; a prospective, randomized study. Spine (Phila Pa 1976). 2011;36(26):2286–92.
33. Sethi R, Tandon MS, Ganjoo P. Neck hematoma causing acute airway and hemodynamic compromise after anterior cervical spine surgery. J Neurosurg Anesthesiol. 2008;20(1):69–70.
34. Krnacik MJ, Heggeness MH. Severe angioedema causing airway obstruction after anterior cervical surgery. Spine (Phila Pa 1976). 1997;22(18):2188–90.
35. Umerani MS, Alzahrani K, Mostafa GA. Hereditary angioedema: a rare presentation after anterior cervical discectomy and fusion. Asian J Neurosurg. 2015;10(3):253–5.

36. Chang HS, Kondo S, Mizuno J, Nakagawa H. Airway obstruction caused by cerebrospinal fluid leakage after anterior cervical spine surgery. A report of two cases. J Bone Jt Surg. 2004;86-A(2):370–2.
37. Roy SP. Acute postoperative neck hematoma. Am J Emerg Med. 1999;17(3):308–9.
38. Quick E, Byard RW. Postoperative cervical soft tissue hemorrhage with acute upper airway obstruction. J Forensic Sci. 2013;58(S1):S264–6.
39. Tang SJ, Rao RD. Perioperative and approach-related complications associated with anterior cervical surgery. Semin Spine Surg. 2009;21:148–55.
40. Skolasky RL, Thorpe RJ, Wegener ST, Riley LH. Complications and mortality in cervical spine surgery: racial differences. Spine (Phila Pa 1976). 2014;39(18):1506–12.
41. Kim M, Choi I, Park JH, Jeon SR, Rhim SC, Roh SW. Airway management protocol after anterior cervical spine surgery. Spine (Phila Pa 1976). 2017;42(18):E1058–66.
42. Basques BA, et al. Gender differences for anterior cervical fusion. Spine (Phila Pa 1976). 2018;43(15):1025–30.
43. Buerba RA, Giles E, Webb ML, Fu MC, Gvozdyev B, Grauer JN. Increased risk of complications after anterior cervical discectomy and fusion in the elderly: an analysis of 6253 patients in the American College of Surgeons National Surgical Quality Improvement Program database. Spine (Phila Pa 1976). 2014;39(25):2062–9.
44. Gwinnutt CL, Walsh GR, Kumar R. Airway obstruction after anterior cervical spine surgery. J Neurosurg Anesthesiol. 1992;4(3):199–202.
45. Kuriloff DB, Blaugrund S, Ryan J, O'Leary P. Delayed neck infection following anterior spine surgery. Laryngoscope. 1987;97(9):1094–8.
46. Penberthy A, Roberts N. Recurrent acute upper airway obstruction after anterior cervical fusion. Anaesth Intensive Care. 1998;26:305–7.
47. Goyal H, Dube SK, Kumar A, Goyal K. An unusual cause of post operative respiratory distress following anterior cervical discectomy and fusion. J Neuroanaesth Crit Care. 2014;1(3):217–8.
48. Skovrlj B, Mascitelli JR, Camins MB, Doshi AH, Qureshi SA. Acute respiratory failure from surgifoam expansion after anterior cervical surgery. J Neurosurg Spine. 2013;19:428–30.
49. Hayashi D, Roemer FW, Mian A, Gharaibeh M, Müller B, Guermazi A. Imaging features of postoperative complications after spinal surgery and instrumentation. Am J Roentgenol. 2012;199(1):123–9.
50. Chen MYM, Bohrer SP. Radiographic measurement of prevertebral soft tissue thickness on lateral radiographs of the neck. Skelet Radiol. 1999;28(8):444–6.
51. Song KJ, Choi BW, Kim HY, Jeon TS, Chang H. Efficacy of postoperative radiograph for evaluating the prevertebral soft tissue swelling after anterior cervical discectomy and fusion. Clin Orthop Surg. 2012;4:77–82.
52. Karasick D, Vaccaro R, Schweitzer ME. Complications of cervical spine fusion: imaging features. Am J Roentgenol. 1997;169:869–74.
53. Emery SE, et al. Steroids and risk factors for airway compromise in multilevel cervical corpectomy patients: a prospective, randomized, double-blind study. Spine (Phila Pa 1976). 2009;34(3):229–32.
54. François B, et al. 12-h Pretreatment with methylprednisolone versus placebo for prevention of postextubation laryngeal oedema: a randomised double-blind trial. Lancet. 2007;369(9567):1083–9.
55. Weinstein J, Schroeder JE, Sama AA, Girardi FP. Effect of steroid placement on a gelatin sponge and soft tissue swelling following anterior cervical discectomy and fusion: a radiological analysis. Spine J. 2014;14(11):S116.
56. Song KJ, Lee SK, Ko JH, Yoo MJ, Kim DY, Lee KB. The clinical efficacy of short-term steroid treatment in multilevel anterior cervical arthrodesis. Spine J. 2014;14:2954–8.
57. Zadegan SA, Jazayeri SB, Abedi A, Bonaki HN, Vaccaro AR, Rahimi-Movaghar V. Corticosteroid administration to prevent complications of anterior cervical spine fusion: a systematic review. Glob Spine J. 2017;8(3):286–302.

58. Weisfeldt ML, Becker LB. Resuscitation after cardiac arrest: a 3-phase time-sensitive model. JAMA J Am Med Assoc. 2002;288(23):3035–8.
59. Vaagenes P, et al. Asphyxiation versus ventricular fibrillation cardiac arrest in dogs. Differences in cerebral resuscitation effects—a preliminary study. Resuscitation. 1997;35(1):41–52.
60. Chen B, et al. Comparison of quantitative characteristics of early post-resuscitation EEG between asphyxial and ventricular fibrillation cardiac arrest in rats. Neurocrit Care. 2017;28(2):247–56.
61. Varvarousis D, Varvarousi G, Iacovidou N, D'Aloja E, Gulati A, Xanthos T. The pathophysiologies of asphyxial vs dysrhythmic cardiac arrest: implications for resuscitation and post-event management. Am J Emerg Med. 2015;33(9):1297–304.
62. Miran K, Križmarić M, Klemen P, Grmec Š. Partial pressure of end-tidal carbon dioxide successful predicts cardiopulmonary resuscitation in the field: a prospective observational study. Crit Care. 2008;12(5):R11.
63. Eastwood GM, Young PJ, Bellomo R. The impact of oxygen and carbon dioxide management on outcome after cardiac arrest. Curr Opin Crit Care. 2014;20:266–72.
64. Petrosoniak A, Ryzynski A, Lebovic G, Woolfrey K. Cricothyroidotomy in situ simulation curriculum (CRIC study): training residents for rare procedures. Simul Healthc. 2017;12(2):76–82.
65. Mutzbauer TS, Munz R, Helm M, Lampl LA, Herrmann M. Emergency cricothyrotomy—puncture or anatomical preparation? Peculiarities of two methods for emergency airway access demonstrated in a cadaver model. Anaesthesist. 2003;52(4):304–10.
66. Brofeldt BT, Panacek EA, Richards JR. An easy cricothyrotomy approach: the rapid four-step technique. Acad Emerg Med. 1996;3(11):1060–3.

Chapter 3
Spine Epidural Hematoma

Callie Herman and Shalin Shah

Introduction

Spinal epidural hematoma (SEH) is a rare condition that accounts for less than 1% of all spinal canal space-occupying lesions [1–3]. It is thought to be most commonly caused by coagulopathies, hypertension, increased venous pressure, or vascular malformations [4, 5]. Spontaneous spinal epidural hematomas (SSEH) result from the accumulation of blood in the epidural space without a known cause and have an incidence of 0.1 in 100,000 per year [2, 3]. Timely and accurate diagnosis is critical for an effective treatment plan and optimal outcome as patients who develop a SEH are at risk for suffering from severe pain and permanent neurological deficits [3, 4]. Since SEH is a rare but serious condition, it is important to highlight the common patient presentations to ensure that physicians at all levels of training are equipped to identify and manage this emergency. Thus, the main purpose of this literature review is to highlight key diagnostic features and treatment strategies for SEH.

C. Herman (✉)
Campbell University School of Osteopathic Medicine, Lillington, NC, USA
e-mail: c_herman0715@email.campbell.edu

S. Shah
Department of Orthopaedic Surgery, Virginia Commonwealth University, Richmond, VA, USA
e-mail: shalin.shah1@vcuhealth.org

W. A. Zuelzer, S. Metikala (eds.), *Unusual Conditions That Every Orthopaedic Surgeon Should Know*, https://doi.org/10.1007/978-3-031-58946-1_3

Clinical Presentation

Typical SEH Presentations

Patients who develop a SEH commonly present with acute onset of severe neck and/or back pain that may radiate into the extremities with symptoms ranging from nerve root irritation to full neurologic impairment [1, 2, 6]. Depending on the level of injury, patients may even experience hyporeflexia and flaccid paralysis due to the insult to lower motor neurons [1]. Risk factors, according to some studies, associate SEH with advanced age, female gender, traumatic and multiple attempts at puncture for neuraxial anesthesia, vascular malformations, anticoagulants, and hypertension [7]. Other studies investigating risk factors for SSEH have suggested that males are slightly more affected than females (1.4:1) [8, 9] and that SSEH typically presents in the fourth and fifth decades of life [2, 6, 9]. Pregnancy has also been identified as a risk factor for SSEH [10]. While SEH has been shown to develop from preexisting medical conditions (e.g. hypertension, vascular malformations) and/or spontaneously, it can also evolve as a secondary complication after invasive procedures. Due to the diverse range of circumstances that can lead to SEH, recognizing key features of the condition is crucial for minimizing the potential long-term neurological sequalae. The following cases highlight key diagnostic features of SEH in patients ranging from elderly adults undergoing total joint arthroplasty to healthy pregnant females and children.

Case Examples

Joint Arthroplasty Postoperative Spinal Epidural Hematoma

In 2009, Kasodekar et al. described an 80-year-old woman who developed a spinal epidural hematoma between 2–4 days after undergoing a left total knee arthroplasty [11]. The patient's medical history was unremarkable except for hypertension and depression. Prior to surgery she received an L4–L5 epidural anesthetic for pain control and discontinued her low molecular weight heparin until postoperative day 1. Thromboprophylaxis was started 24 h after the epidural injection and by postoperative day two she had been weaned to an epidural infusion of 2 mL/h and 1 mg of oral hydromorphone every 4 h.

By the evening of day 2, the patient was unable to move her feet or lift her right leg. Vitals were normal, coagulation and blood count were normal, and she did not complain of back pain or fecal incontinence. Her medications were temporarily paused and by the next morning she was able to move her feet and right leg but was unable to flex at the hips. MRI results revealed a finding suggestive of an epidural hematoma at T12–L4 and she was transferred for surgical care of her spine. Upon her admittance, her neurological exam had normalized and thus decompression surgery was deferred. Later that evening the patient began experiencing fecal incontinence and she had diminished rectal tone. A follow-up MRI showed a larger lesion at T12–L4 and decompression surgery was performed on postoperative day 4. Following surgery, the patient made a full recovery in both sensory and motor function. Though this patient did not experience acute-onset pain, her neurological deficits were sufficient to warrant further imaging that confirmed the presence of SEH.

Makris et al. described similar case of a 64-year-old female who developed a postoperative SEH following an elective total left knee arthroplasty [12, 13]. The patient had an unremarkable medical history, received spinal anesthesia via an L2–L3 lumbar puncture, and underwent a successful surgery without complications. On postoperative day 3, 4 h after receiving her daily postoperative dose of bemiparin (low weight molecular heparin), she experienced an acute onset of bilateral shoulder and upper extremity pain. Twenty minutes after the onset of pain, she reported upper extremity paresis and later experienced sensory loss below T10, which progressed to paralysis of the lower extremities. MRI revealed a hematoma at C2–C3 that was primarily compressing the C5–C7 spinal levels. Following the MRI, the patient's symptoms began to improve and conservative treatment was implemented (bemiparin replaced by calf compressions). The patient progressively regained full neurological function and was discharged 9 days later.

More recently in 2020, Moorthy et al. presented a case of a 56-year-old man who underwent a complete L1 and partial T12 laminectomy, T11–L3 stabilization and posterior lateral and inter-facet fusion due to neurological complications related to renal cell carcinoma metastasis [14]. From postoperative days 1–6, the patient showed great improvement in lower limb neurological function. The patient was kept on thromboprophylaxis therapy daily following his surgery. In the evening of postoperative day 8, the patient was readmitted for progressive paralysis in his lower limbs. L2–L3 had a motor power grade of 1, and a motor power grade of 0 for L4–S1 with paresthesia over the left L3–L5 dermatome. Bilateral plantar reflexes were upgoing and there was perianal anesthesia and lax tone. MRI indicated a large posterior epidural and subcutaneous hematoma. The patient underwent urgent decompression surgery and by his discharge date, power of the right lower limb had gradually improved to 4/5 but hemiparesis was still present in the left lower limb.

All three cases highlight the need for physicians to consider multiple aspects of a patient's current and past medical history to reach a timely and accurate diagnose of SEH. In all three patients, the sudden onset of pain and/or loss of motor and sensory function, without an immediate neurological insult, served as key indicators for a potential SEH. Although these examples show how preexisting health conditions and postoperative risk factors can influence a suspicion of SEH, some patients initially present with more ambiguity.

Spontaneous Spinal Epidural Hematoma (SSEH)

Raasck et al. in 2017 conducted a literature review of novel case studies from January 2000 to April 2015 to advance the current understanding of SSEH [15]. For the 65 cases included, the mean age at the time of SSEH was 53.2 ± 23 years. Of the 6 case reports included, 4 patients had a history of hypertension, atrial fibrillation, and anticoagulation therapy, and the remaining 2 patients had unremarkable medical histories. Four of the 6 patients presented to the emergency room for severe neck or upper thoracic region pain while the other two patients were originally admitted for treatment of fever and leukopenia and pneumonia. All 6 patients experienced progressive muscle weakness and sensory loss. Overall, this literature review offered further support for the risk factors and diagnostic features that have been previously associated with SEH and highlighted how SSEH can present in patients of varying health backgrounds.

Figueroa et al. later conducted a literature review on SSEH and provided the case of a 42-year-old man presenting to the hospital with "pain all over" and "muscle spasms" [3]. The patient's only significant medical history was a vertical sleeve gastrectomy for obesity management approximately 1 year prior to his presentation, intranasal crystal methamphetamine abuse, and a tooth extraction 8 days prior to his newly developed symptoms. One week before his presentation he had put his backpack on his right shoulder and felt a popping sensation in his back that resembled "pulling a muscle". Within 3 days of that pop, he experienced stabbing pain in his thoracic and lumbar spine regions and subsequently right lower extremity numbness and unsteady gait while dismounting his motorcycle.

Upon admittance to the emergency room, physicians determined that his only neurological deficit was urinary retention. MRI identified a small paracentral herniated nucleus pulposus at L5–S1 that was not impinging the exiting nerve root. The patient was discharged with an at-home treatment for prostatitis and within 8 h began experiencing stabbing back pain accompanied by headache, nausea, neck pain, stomachache, and thigh pain. Following readmittance he complained of saddle anesthesia and had diminished neck range of motion and motor strength (4/5) of the right iliopsoas. A follow-up MRI of the entire neuroaxis revealed a T1-weighted image with a hyperintense lesion of the epidural space from T3–T11 that was hypointense on T2-weighted imaging and did not enhance with gadolinium. An epidural hematoma was suspected and decompression surgery was performed. Six weeks after surgery, the patient was neurologically intact and had regained full bladder function.

As in the cases mentioned above, sudden, sharp pain and loss of sensation were key symptoms present throughout the progression of this patient's SEH. Yet, without a direct insult to the spine or medications impacting blood flow (e.g., anticoagulants), the differential for this patient was initially subject to wider interpretation. Thus, a strong understanding of the risk factors associated with SEH and SSEH and circumstances in which these medical emergencies may arise is critical for early diagnosis and optimal prognosis.

Pregnancy-Related Spinal Epidural Hematoma

In 2020, Zheng et al. conducted a literature review of the available postpartum SSEH cases [16]. All SSEH were located in the cervical or thoracic level and on the dorsal side of the spinal cord. Paralysis occurred during labor or within 3 h of delivery. Four of the seven patients received epidural or spinal anesthesia for pain management. In addition to the literature review, Zheng et al. included another case report outlining the symptoms experienced by a healthy postpartum female [16]. A 28-year-old female, with two uneventful previous spontaneous deliveries, had a third normal spontaneous delivery under epidural anesthesia and developed interscapular pain and bilateral lower limb flaccid paralysis with loss of sensation 12.5 h after delivery. MRI showed a spinal epidural hematoma with severe spinal cord stenosis at spinal levels T2–T5 with no evidence of vascular abnormality. Emergency surgery to evacuate the SEH was performed and following surgery, lower limb strength improved to 1/5 and sensation gradually improved over the first 22 postoperative days. Lower limb muscle strength returned to normal after 3 months. Since pregnancy is a known risk factor for SSEH, clinicians should closely monitor postpartum patients for the return of pain and/or loss of sensation that may have been overshadowed by active labor.

Atypical SEH Presentations

Just as it is important to recognize the typical presentation and risk factors of SEH, it is also beneficial to be cognizant of atypical presentations of epidural hematomas. Examples of atypical presentations include younger adults with no identifiable risk factors and children. Thus, physicians must be familiar with the spectrum of possible SEH presentations in order to diagnose a neurological emergency.

Shah et al. in 2020 conducted a case report on a 33-year-old African American woman with no identifiable risk factors who initially presented to the emergency room with severe neurological compromise [5]. The patient presented after awakening with acute-onset neck and left arm pain with subsequent paresthesia and profound weakness in her left upper and lower extremities. CT revealed a severe spinal canal stenosis at levels C5–C6 and MRI indicated a heterogenous collection within the dorsal epidural space on the left extending from C4 through C7. The patient was taken for emergency surgery and a large left-sided congealed epidural hematoma was revealed that required bilateral and dome laminectomies from C4–6 and C7, respectively. By postoperative day 9, the patient had demonstrated dramatic improvements in her neurological function and by her 1-month follow-up had largely returned to baseline strength in all extremities except for her left tibialis anterior and extensor hallucis longus (4/5 strength).

SSEH is extremely rare in children, but a few cases have been noted in patients diagnosed with hemophilia [13]. For example, Crumm et al. provided a case of a 3-month-old boy, with an initially unremarkable medical history, experiencing persistent irritability and sudden crying after being removed from a car seat. Upon examination at an urgent care facility, no signs of trauma or abuse were found and the only concerning finding was nuchal rigidity. The infant was transferred to the emergency department for concerns of meningitis. He had no focal neurological deficits, symmetrical muscle tone, and kept his neck tense with pull-to-sit. Complete blood count, blood cultures, and urine analysis were unremarkable. CT of the abdomen and a skull MRI were unremarkable, but a spine MRI revealed a right eccentric dorsal epidural hematoma extending from C2–T12. Nonaccidental trauma and coagulation lab results had initially been normal upon admittance, but 24 h after these initial tests, coagulation labs indicated hemophilia. The infant was started on plasma-derived Von Willebrand factor contain factor VIII. No surgical treatment was needed and the spinal accumulation gradually resolved [13].

Though SSEH is uncommon among young individuals with no apparent risk factors, physicians should be suspect of SEH whenever acute neck and/or back pain and motor strength deficits are observed. In young children who may be unable to articulate their symptoms, imaging and extensive nonaccidental trauma workup and blood panels should be conducted to properly confirm a suspected SEH and further identify the cause of hemorrhage.

Recognition

The diagnosis of spinal epidural hematoma begins with understanding the pathology and having a low index of suspicion. SEH is a rare condition that can affect a diverse range of individuals. Physicians should have a strong suspicion in patients who present with sudden neck and/or back pain, motor strength deficits, and without obvious trauma to the spine. Important risk factors to consider include age, female gender, multiple attempts at a spinal puncture (e.g. lumbar puncture for pain management), hypertension, anticoagulant therapies, and pregnancy.

Beginning with the history, it is important to clarify the time of onset of the symptoms, duration, and any associated symptoms. Basic demographics may also be useful including patient age, gender, and medical history including medications, particularly the use of anticoagulants. The patient's family history may also be useful in suggesting any potential coagulopathies or other risk factors.

After a detailed history is obtained, a thorough neurologic exam is essential for appropriate diagnosis. This includes an assessment of sensory and motor responses including reflexes to determine the competence of the nervous system. Muscle strength should be graded on a scale from 0 to 5 with a muscle group determined to be 0 grade meaning no muscle activation, and 5 meaning normal muscle activation against resistance with full range of motion. A grade of 1 will represent a slight twitch or trace muscle activation. Grade 2 represents muscle activation with appropriate range of motion with gravity eliminated. Grade 3 represents muscle activation against gravity. And grade 4 represents muscle activation against some resistance (Table 3.1). Commonly tested muscles include the shoulder abductors, elbow flexors, elbow extensors, wrist extensors, finger flexors, hand intrinsics, hip flexors, knee extensors, dorsiflexors, great toe extensor, and plantar flexors. Assessing the muscle tone for signs of rigidity and spasticity may also suggest dysfunction in the neurologic system. Sensory testing involves the assessment of fine touch, pain and temperature. This can be performed with a monofilament test and requires the understanding of dermatomes and may identify a sensory level (Image 3.1).

The physician must understand spinal anatomy, physiology and differentiate between upper motor neuron and lower motor neuron dysfunction. This will be done by a combination of examining deep tendon reflexes along with assessment for a Hoffman's sign, Babinski sign, and sustained clonus. Brisk reflexes typically suggest an abnormality of the upper motor neuron tract, while decreased reflexes suggest abnormality in the anterior horn, or lower motor neuron tract. This should be done with a reflex hammer and graded and documented appropriately. After a detailed history and neurologic examination, prompt neuroimaging, including CT and MRI may provide useful in identifying and localizing compressive epidural lesions.

Table 3.1 Manual muscle testing grade

Grade	Description
0	No visible or palpable contraction
1	Flicker/trace contraction
2	Active movement ***with gravity eliminated***
3	Active movement ***against gravity***
4	Active movement against gravity with moderate resistance
5	Active movement against gravity with maximal resistance

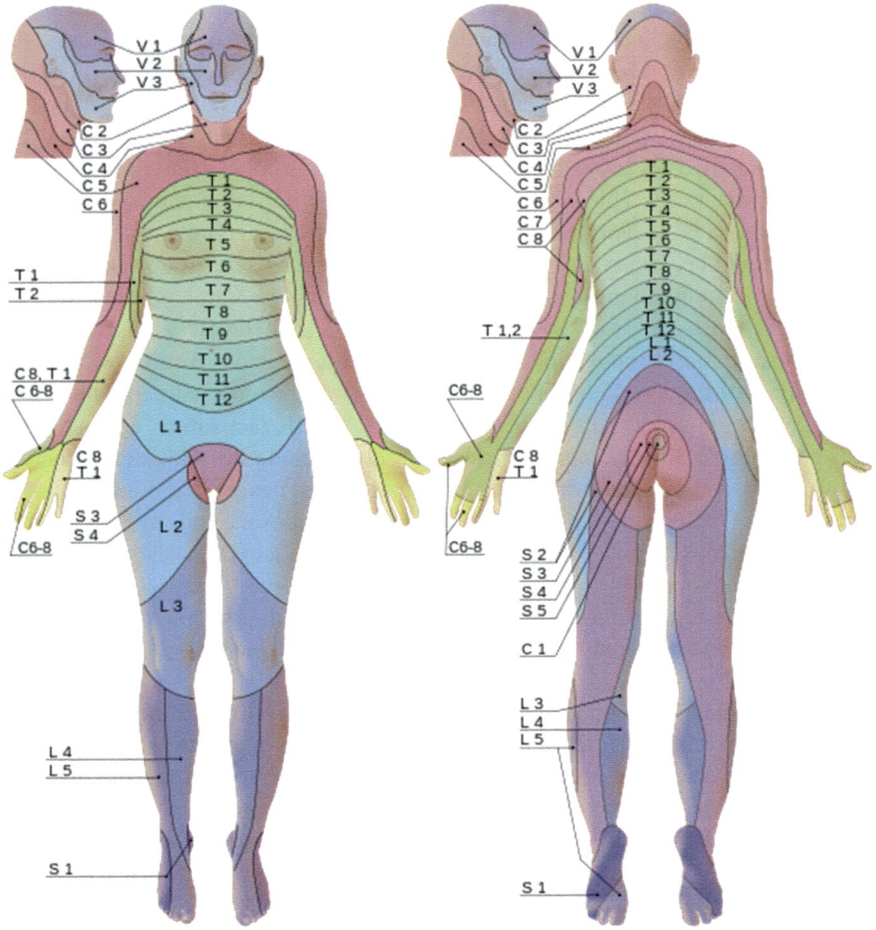

Image 3.1 Dermatome map. (https://upload.wikimedia.org/wikipedia/commons/5/55/Dermatomes_labeled%2C_female_front-back_3d-shaded.svg)

Treatment Strategies

Currently, there is no consensus on the most effective treatment method for SEH. Due to the low incidence and wide variation in presentation, the spectrum of severity is too wide for one general treatment. As recognized in the cases above, surgery and conservative measures are the two most common management strategies for SEH. However, these methods are considered sub-optimal due to the 5.7% related mortality and the fact that over 50% of patients continue to have some level of sensorimotor deficits following treatment [15]. Therefore, these treatment modalities and their relative successes among various patient presentations will be discussed to help further define when surgery and/or conservative strategies may be most effective.

Surgical Intervention

Per the literature review by Raasck et al. in 2017, decompression laminectomy and hematoma evacuation are the standard surgical procedures for SSEH [15]. Further, the degree of pre-operative neurological deficits and the timing between onset of symptoms and surgery play a major role in the success of these two procedures [17]. Literature reviews conducted by Gopalkrishnan et al. in 2012 and Raasck et al. in 2017 both included case series and evaluations of current treatment methods for SEH and indicated that pre-operative American Spinal Injury Association (ASIA) impairment scores can be indicative of post-operative success [15, 17]. Of the 12 case studies from Gopalkrishnan et al. 30% of patients who presented with an ASIA score of A did not improve with surgery but patients presenting with a C or D score improved after surgery [17]. These findings were later supported by Raasck et al. who observed that one of their two patients with an ASIA score of A did not improve with surgery but those with pre-operative scores of C and D all improved [15]. These reviews provide evidence for how pre-operative neurological deficits can be indicative of surgical success.

In addition to pre-operative neurological deficits, timing of surgical intervention has been shown to impact recovery patterns. Lawton et al. provided support that the chance of improvement decreases with time [18]. Fifty-two percent of patients who received surgical intervention within 12 h of neurological deficits had a complete recovery while only 25% of patients undergoing surgery between 12–24 h after initial deficits experienced a full recovery. Overall, they determined that patients treated within 12–36 h of deficit onset had similar outcomes to those treated ≥36 h after symptoms began. Later in 2006, Shin et al. also found that patients who were operated within 12 h of symptom onset scored significantly higher (84%) on a recovery scale set by the Japanese Orthopaedic Association than those who underwent surgery between 12 and 24 h (64%) and ≥24 h (47%) following initial signs of deficits [19]. More recently in 2019, Baeesa et al. conducted a literature review on SSEH management and evaluated long term improvement of patients who underwent surgical treatment [20]. All 14 patients received multilevel decompressive laminectomies and hematoma evacuations. The average interval of time from initial presentation to surgery was 21.29 ± 10.2 h. All patients had improved from the time-of-surgery to the 1-year follow up per ASIA scores. At the 6-month post-operative follow up appointment, a weak negative relationship was found between time-to-surgery and change in ASIA score. Furthermore, a weak positive relationship was found between the two variables at the 1-year follow up appointment. Based on the existing evidence, early surgical intervention is critical for patients with prominent initial neurological deficits.

Conservative Treatment

Despite the increasing number of SSEH cases being reported as managed with conservative treatment (non-surgical modalities), the factors that contribute to the decision to use conservative treatment and the overall benefit are poorly understood. Raasck et al. reported that several studies and reviews have offered support for the use of conservative measures, but that success rates may be due in part to patients having minor pre-operative neurological deficits and small lesions [15]. For example, Groen et al. had reported that 84% of patients treated non-operatively experienced a complete recovery [10]. Yet, patients treated conservatively were 3 times as likely to have an ASIA score of D, the least severe score for neurological deficits. Thus, conservative measures may be beneficial in patients experiencing minor deficits with small, localized spinal epidural hematomas.

An important aspect of conservative treatment to monitor the patient for increase in size of the hematoma and for progressive neurological deficits. Previous research has shown that cases initially treated conservatively ultimately required surgery due to the patient's neurological deterioration [21]. An example was described earlier in the case of an 80-year-old female experiencing a SEH 2–4 days following a total knee arthroplasty. In this patient's case, her symptoms began to improve after an initial MRI and transfer to a neurological care center, so decompression surgery was deferred. Yet within hours of arriving to the new care facility, her neurological deficits had progressed to the point where surgical intervention was required [11]. Figueroa et al. conducted a retrospective medical chart review on seven SSEH patients and found that that the two patients had recovered to a D score within hours of admission and were therefore treated conservatively [4]. Despite the minor deficits prior to treatment, these patients were still experiencing gait disturbances, clumsiness, and bladder and bowel dysfunction, approximately 25 months after intervention. Based on the contradicting findings and potential for patient deterioration and long-term sequalae, conservative treatment should be used with caution in patients with very mild neurological deficits and lesions. Patients undergoing conservative management should also be closely monitored for worsening pain and/or neurological impairment.

Summary

Overall, surgical decompression appears to offer the most benefit for patients with significant neurologic deficit suffering from SEH. Rapid surgical intervention shows the most promise for minimizing the long-term neurological sequelae. Lastly, conservative treatment should be reserved for patients with mild deficits and small lesions with a low risk of spread and these patients must be closely monitored for signs of SEH progression.

Questions

1. Which two features are most predictable of positive neurologic outcome in patients with spontaneous epidural hematomas?

    (a) When a patient is diagnosed with an epidural hematoma, it is most important to understand their neurologic status as they often may present with deficits in motor strength, sensation, or both. If patients do have neurologic deficits, then surgical decompression is often indicated to relieve pressure off of the neural elements. The extent of their preoperative neurological deficit, often measured by their ASIA impairment score, may predict their postoperative outcomes. For example, if patient comes in as an ASIA A, with complete motor and sensory loss, then they have a lesser likelihood of recovery compared to an ASIA B. Additionally, the timing between onset of neurologic deficit and decompression correlates with outcomes, with quicker time to decompression, ideally within 12 h, portends a more favorable prognosis.

2. Which symptoms and examination findings are suggestive of upper motor neuron pathology?

    (a) Upper motor neuron signs consist of a characteristic set of clinical findings. Patients may present with weakness, spasticity, brisk reflexes, sustained clonus, downgoing Babinski, positive Hoffman's, or rigidity.

3. If a patient presents with sensory deficits and associated physical exam findings of the ability to dorsiflex the ankle with gravity eliminated, but NOT anti-gravity, which motor grade would it be assigned?

    (a) It is imperative to examine and appropriately document a patient's motor strength and sensation for patients with suspected or diagnosed spinal epidural hematomas. This involves testing key muscles. A patient with the ability to perform full range of motion with gravity eliminated would be considered a Grade 2. This is contrast to Grade 3 which implies muscle activation against gravity, or Grade 4 which is muscle activation against moderate resistance. (See Table 3.1).

References

1. Al-Mutair A, Bednar DA. Spinal epidural hematoma. JAAOS J Am Acad Orthop Surg. 2010;18(8):494–502.
2. Bhat KJ, Kapoor S, Watali YZ, Sharma JR. Spontaneous epidural hematoma of spine associated with clopidogrel: a case study and review of the literature. Asian J Neurosurg. 2015;10(1):54.
3. Figueroa J, DeVine JG. Spontaneous spinal epidural hematoma: literature review. J Spine Surg. 2017;3(1):58.
4. Matsumura A, Namikawa T, Hashimoto R, Okamoto T, Yanagida I, Hoshi M, Takami M. Clinical management for spontaneous spinal epidural hematoma: diagnosis and treatment. Spine J. 2008;8(3):534–7.

5. Shah JA, Patel NN, Michael KW. Spontaneous spinal epidural hematoma: an atypical clinical presentation and discussion of management. Int J Spine Surg. 2020;14(2):158–61.
6. Babayev R, Ekşi MŞ. Spontaneous thoracic epidural hematoma: a case report and literature review. Childs Nerv Syst. 2016;32(1):181–7.
7. Kreppel D, Antoniadis G, Seeling W. Spinal hematoma: a literature survey with meta-analysis of 613 patients. Neurosurg Rev. 2003;26(1):1–49.
8. Dziedzic T, Kunert P, Krych P, Marchel A. Management and neurological outcome of spontaneous spinal epidural hematoma. J Clin Neurosci. 2015;22(4):726–9.
9. Zhong W, Chen H, You C, Li J, Liu Y, Huang S. Spontaneous spinal epidural hematoma. J Clin Neurosci. 2011;18(11):1490–4.
10. Groen RJM. Non-operative treatment of spontaneous spinal epidural hematomas: a review of the literature and a comparison with operative cases. Acta Neurochir. 2004;146(2):103–10.
11. Kasodekar SV, Goldszmidt E, Davies SR. Atypical presentation of an epidural hematoma in a patient receiving aspirin and low molecular weight heparin. Was epidural analgesia the right choice? J Clin Anesth. 2009;21(8):595–8.
12. Makris A, Gkliatis E, Diakomi M, Karmaniolou I, Mela A. Delayed spinal epidural hematoma following spinal anesthesia, far from needle puncture site. Spinal Cord. 2014;52(1):S14–6.
13. Crumm CE, Crotty EE, Albert CM, Blair AB, Otjen JP, Feldman KW. Atraumatic spinal epidural hematoma as initial presentation of hemophilia a in an infant. Pediatr Emerg Care. 2021;37(11):e772–4.
14. Moorthy V, Wang JX, Tang JH, Oh JYL. Postoperative spinal epidural hematoma following therapeutic anticoagulation: case report and review of literature. J Spine Surg. 2020;6(4):743.
15. Raasck K, Habis AA, Aoude A, Simões L, Barros F, Reindl R, Jarzem P. Spontaneous spinal epidural hematoma management: a case series and literature review. Spinal Cord Ser Cases. 2017;3(1):1–6.
16. Zheng HX, Nyam TTE, Liu CA, Lee YL, Kuo JR, Sung KC. Spontaneous spinal epidural hematoma after normal spontaneous delivery with epidural analgesia: case report and literature review. World Neurosurg. 2020;137:214–7.
17. Gopalkrishnan CV, Dhakoji A, Nair S. Spontaneous cervical epidural hematoma of idiopathic etiology: case report and review of literature. J Spinal Cord Med. 2012;35(2):113–7.
18. Lawton MT, Porter RW, Heiserman JE, Jacobowitz R, Sonntag VK, Dickman CA. Surgical management of spinal epidural hematoma: relationship between surgical timing and neurological outcome. J Neurosurg. 1995;83(1):1–7.
19. Shin JJ, Kuh SU, Cho YE. Surgical management of spontaneous spinal epidural hematoma. Eur Spine J. 2006;15(6):998–1004.
20. Baeesa S, Jarzem P, Mansi M, Bokhari R, Bassi M. Spontaneous spinal epidural hematoma: correlation of timing of surgical decompression and MRI findings with functional neurological outcome. World Neurosurg. 2019;122:e241–7.
21. Duffill J, Sparrow OC, Millar J, Barker CS. Can spontaneous spinal epidural haematoma be managed safely without operation? A report of four cases. J Neurol Neurosurg Psychiatry. 2000;69(6):816–9.

Chapter 4
Popliteal Entrapment Syndrome

William Rothstein, Syeda Farooq, and Daniel H. Newton

Clinical Vignette

A 30-year-old physically active and otherwise healthy male presented with worsening unilateral calf pain which began years prior. His pain would start after a few minutes of running or prolonged walking, progressively increasing until it forced him to rest. The pain was relieved fully with rest. On exam, he had normal palpable dorsalis pedis and posterior tibial pulses. Plain radiographs were unremarkable, and arterial-brachial indices were normal as well. An MRI was obtained which was unremarkable but for a possible accessory slip of the lateral head of the gastrocnemius. An angiogram was performed (Fig. 4.1), showing occlusion and lateral displacement of the popliteal artery with dorsiflexion of the foot.

The patient underwent exploration of the popliteal artery from the posterior approach. A thin band of muscle was noted tethering the popliteal artery, which was divided. The patient recovered without complication and was able to return to his prior activities without pain.

This chapter will review popliteal entrapment syndrome, with emphasis on the early recognition and anatomical considerations of this difficult to diagnose pathology.

Questions

1. What are the anatomical variants that cause popliteal entrapment syndrome?
2. What are the presenting symptoms that merit evaluation?
3. What are the appropriate treatments?

W. Rothstein
Division of Vascular Surgery and Endovascular Therapy, University of Pennsylvania, Philadelphia, PA, USA
e-mail: william.rothstein@pennmedicine.org

S. Farooq · D. H. Newton (✉)
Division of Vascular Surgery, Virginia Commonwealth University, Richmond, VA, USA
e-mail: daniel.newton@vcuhealth.org; syeda.farooq@vcuhealth.org

W. A. Zuelzer, S. Metikala (eds.), *Unusual Conditions That Every Orthopaedic Surgeon Should Know*, https://doi.org/10.1007/978-3-031-58946-1_4

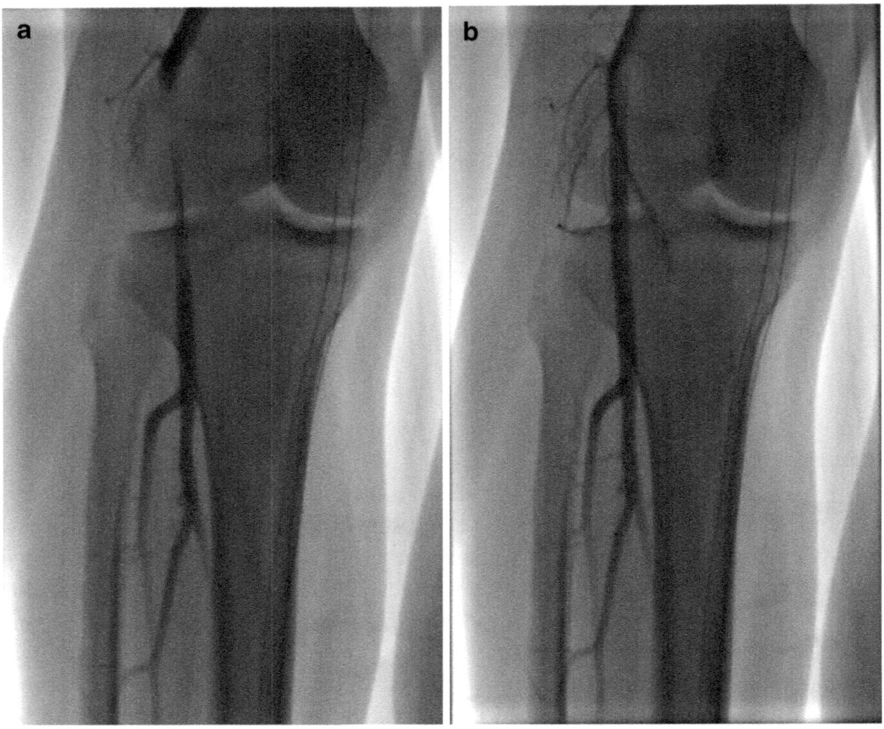

Fig. 4.1 Arteriography showing occlusion of the popliteal artery with plantarflexion of the foot (**a**) and restoration of normal flow with relaxation (**b**)

Introduction

Popliteal entrapment syndrome (PES) is a rare condition characterized by compression or entrapment of the popliteal artery in the area behind the knee. This can lead to restricted blood flow distally, resulting in pain and other symptoms. Stenotic, aneurysmal, and thromboembolic sequelae may develop from repeated arterial trauma. The condition is usually caused by anatomical abnormalities in the popliteal artery or surrounding structures, such as muscle or fibrous tissue, which can impinge upon the artery and cause compression.

Symptoms of PES can vary from mild discomfort to severe pain and swelling in the affected leg. In some cases, patients may also experience numbness or mild paresthesias, and the affected leg may feel weak or tired. Diagnosis is notoriously difficult and relies on an attentive history coupled with imaging studies, such as ultrasound or MRI. Treatment for PES depends on the underlying anatomic abnormality and the health of the involved vessel. Management may include conservative measures such as rest and physical therapy. Thrombolysis or thrombectomy may be required for thromboembolic complications. In some cases, surgery may be necessary to restore distal perfusion, by relieving the compression or bypassing the native vessel.

Embryology and Clinical Anatomy

Embryology

Understanding the pathophysiology of popliteal entrapment syndrome requires an understanding of the embryological development of the popliteal fossa. The primitive root of the lower limb, the axial artery, forms from the dorsal root of the umbilical artery and runs deep to the popliteus muscle. The popliteal artery forms relatively late in development as a bridging vessel joining the axial artery and the separately developing femoral artery at the adductor hiatus [1–3]. The portion of the axial artery deep to the popliteus muscle typically obliterates [1, 2].

As development progresses, the medial head of the gastrocnemius moves more proximally relative to the lateral head from their common origin on the femoral metaphysis. The medial head of the gastrocnemius moves laterally through the popliteal fossa; the popliteal artery moves with it, remaining lateral to the medial head in its final anatomic configuration [1, 2].

Several developmental abnormalities may result in popliteal entrapment syndrome. Failure of the portion of the axial artery deep to the popliteus muscle to obliterate results in a popliteal artery variant deep to the popliteus. Excessive migration of the medial head of the gastrocnemius can lead to it crossing the popliteal artery, leading to a final configuration in which the popliteal artery lies medially to or within the muscle [1].

Clinical Anatomy

Multiple classification schema exist for popliteal entrapment syndrome, the most widely used proposed by Rich et al. as a modification to the system originally reported by Insua et al. (Fig. 4.2) [4–8].

Type I—the popliteal artery is positioned medially to the normally positioned medial head of the gastrocnemius.

Type II—the medial head of the gastrocnemius is located excessively laterally relative to a normally positioned popliteal artery.

Type III—an accessory or abnormal muscle bundle from the gastrocnemius compresses a normally positioned popliteal artery.

Type IV—the popliteal artery is located deep to the popliteus muscle.

Type V—any of type I–IV that also includes compression of the popliteal vein.

Type VI—added by Rich et al. to the original taxonomy from Insua et al. consisting of patients with normal anatomy but functional compression of the popliteal artery during exercise secondary to hypertrophic musculature.

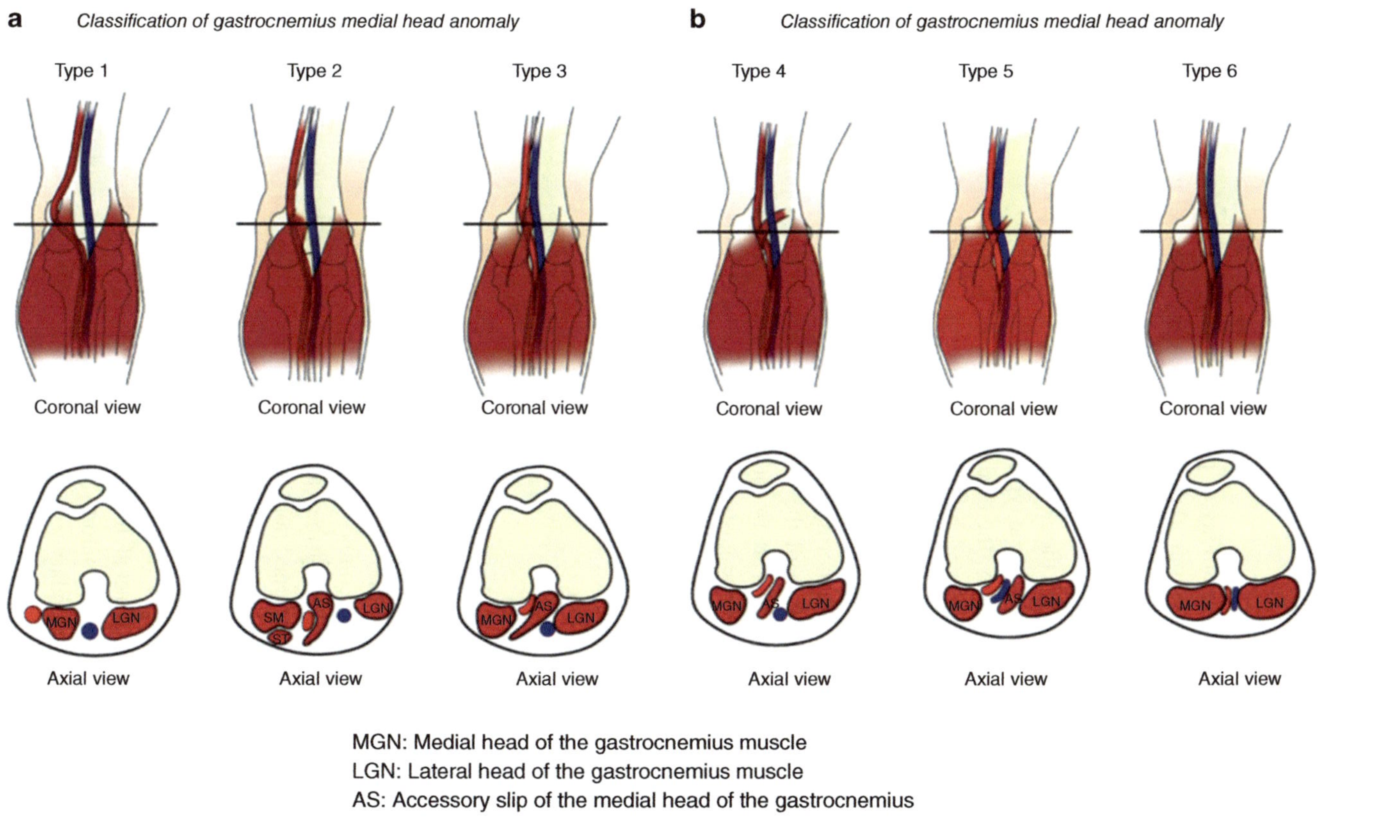

Fig. 4.2 (**a**) Popliteal entrapment types I, II, III [4]. *MGN* medial head of the gastrocnemius muscle, *LGN* lateral head of the gastrocnemius muscle, *AS* accessory slip of the medial head of the gastrocnemius. (**b**) Popliteal entrapment types IV, V, VI [4]. *MGN* medial head of the gastrocnemius muscle, *LGN* lateral head of the gastrocnemius muscle, *AS* accessory slip of the medial head of the gastrocnemius

Clinical Presentation

Various studies have reported incidence rates ranging from 0.17 to 3.5% [9]. The clinical features and symptomatology of popliteal artery entrapment are variable and depend upon the chronicity and extent of the pathology. Often, the condition affects young, athletic male individuals with no atherosclerotic risk factors. For example, a recent study found that among patients undergoing surgery for popliteal artery entrapment syndrome (PAES), the majority were male (78%), with a mean age of 36 years. Intermittent claudication was noted to be the most common symptom, affecting 9 in 10 patients [10]. Unfortunately, PAES can also present with acute arterial occlusion and limb ischemia. In fact, a study found that nearly 20% of affected extremities were presented with limb-threatening ischemia. The authors noted that given the young age of onset and potentially debilitating disease course, prompt diagnostic workup is warranted [11]. Interestingly, over two-thirds of patients have bilateral popliteal artery entrapment, with nearly four-fifths of individuals having chronically elevated compartment pressures [12].

Exercise Induced Claudication

Chronic lower leg pain is a common condition among young athletic people with numerous causes [13]. As such, the ambiguity of presenting symptoms makes the diagnosis challenging. Popliteal entrapment most frequently presents as exertional lower extremity claudication typically in young athletes and soldiers [11]. Patients report cramp-like pain in the calf or feet occurring during lower limb exercise. These symptoms often mimic and are mistaken for arterial insufficiency as well as other musculoskeletal conditions. Importantly, patients with peripheral arterial disease tend to have multiple atherosclerotic risk factors leading to physical exam findings such as nonpalpable distal pulses and a resting ankle-brachial index <0.9. Conversely, patients with PAES tend to be healthy at baseline with normal pulses and ABIs at rest.

Thromboembolic Complications and Acute Limb Ischemia

With chronic damage to the popliteal artery caused by its compression, patients can develop a fixed stenosis, no longer dependent on the extrinsic compression. The area of damaged artery can go on to occlude completely in up to 9% of patients [14]. When this occurs acutely, the patient may present with a pale, cold extremity with loss of sensation and motor function. For instance, in an analysis of 31 patients undergoing surgery for PAES, 2 (6%) patients presented with acute limb ischemia [15]. Chronic arterial entrapment can also cause progressive degeneration of the vessel wall, often leading to aneurysm formation. In the later stages of the disease, embolization can occur, thereby occluding the distal tibial arteries and negatively impacting the patency of any vascular reconstruction. In other cases, an aneurysmal popliteal artery can acutely thrombose. Limb loss has been reported to be uncommon among patients with PAES as pathophysiology is insidious and chronic, thereby allowing collateral formation. In fact, a study reported that among 38 patients treated surgically for this condition, no limb loss occurred and the patients were cured of their symptoms at a median follow-up of 34 months [16]. However, a small minority of patients may present with irreversible ischemia requiring an amputation. This makes it important to consider PAES as a possible differential among patients with no atherosclerotic risk factors who present with ischemic symptoms of the lower extremity [17].

Differential Diagnosis

Popliteal entrapment is a rare but important cause of peripheral vascular insufficiency among young patients. Of note, it may present in a similar fashion to certain other musculoskeletal conditions. For example, adventitial cystic disease is a non-atherosclerotic disorder characterized by the formation of cysts between the adventitia and the media layers. This rare, putatively embryologic disease, primarily affects the popliteal artery. Patients most often report unilateral lower leg claudication. Imaging with duplex ultrasound, MRI, or CT angiography will readily identify the cystic structure surrounding the popliteal artery (Fig. 4.3) [18, 19].

Lower extremity pain is a common problem among athletes. Medial tibial stress syndrome also known as shin splints is typically seen in female runners and has an incidence ranging from 13 to 42%. As such, it is associated with a stress reaction occurring in the periosteum and the bone. Patients report mid to distal tibial pain and tenderness and have a 12-fold increased risk of fractures [17]. Similarly, tibial stress injuries are also frequently encountered among athletes and military personnel. These occur as a result of repeated stress to a normal bone resulting in periosteal inflammation as well as cortical fractures. Although, stress-related microfractures may not be visible on imaging in the early stages, periosteal reaction later in the symptomatic region usually indicates the diagnosis [20].

Chronic exertional compartment syndrome is the second most common cause of lower extremity pain seen in athletes. Exercise causes muscle volume expansion within a closed fibro-osseous space, thereby leading to decreased tissue perfusion and ischemic pain. Perhaps unsurprisingly, the anterior compartment is most frequently affected; however, the pain usually subsides with cessation of exercise. Moreover, compartment pressures are found to be elevated and remain elevated up to 30 min post-exercise. If the athlete continues to compete despite the pain, CECS may progress to acute compartment syndrome [21].

Another condition similar to PES is the soleal sling syndrome where the tibial nerve can be compressed as it passes under the soleal sling in the posterior knee. Interestingly, the patients tend to experience calf pain as well as plantar foot

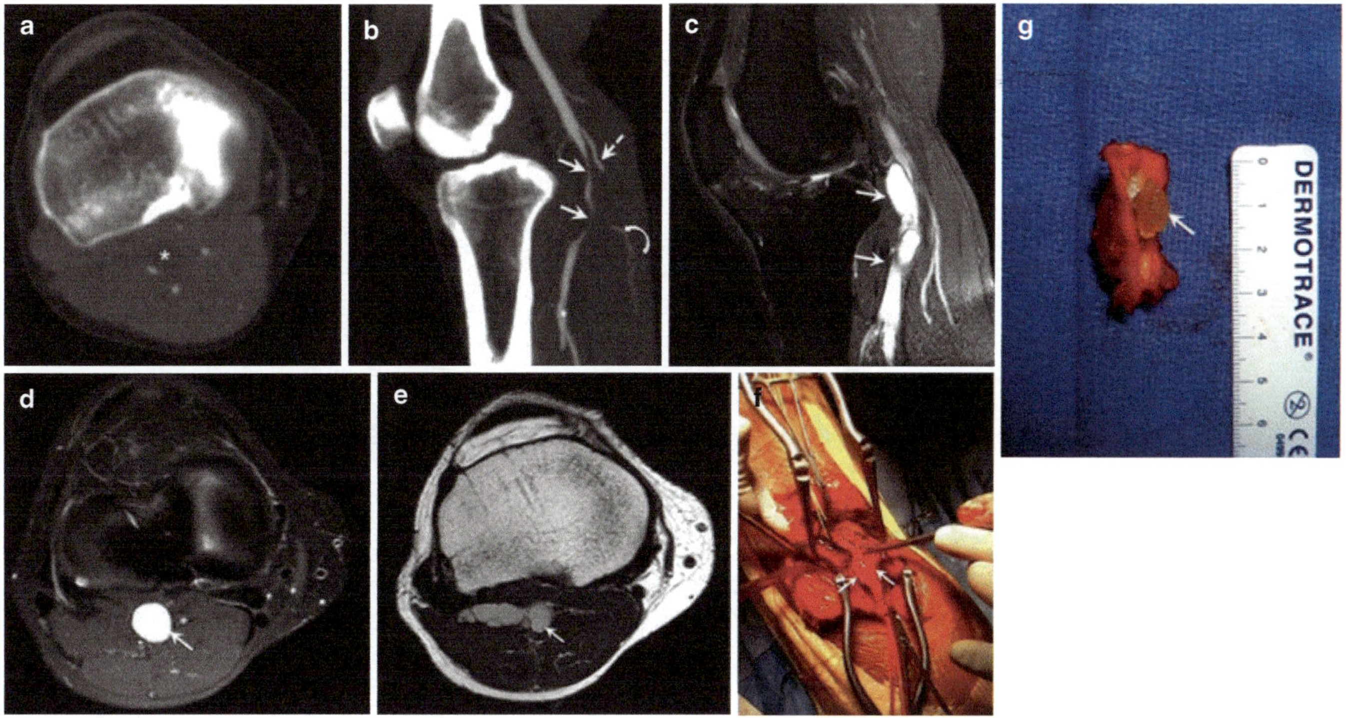

Fig. 4.3 CT and MRI depiction of cystic adventitial disease of the popliteal artery [18]. A case of adventitial cystic disease. (**a**) CT demonstrates a fluid-filled lesion within the popliteal fossa (asterisk) compressing the popliteal artery. (**b**) Sagittal reconstruction of the CT showing stenosis of the popliteal artery (solid arrows) with prominent collateral vessels (curved and dashed arrows). (**c, d**) T2-weighted MR images—a fluid-filled cyst compressing the lumen of the popliteal artery (arrows). (**e**) Axial T1-weighted MR image—the adventitial cyst (arrow). (**f**) Intraoperative photo showing the adventitial cyst in the wall of the popliteal artery (arrows). (**g**) Demonstrated clearly (arrow) the resected specimen

tightness; however, claudication is absent. Patients have a positive Tinel's sign, i.e., pain on palpation of the tibial nerve as it courses under the soleus in the popliteal region [22].

Arterial endofibrosis is a flow-limiting condition of the external iliac artery and is mainly seen in endurance athletes including cyclists and marathon runners. It is thought to occur secondary to repetitive increases in the hemodynamic load within the artery leading to increased myofibroblast activity and deposition of elastin and collagen within the tunica intima [23]. The condition presents as leg weakness and thigh pain during exercise [24].

Imaging

Duplex Ultrasound

Duplex ultrasonography is often the first imaging modality obtained to assess suspected popliteal entrapment syndrome and may demonstrate vascular compression elicited by plantar and dorsiflexion of the feet when performed by an experienced technician [25–27]. Some authors have argued that compression of the popliteal artery during plantar and dorsiflexion of the foot is a normal physiologic phenomenon and lacks specificity in diagnosing popliteal entrapment syndrome [25]. Sonography may also reveal popliteal artery aneurysm or occlusion [27].

CT Angiography

CT, as well as MRI, is advantageous over digital subtraction angiography in that they are non-invasive, and reveals anatomic details of the soft tissue structures around the popliteal artery [28–30].

CT angiography can demonstrate aberrant muscular and fibrous structures responsible for popliteal entrapment syndrome pathology, although in less detail compared to MRI [6, 30]. However, morphologic features of the vessel itself, including displacement, aneurysm, occlusion, and stenosis, can be easily interpreted by the surgeon [28, 30]. Three-dimensional reconstruction can also assist with understanding the patient's anatomy and facilitate surgical planning [30].

Magnetic Resonance Imaging

MRI provides superior resolution of soft tissue anatomy and additionally spares patients exposure to ionizing radiation and iodinated contrast [27, 31]. MR angiography can demonstrate dynamic compression during provocative maneuvers, as well as flow abnormalities [27, 31, 32], in addition to morphologic features of the vessel. It can demonstrate changes in the relative positions of the gastrocnemius and popliteal artery during provocative maneuvers, providing dynamic images [32].

Angiography

Conventional digital subtraction angiography is classically the diagnostic test of choice [27]. The morphological features of the artery, such as aneurysm and occlusion, may be demonstrated. Dynamic compression may also be observed, but are subject to the same caveats as in duplex sonography [25, 27].

Treatment

The therapeutic approach depends on the culprit anatomical abnormality and the health of the vessel [1]. Surgical decompression is the default treatment for popliteal entrapment. Resolving the compression will improve symptoms and prevent chronic injury to the popliteal artery. For patients with significant stenosis or aneurysmal degeneration, arterial reconstruction or bypass may be required as well. Nonoperative management has been chosen by some patients with mild symptoms or those with Type VI (function) popliteal entrapment and should be accompanied by surveillance, usually with duplex ultrasound, to monitor for the development of stenosis or aneurysmal degeneration.

Surgical Approach

Multiple approaches may be used to expose the popliteal artery and must be individualized based on the patient's anatomy and the therapeutic strategy.

A direct posterior approach facilitates access to popliteal artery pathology when bypass is not required. The patient is positioned prone with the knee in slight flexion, and an s-shaped incision is made with a superormedial longitudinal incision on the posterior thigh, brought laterally across the flexion crease, and continued as an inferolateral longitudinal incision on the posterior calf [33]. The lesser saphenous vein is encountered and divided prior to longitudinally incising the deep fascia. The contents of the popliteal fossa may be exposed by retracting the heads of the gastrocnemius apart. The most superficial structure is the tibial nerve, which is retracted medially to reveal the sheath containing the popliteal vessels. When the sheath is opened, the popliteal artery is deep and medial to the popliteal vein.

When a longer bypass is required for treatment, the popliteal artery is most commonly exposed from a medial approach to its suprageniculate and infrageniculate segments. The patient is positioned supine with the knee in slight flexion. The suprageniculate popliteal artery is exposed through a longitudinal incision on the distal thigh along the anterior border of the sartorius muscle. The fascia of the sartorius is incised. The sheath containing popliteal vessels may be seen by retracting the sartorius inferiorly, and the vastus medialis anteriorly.

The infrageniculate popliteal artery may be exposed through a longitudinal incision 1 cm posterior to the proximal tibia. The proximal neurovascular bundle may be found by making a longitudinal incision in the fascia and retracting the medial head of the gastrocnemius inferiorly. Upon incising the vascular sheath, the popliteal vein is encountered medially. The popliteal artery may be elevated into view with vessel loops. Care must be taken to avoid injury to the neighboring tibial nerve.

The exposure may need to be modified depending on the patient's pathologic anatomy.

Lateral approaches to both the suprageniculate and infrageniculate popliteal arteries have been described, but are beyond the scope of this chapter.

Pearls and Pitfalls

- Popliteal entrapment should be considered when a patient without atherosclerotic risk factors presents with exertional calf pain.
- Workup for popliteal entrapment includes, most commonly, MRI and vascular imaging such as duplex or angiography which can demonstrate vascular compression during provocative maneuvers. Popliteal compression alone, however, is not diagnostic of the syndrome and may be seen in asymptomatic individuals.
- The anatomic abnormalities leading to popliteal entrapment can be classified depending on the compressing musculature.
- Untreated, popliteal entrapment can lead to a fixed stenosis or aneurysmal degeneration of the vessel, placing the patient at risk for more ischemic events, or even amputation.
- Surgical decompression is performed via a posterior approach. Aneurysmal degeneration or severe stenosis or occlusion may require arterial bypass, often done via a medial approach.

Conclusion

Presenting as calf claudication in an otherwise healthy young person, popliteal entrapment may be easily dismissed or misdiagnosed by providers unfamiliar with its possible etiologies. Awareness of this rare syndrome is critical to identifying this potentially debilitating and treatable condition. In rare circumstances, the condition may progress to more critical vascular compromise.

Questions

1. What are the anatomical variants that cause popliteal entrapment syndrome?

   Popliteal entrapment is caused by compression of the popliteal artery (or neurovascular bundle) by an abnormal anatomic relationship with the medial head of gastrocnemius or popliteus muscle. In the most common anatomic variants, the popliteal artery takes a course unusually medial to at least a portion of the medial head of the gastrocnemius muscle.

2. What are the presenting symptoms that merit evaluation?

   Popliteal entrapment usually presents as exercise induced pain that resolves quickly with rest (claudication). Rarely, it can present as acute limb ischemia. Because popliteal entrapment can progress to a fixed stenosis or occlusion and therefore further vascular-focused imaging (usually MRI), and expert consultation should be considered when there is no orthopaedic cause for the pain identified.

3. What are the appropriate treatments?

   Treatment typically requires exploration of the popliteal fossa and release of compressing tissue bands, with reconstruction of the artery if necessary.

References

1. Lambert AW, Wilkins DC. Popliteal artery entrapment syndrome. Br J Surg. 1999;86(11):1365–70. https://doi.org/10.1046/j.1365-2168.1999.01257.x.
2. Rosset E, Hartung O, Brunet C, Roche PH, Magnan PE, Mathieu JP, Branchereau A, Farisse J. Popliteal artery entrapment syndrome. Anatomic and embryologic bases, diagnostic and therapeutic considerations following a series of 15 cases with a review of the literature. Surg Radiol Anat. 1995;17(2):161–9. https://doi.org/10.1007/bf01627578.
3. Senior HD. The development of the arteries of the human lower extremity. Am J Anat. 1919;25(1):54–95.
4. Kim HK, Shin MJ, Kim SM, Lee SH, Hong HJ. Popliteal artery entrapment syndrome: morphological classification utilizing MR imaging. Skelet Radiol. 2006;35(9):648–58. https://doi.org/10.1007/s00256-006-0158-5.
5. Insua JA, Young JR, Humphries AW. Popliteal artery entrapment syndrome. Arch Surg. 1970;101(6):771–5. https://doi.org/10.1001/archsurg.1970.01340300127021.
6. Rich NM, Collins GJ Jr, McDonald PT, Kozloff L, Clagett GP, Collins JT. Popliteal vascular entrapment. Its increasing interest. Arch Surg. 1979;114(12):1377–84. https://doi.org/10.1001/archsurg.1979.01370360031004.
7. Schweizer M, Hügli R, Koella C, Jeanneret C. Popliteal entrapment syndrome and age. Vasa. 2012;41(4):262–8. https://doi.org/10.1024/0301-1526/a000201.
8. Tercan F, Oğuzkurt L, Kizilkiliç O, Yeniocak A, Gülcan O. Popliteal artery entrapment syndrome. Diagn Interv Radiol. 2005;11(4):222–4.
9. Gibson MH, Mills JG, Johnson GE, Downs AR. Popliteal entrapment syndrome. Ann Surg. 1977;185(3):341–8. https://doi.org/10.1097/00000658-197703000-00016.
10. Fujimura N, Obara H, Takahashi A, Miyata H, Hosaka A, Obitsu Y, Zempo N, Miyata T, Azuma N, Komori K, Japanese Society for Vascular Surgery Database Management Committee. Surgical treatment for popliteal artery entrapment syndrome in Japan: a retrospective, multicentre study using a National Clinical Registry. Eur J Vasc Endovasc Surg. 2023;66(23):381–8. https://doi.org/10.1016/j.ejvs.2023.05.031.
11. Levien LJ, Veller MG. Popliteal artery entrapment syndrome: more common than previously recognized. J Vasc Surg. 1999;30(4):587–98. https://doi.org/10.1016/s0741-5214(99)70098-4.
12. Corneloup L, Labanère C, Chevalier L, Jaussaud J, Mignot A, Gencel L, Corneloup O, Midy D. Presentation, diagnosis, and management of popliteal artery entrapment syndrome: 11

years of experience with 61 legs. Scand J Med Sci Sports. 2018;28(2):517–23. https://doi.org/10.1111/sms.12918.
13. Brewer RB, Gregory AJM. Chronic lower leg pain in athletes: a guide for the differential diagnosis, evaluation, and treatment. Sports Health. 2012;4(2):121–7. https://doi.org/10.1177/1941738111426115.
14. Lavingia KS, Dua A, Rothenberg KA, Fredericson M, Lee JT. Surgical management of functional popliteal entrapment syndrome in athletes. J Vasc Surg. 2019;70(5):1555–62. https://doi.org/10.1016/j.jvs.2019.01.068.
15. Altinsoy HB, Alatas O, Khalil E, Kara KA, Okten CC, Dogan OF. A very rare cause of lower limb ischemia in young people: popliteal artery entrapment. Open Cardiovasc Med J. 2018;12:18–28. https://doi.org/10.2174/1874192401812010018.
16. Gourgiotis S, Aggelakas J, Salemis N, Elias C, Georgiou C. Diagnosis and surgical approach of popliteal artery entrapment syndrome: a retrospective study. Vasc Health Risk Manag. 2008;4(1):83–8. https://doi.org/10.2147/vhrm.2008.04.01.83.
17. Goh BKP, Tay K-H, Tan S-G. Diagnosis and surgical management of popliteal artery entrapment syndrome. ANZ J Surg. 2005;75(10):869–73. https://doi.org/10.1111/j.1445-2197.2005.03555.x.
18. Jarraya M, Simmons S, Farber A, Teytelboym O, Naggara N, Guermazi A. Uncommon diseases of the popliteal artery: a pictorial review. Insights Imaging. 2016;7(5):679–88. https://doi.org/10.1007/s13244-016-0513-6.
19. Veraldi GF, Scudo G, Scorsone L, Mezzetto L, Castellani RL. Cystic adventitial disease of the popliteal artery: report of two cases and review of the literature. G Chir. 2014;35(9–10):229–34.
20. Bresler M, Mar W, Toman J. Diagnostic imaging in the evaluation of leg pain in athletes. Clin Sports Med. 2012;31(2):217–45. https://doi.org/10.1016/j.csm.2011.09.006.
21. George CA, Hutchinson MR. Chronic exertional compartment syndrome. Clin Sports Med. 2012;31(2):307–19. https://doi.org/10.1016/j.csm.2011.09.013.
22. Gaunder C, McKinney B, Rivera J. Popliteal artery entrapment or chronic exertional compartment syndrome? Case Rep Med. 2017;2017:6981047. https://doi.org/10.1155/2017/6981047.
23. Posthuma JJ, Posma JJN, Schep G, Bender MMH, van Oerle R, van der Wal AC, Ten Cate H, Spronk HMH. Protease-activated receptors are potential regulators in the development of arterial endofibrosis in high-performance athletes. J Vasc Surg. 2019;69(4):1243–50. https://doi.org/10.1016/j.jvs.2018.05.220.
24. van Hooff M, Colenbrander FFC, Bender MHM, Loos MMJA, Brini A, Savelberg HHHCM, Scheltinga MR, Schep G. Short- and long-term outcomes after endarterectomy with autologous patching in endurance athletes with iliac artery endofibrosis. J Vasc Surg. 2023;78(2):514–524.e2. https://doi.org/10.1016/j.jvs.2023.03.501.
25. Akkersdijk WL, de Ruyter JW, Lapham R, Mali W, Eikelboom BC. Colour duplex ultrasonographic imaging and provocation of popliteal artery compression. Eur J Vasc Endovasc Surg. 1995;10(3):342–5. https://doi.org/10.1016/s1078-5884(05)80054-1.
26. di Marzo L, Cavallaro A, Sciacca V, Lepidi S, Marmorale A, Tamburelli A, Stipa S. Diagnosis of popliteal artery entrapment syndrome: the role of duplex scanning. J Vasc Surg. 1991;13(3):434–8. https://doi.org/10.1067/mva.1991.26375.
27. Macedo TA, Johnson CM, Hallett JW Jr, Breen JF. Popliteal artery entrapment syndrome: role of imaging in the diagnosis. AJR Am J Roentgenol. 2003;181(5):1259–65. https://doi.org/10.2214/ajr.181.5.1811259.
28. Hai Z, Guangrui S, Yuan Z, Zhuodong X, Cheng L, Jingmin L, Yun S. CT angiography and MRI in patients with popliteal artery entrapment syndrome. AJR Am J Roentgenol. 2008;191(6):1760–6. https://doi.org/10.2214/AJR.07.4012.
29. Müller N, Morris DC, Nichols DM. Popliteal artery entrapment demonstrated by CT. Radiology. 1984;151(1):157–8. https://doi.org/10.1148/radiology.151.1.6701307.
30. Zhong H, Gan J, Zhao Y, Xu Z, Liu C, Shao G, Wu X. Role of CT angiography in the diagnosis and treatment of popliteal vascular entrapment syndrome. AJR Am J Roentgenol. 2011;197(6):W1147–54. https://doi.org/10.2214/AJR.11.6789.

31. McGuinness G, Durham JD, Rutherford RB, Thickman D, Kumpe DA. Popliteal artery entrapment: findings at MR imaging. J Vasc Interv Radiol. 1991;2(2):241–5. https://doi.org/10.1016/s1051-0443(91)72289-6.
32. Di Cesare E, Marsili L, Marino G, Masciocchi C, Morettini G, Spartera C, Lupattelli L, Passariello R. Stress MR imaging for evaluation of popliteal artery entrapment. J Magn Reson Imaging. 1994;4(4):617–22. https://doi.org/10.1002/jmri.1880040418.
33. Wind GG, James Valentine R. Anatomic exposures in vascular surgery. Lippincott Williams & Wilkins; 2013. https://play.google.com/store/books/details?id=R-XxQ2OH5MgC.

Chapter 5
Charcot Arthropathy of the Shoulder

Sreenivasulu Metikala, Dirk W. Verheul, Megan Rajagopal, Neel Dixit, Jennifer L. Vanderbeck, R. Scott Graham, and Wilhelm A. Zuelzer

Clinical Vignette 1

A 23-year-old man came to the orthopaedic clinic with a 2-month history of dull pain in his dominant right shoulder. The pain started when he overstretched his arm during yard work and was accompanied by an immediate popping sensation. The patient reported no prior traumatic events, systemic symptoms, or significant past medical conditions and was not taking any prescribed medications.

Physical examination revealed diffuse swelling of the right shoulder with mild tenderness in the biceps groove. The range of motion (ROM) included 160° forward elevation, 5° external rotation, and internal rotation up to the lower thoracic region. On manual muscle testing, the superior rotator cuff was found to be weak, with a 4/5 grade. The Spurling test was negative, and his distal neurovascular status was intact. Plain radiographs (Fig. 5.1) revealed narrowing of the acromioclavicular interval with down-sloping of the anterolateral acromion, loose body at the glenoid neck, and os acromiale.

S. Metikala (✉) · D. W. Verheul · J. L. Vanderbeck
Department of Orthopaedic Surgery, Virginia Commonwealth University School of Medicine, Richmond, VA, USA
e-mail: sreenivasulu.metikala@vcuhealth.org; dirk.verheul1@vcuhealth.org; jennifer.vanderbeck@vcuhealth.org

W. A. Zuelzer
Orthopaedic Surgery, Virginia Commonwealth University Medical School, Richmond, VA, USA
e-mail: wilhelm.zuelzer@vcuhealth.org

M. Rajagopal · R. S. Graham
Department of Neurosurgery, Virginia Commonwealth University, Richmond, VA, USA
e-mail: megan.rajagopal@vcuhealth.org; robert.graham@vcuhealth.org

N. Dixit
Department of Neurology, Virginia Commonwealth University, Richmond, VA, USA
e-mail: neel.dixit@vcuhealth.org

W. A. Zuelzer, S. Metikala (eds.), *Unusual Conditions That Every Orthopaedic Surgeon Should Know*, https://doi.org/10.1007/978-3-031-58946-1_5

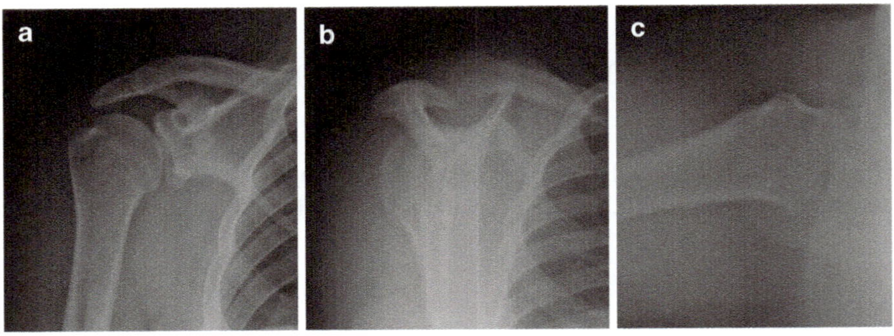

Fig. 5.1 Plain radiographs of the right shoulder: (**a**) Grashey view presenting diminished acromio-humeral distance and loose body adjacent to the glenoid neck. (**b**) Scapular-Y view with down-sloping of the anterior acromion. (**c**) Axillary lateral view showing os acromiale

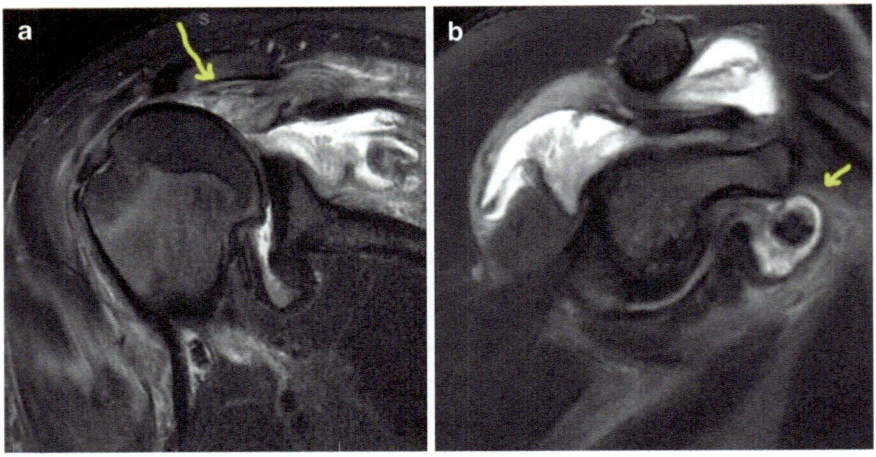

Fig. 5.2 Right shoulder MRI scan obtained without contrast. (**a**) Coronal T2-weighted image depicting a massive superior rotator cuff tear with medial retraction and proximal migration of humeral head. (**b**) Sagittal T2-weighted image showing effusion and loose body in superior subscapularis recess

A subsequent magnetic resonance image (MRI) scan (Fig. 5.2) showed a massive, retracted tear of supraspinatus and infraspinatus with mild atrophy, proximal humeral head migration, loose bodies, and a large effusion.

Given the age and activity levels, surgical repair of his rotator cuff tear was recommended. Infection was excluded through preoperative inflammatory indices and negative microbiology of joint aspirate analysis. The patient then underwent arthroscopic rotator cuff repair by the standard double-row suture anchor technique, augmented with a bioinductive patch due to poor tissue quality and retraction. During the procedure, it was necessary to medialize the footprint and perform interval slides to obtain adequate mobility and a tension-free repair interface. He was apparently well until 6 weeks after the surgery, when he experienced a painless effusion that yielded 15 mL of opaque red fluid upon arthrocentesis. The aspirate analysis showed 70,073/cm total nucleated cells with 94% polymorphs and 80,418/cm red cells. His ESR and CRP were also elevated at 83 mm and 3.9 mg/dL, respectively. Further imaging by CT scan with intravenous (IV) contrast revealed peripherally enhancing fluid collections with superior subluxation of the humeral head and erosive changes in the anterosuperior glenoid, concerning septic arthritis. The patient underwent a second surgery, through an open deltopectoral approach, which revealed a large amount of purulent joint fluid, phlegmon, and complete detachment of the previous rotator cuff repair. A thorough debridement was performed, explanting the previous suture anchors and the bioinductive patch. The surgical wound was closed over a drain that was removed after 48 h. The intraoperative cultures yielded *Cutibacterium acnes* and *Staphylococcus saccharolyticus*. Following susceptibility testing, the patient was given IV Ceftriaxone for 4 weeks, which led to healing of surgical incision and subsequent improvement in his shoulder symptoms.

During the hospital stay, it was later discovered that the patient previously suffered from chronic neck pain with arm weakness due to an underlying Arnold-Chiari malformation with cervical cord syrinx. It was then managed by suboccipital decompression craniectomy and C1 posterior arch resection with eventual resolution of symptoms. The current shoulder issues surfaced about 5 years after the above neurosurgical procedure was carried out. A re-evaluation of nervous system at this point revealed normal responses to light touch, temperature, and pain sensations in all extremities, with the cranial nerves intact. There was no hyperreflexia or clonus, and the Hoffmann sign was negative. Following a whole spine MRI scan, the patient was now diagnosed with a large cervicothoracic syrinx that extended to T10, the most significant area being from C7 to T2. It was accompanied by low-lying cerebellar tonsils below the foramen magnum, findings consistent with Chiari 1 malformation (Fig. 5.3).

Considering the patient's remarkable past surgical history (revealed in hindsight) and the recent emergence of atraumatic massive rotator cuff tear without any major pain, the diagnosis of Charcot shoulder arthropathy was established. Afterwards, a

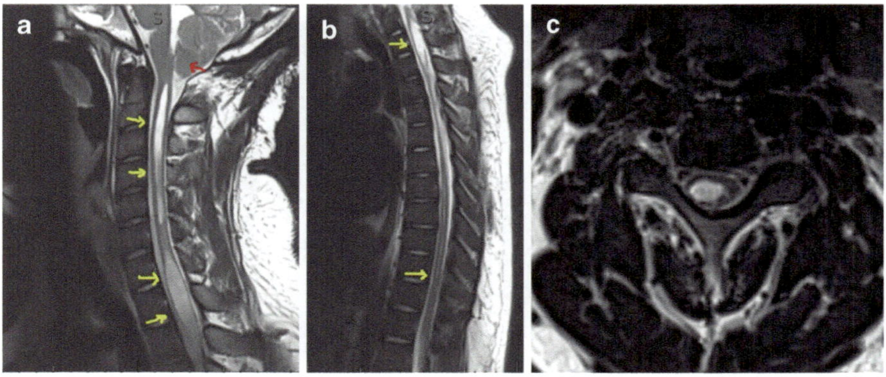

Fig. 5.3 MRI spine images. (**a**) Sagittal T2-weighted cervical and (**b**) thoracic spine images, including (**c**) axial section showing an expansile syrinx of cervical cord extending to the T10 endplate (yellow arrows) and low-lying cerebellar tonsils (red arrow)

neurosurgical consultation was sought to determine the next steps for the syrinx management. As the syrinx characteristics had not changed since the last imaging studies, no further neurosurgical intervention was deemed necessary. It was concluded that the preexistent syrinx had already triggered spinal cord damage prior to the cranial decompression surgery, which eventually led to a Charcot shoulder.

Regarding the right shoulder 6 weeks post-surgery, there was a significant limitation of active forward flexion, and external rotation although the passive motion was full. Despite all, the patient did not have any major pain in his shoulder, a finding consistent with an established Charcot joint. No further orthopaedic surgeries were planned at this time due to potential surgical risks. The patient was educated about joint protection tactics, and physical therapy was continued to optimize overall shoulder function.

Clinical Vignette 2

A 25-year-old woman visited the clinic due to sharp pain and swelling in her right shoulder, which is her dominant arm. She has been experiencing this for the past 2 days since waking up from sleep. There was no history of trauma, previous shoulder issues, pain in other joints, intravenous drug abuse, recent steroid use, or systemic symptoms. The patient's prior medical records indicated bilateral carpal tunnel syndrome, with the left side being operated a year ago. Upon examination, the shoulder was found to be warm, swollen, and stiff with diffuse tenderness and marked weakness of the rotator cuff. Her neurological examination was normal, and the vitals were otherwise stable. The plain radiographs demonstrated soft tissue swelling with the widening of acromiohumeral distance, calcific density adjacent to the lateral acromion, and pseudosubluxation of the humeral head in the glenoid fossa (Fig. 5.4).

Further evaluation by a magnetic resonance imaging (MRI) scan revealed a large effusion, flattening of the humeral head with bone marrow edema, and widespread glenohumeral chondrolysis. Also, there were massive full-thickness retracted tears of the supraspinatus and infraspinatus tendons with moderate atrophy (Fig. 5.5).

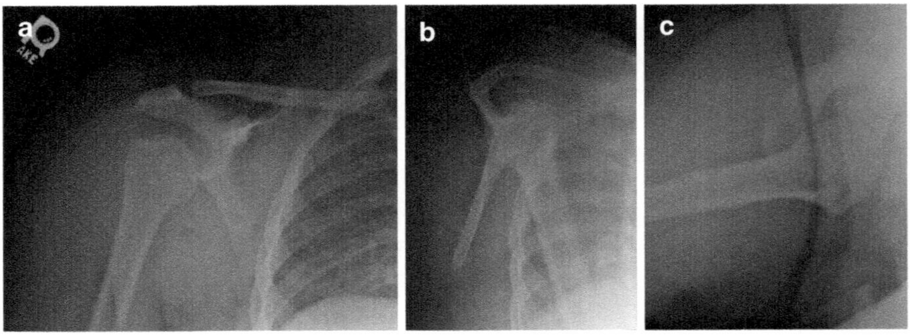

Fig. 5.4 Plain radiographs of the right shoulder, including anteroposterior (**a**), scapular-Y (**b**), and axillary lateral (**c**) views, showing widening acromiohumeral distance, calcific density adjacent to the lateral acromion, and pseudosubluxation of the humeral head

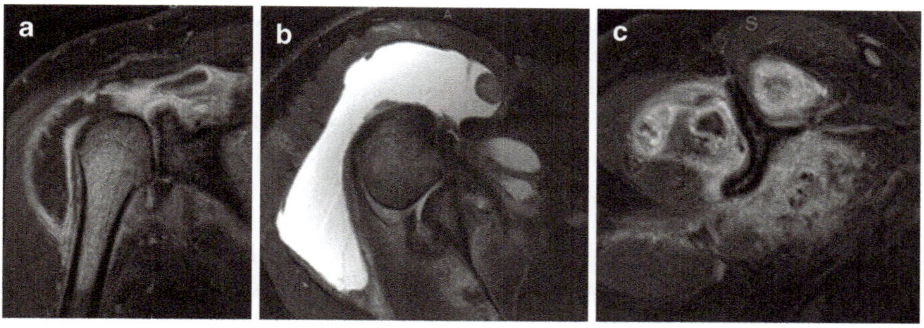

Fig. 5.5 MRI of the right shoulder without contrast. (**a**) Coronal T2-weighted image showing full-thickness rotator cuff tear with flattening of the humeral head and cartilage loss. (**b**) Axial T2-weighted image with gross effusion. (**c**) Sagittal T2-weighted image displaying widespread atrophy of rotator cuff

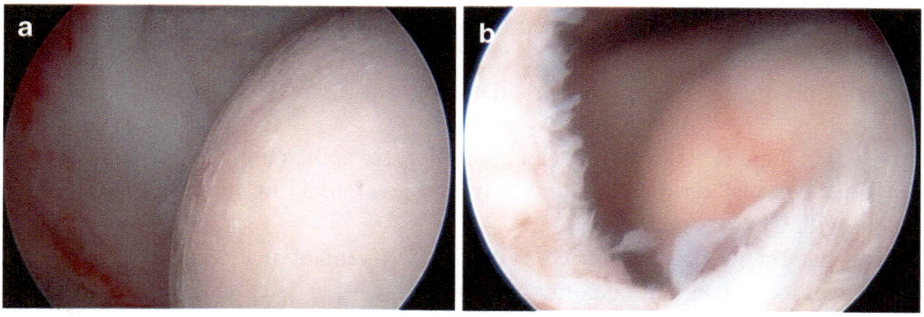

Fig. 5.6 Arthroscopic right shoulder posterior glenohumeral portal view (**a**) showing widespread grade 4 chondrosis of humeral head and glenoid. Posterior subacromial portal view (**b**) showing the massive, retracted tear of the supraspinatus and infraspinatus tendons

Based on the acute presentation and corresponding imaging studies, septic shoulder was considered as the provisional diagnosis. A subsequent arthroscopic shoulder procedure showed a large amount of cloudy, red-tinged synovial fluid with no obvious purulence. Joint irrigation and debridement of the rotator cuff tears were performed without any surgical repair in the context of suspected infection. The patient was discharged home on provisional antibiotics which were later discontinued as the intraoperative cultures yielded no microbial growth even after an extended incubation. At the 2-month mark post-surgery, the acute shoulder symptoms had subsided without any pain or systemic symptoms. However, this dominant arm was lacking strength due to a massive rotator cuff tear, and so further surgical procedure was planned for a potential repair. During this second arthroscopic surgery, diffuse grade 4 cartilage lesions were evident in the humeral head and glenoid with a large amount of clear synovial fluid. Massive tears of the supraspinatus and infraspinatus tendons were observed with medial retraction to the level of the glenoid (Fig. 5.6).

The situation was deemed "non-repairable" due to the extensive atrophy and lack of tendon mobility despite adequate releases and interval slides. Therefore, gentle debridement was done without any repair. The intraoperative cultures, once again, were negative for microorganisms, including acid-fast bacilli, bacteria, and fungi. Histopathology report showed features of granulation tissue and negative Congo red staining for amyloid. A right carpal tunnel release was performed under the same anesthesia to address her sensory symptoms in the hand and digits.

Following the second surgery, she developed recurrent painless shoulder effusion yielding about 300 mL of clear synovial fluid and particulate debris upon arthrocentesis. The patient's vital signs were steady, and there were no systemic manifestations. During a subsequent rheumatology assessment, the antistreptolysin O (ASO) titers were elevated at 400 IU/mL, and the ESR and CRP levels were determined to be 55 mm and 2.1 mg/dL, respectively. The patient was prescribed oral sulfasalazine initially, followed by adalimumab (Humira) injections, which ultimately resolved the shoulder effusions. No further shoulder surgeries were planned, and the patient was recommended to continue with outpatient PT to optimize shoulder function.

About a year later, the patient presented to the emergency department with a severe headache. Further evaluation by CT and MRI scans of the head (Fig. 5.7a) showed chronic severe ventricular dilatation with a small posterior cranial fossa (Fig. 5.7b).

A subsequent MRI of the cervical and thoracic spine (Fig. 5.8) revealed hydrocephalus, cervical syrinx extending to the T4 level, and low-lying cerebellum consistent with Chiari 2 malformation.

The patient was then referred to the department of neurosurgery, where she underwent a cervical laminectomy with posterior fossa decompression.

Repeat orthopaedic evaluation, at this point, showed right shoulder effusion with minimal discomfort and weakness of rotator cuff. The active forward elevation,

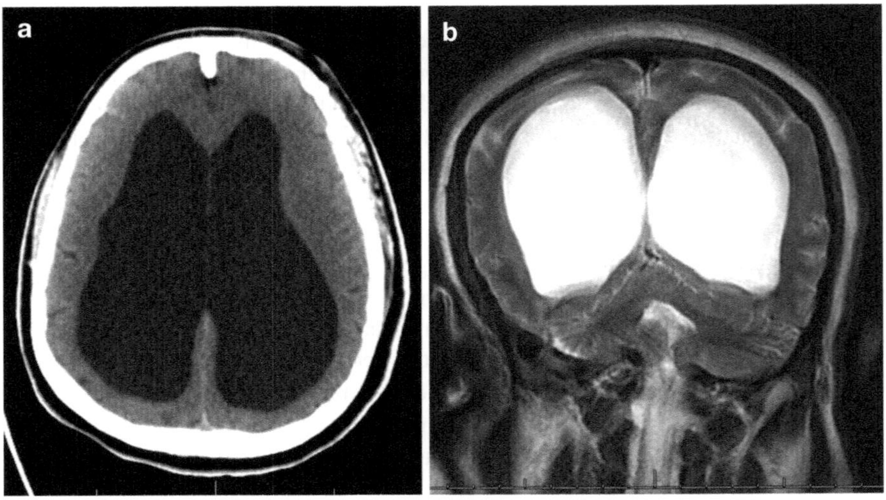

Fig. 5.7 Axial non-contrast CT (**a**) and coronal T2 MRI (**b**) images showing hydrocephalus

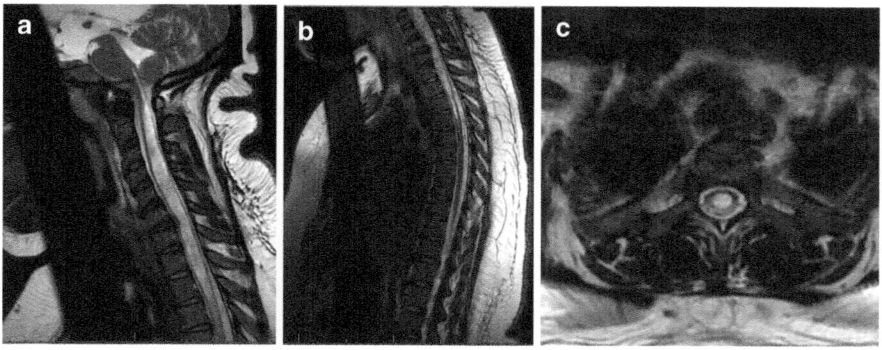

Fig. 5.8 MRI study. Sagittal T2-weighted images of the cervical (**a**) and thoracic spine (**b**, **c**) depicting an expansile syrinx of the cervical cord up to the level of T4, along with hydrocephalus and downward displacement of the cerebellum

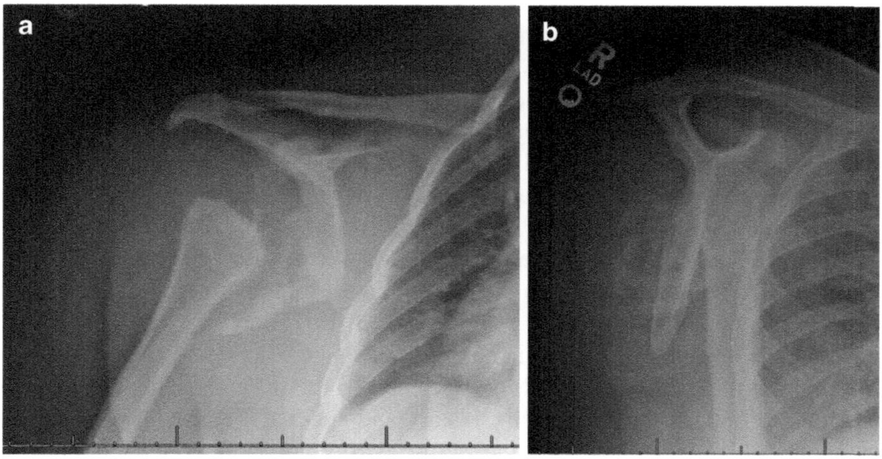

Fig. 5.9 Plain radiographs of the right shoulder, anteroposterior (**a**), and scapular-Y (**b**) views depicting resorption of the humeral head, glenoid erosions, bony fragmentation, and significant soft tissue swelling, suggestive of progressive neuropathic arthropathy

abduction, and external rotation were markedly limited, while the passive ROM was preserved. The sensations of light touch were diminished throughout the upper extremity. Plain radiographs (Fig. 5.9), unlike before, demonstrated severe destruction of the glenohumeral joint compared to the images taken 2 years ago, along with significant soft tissue swelling consistent with the Charcot joint.

Given the established Charcot changes in the shoulder with underlying Chiari 2 malformation, no further shoulder surgical procedures were recommended due to the potential for infection and surgical complications. Therefore, patient was recommended to continue PT and home exercises to optimize shoulder function.

Questions

1. What are the lessons learned?
2. What could have been done differently (in retrospect)?
3. What would be the preferred treatment for rotator cuff tear in an established Charcot shoulder?

Introduction

Charcot arthropathy (CA), also known as neuropathic arthropathy of the shoulder, is an unusual chronic degenerative disease characterized by progressive destruction of the joint and periarticular tissues. CA, in general, develops due to loss of pain sensation of the affected joint caused by an underlying neurological disorder such as tabes dorsalis, leprosy, diabetes mellitus, or syringomyelia [1–3]. The other causes include peripheral neuropathy, intra-articular steroid injections, myelomeningocele, chronic alcoholism, multiple sclerosis, congenital insensitivity to pain, myelodysplasia, and amyloidosis [4–6]. With regard to CA affecting the shoulder joint, cervical syringomyelia is the most common underlying disease in almost 80% of cases [4, 7, 8]. In syringomyelia, a central fluid-filled cavity (syrinx), develops in the spinal cord, causing neuronal compression with abnormal nerve conduction of fibers carrying pain and temperature sensations, leading to progressive shoulder joint destruction.

Typically, the neurological manifestations of the cervical syrinx are occult and often overshadowed by the shoulder symptoms, resulting in misdiagnosis and delayed diagnosis of the primary pathology [4, 9, 10]. Therefore, when the patient has shoulder swelling with profound loss of active range of motion (ROM) but with a minimal-to-no pain, CA should be included in the differential diagnosis. It is essential to obtain a comprehensive history and conduct a thorough neurological assessment [3, 8]. The imaging studies of the affected shoulder, notably an MRI scan, reveal significant joint destruction that is clearly more than what would be expected from the shoulder discomfort. A subsequent cervical spine MRI is an absolute necessity for assessing syringomyelia when a CA shoulder is suspected. When evident, a prompt referral to the neurosurgery department for the treatment of syrinx should be given precedence over orthopaedic management to successfully stabilize and treat this degenerative process. Historically, a conservative approach has been advocated in the management of CA shoulder because of unfavorable outcomes with surgical interventions. Although recent literature suggests shoulder reconstruction in a select subset of patients, the indications remain unclear. This review aims to summarize the current knowledge about pathogenesis and clinical presentation of CA shoulder and highlight the general lines of management with the description of the above two case examples.

History

In 1703, William Musgrave gave the first clinical description of neuropathic arthropathy in a patient with flaccid paralysis [11]. John Kearsley Mitchell, in 1831, reported an association of spinal cord paralysis with arthritis of the foot and ankle joints. The eponym Charcot arthropathy was named after French neurologist Jean-Martin Charcot, who first published the neuropathic nature of the disease in tabes dorsalis in 1868 [2]. Later, in the year 1881, he gave a presentation of his findings at the seventh International Medical Congress in London. Since then, the attribution of neuropathic arthropathies to Charcot has remained independent of etiology. However, the association between syringomyelia and the development of upper extremity neuropathic arthropathy was not reported until 1892 by Sokoloff [3].

Etiopathology

Charcot shoulder is most often associated with cervical syringomyelia, though it is seen in many neurological disorders. Overall, syringomyelia contributes up to 25% of all CA cases, and 80% of them happen in the upper extremity [1, 2, 8, 9]. The involvement of multiple joints is seen in up to 20% of cases [10]. After the shoulder, the elbow is the most affected joint in syringomyelia, followed by the wrist and the hand [4, 12–15].

Syringomyelia is a chronic progressive disease characterized by the development of longitudinal cavitations (syrinx) containing cerebrospinal fluid (CSF) within the substance of the spinal cord. The syrinx starts centrally and then enlarges outward, damaging the adjacent neurons. The disease is primarily congenital. It is seen in 80% of patients with a Chiari malformation, which is characterized by herniation of the cerebellar tonsils into the foramen magnum with the CSF outflow obstruction leading to cavitations in the spinal cord and hydrocephalus. Syringomyelia can also be acquired by any condition that blocks the CSF flow within the central canal or damages the spinal cord, such as trauma, tumor, or abscess. Regardless of the etiology, since the neuronal compression starts close to the midline, the decussating fibers of the spinothalamic tract are the first structures to be damaged, sparing dorsal columns. As a result, dissociative sensory loss ensues with selective loss of pain and temperature, sparing proprioception. This abnormal innervation subsequently affects the peripheral joint or joints with loss of protective pain sensation. Eventually, the expansion of the syrinx disrupts dorsal column fibers and the anterior horn's lower motor neurons, resulting in muscle atrophy, areflexia, and loss of proprioception with progressive joint destruction.

Pathogenesis

While the literature contains descriptions of it, the exact pathophysiology of CA development is not well understood and has been the subject of much debate. It generally revolves around the following theories.

Neurovascular Theory

Referred to as the French theory, advocated by Mitchell and Charcot, which speculates that the sensory deficits disrupt the trophic centers that control bone and joint nutrition, leading to increased blood flow, greater delivery of osteoclasts, and subsequent bone resorption. These trophic centers are now understood as autonomic nerves that regulate the arterial smooth muscle affecting the blood flow [16–20].

Neurotraumatic Theory

Volkmann and Virchow later proposed neurotraumatic theory, also known as German theory, which emphasizes the loss of protective joint sensation as the root cause of CA. An insensate joint has disrupted somatic muscle reflexes, which would otherwise safeguard it from exceeding the safe limits of the ROM, resulting in recurrent subclinical trauma, subsequent cartilage damage, and ultimately progressive joint destruction [17, 19, 21–23]. However, it can be observed that spinal cord-injured patients who do not suffer from such repeated microtrauma also develop CA, which refutes the above mechanical basis. This led to the current widely accepted theory that the neurovascular process may play the initial role of inducing bone osteolysis, which subsequently results in progressive damage of joints and periarticular tissues due to continued low-grade neurotraumatic processes [17, 24].

Molecular Biology

Regardless of the etiology, chronic tissue injury and the resultant inflammation appear to be the drivers in the development of CA. The release of pro-inflammatory cytokines such as interleukin-1β, interleukin-6, and tumor necrotic factor-α (TNF-α) [25] activates the T-cells resulting in the expression of receptor activator of nuclear factor κβ ligand (RANK-L) on the surface of osteoblastic stromal cells. This ligand binds to the RANK receptor on the osteoclast precursor leading to a cascade of events comprising induction of gene transcription through nuclear factor κβ, maturation of osteoclasts, and subsequent bone resorption. The above process is

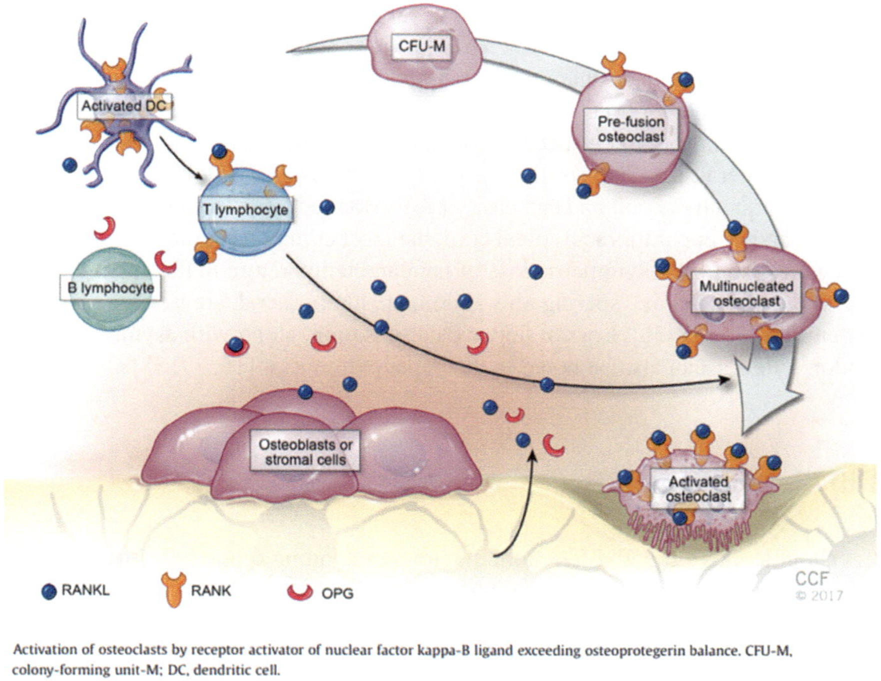

Fig. 5.10 Molecular biology signaling pathway associated with Charcot joint. *RANK* receptor activator of nuclear factor kappa-B, *RANK-L* receptor activator of nuclear factor kappa-B ligand, *OPG* osteoprotegerin. [Reproduced with permission from Connors JC, Hardy MA, Kishman LL, Botek GG, Verdin CJ, Rao NM, Kingsley JD. Charcot Pathogenesis: A Study of In Vivo Gene Expression. J Foot Ankle Surg. 2018 Nov-Dec;57(6):1067–1072.]

naturally regulated by osteoprotegerin (OPG), also known as osteoclastogenesis inhibitory factor, which binds the RANK receptor and inhibits RANK-RANKL mediated differentiation of osteoclast precursors to mature osteoclasts (Fig. 5.10). Denosumab, a pharmacological agent, also has a similar mechanism but inhibits RANK-L of osteoblastic stromal cells and is thought to help arrest the disease progression [26, 27]. The overproduction of RANK-L and lack of regulation by OPG have been implicated in enhanced osteoclastogenesis among CA patients [28–32].

Presentation

Although the primary pathology is neurologic, the shoulder symptoms manifest early, so patients typically consult orthopaedic offices, often with a history of trivial trauma. The common presenting features include a painful or painless shoulder, joint swelling, and loss of ROM accompanied by strange noises heard from the joint. Clinical examination findings can be variable based on the stage of joint degeneration. Generalized effusion with variable amounts of tenderness, often accompanied by erythema and local warmth, are some of the characteristic findings. Loss of active ROM and rotator cuff strength are also evident with reasonable preservation of passive motion. Joint destruction advances slowly over time, although rapid deterioration is likely because of direct or indirect trauma. CA shoulder is mostly unilateral; it is rare for it to involve both sides [33, 34]. Neurological findings are frequently occult and can easily be overlooked. Syringomyelia of the lower cervical and/or upper thoracic spinal cord, the most common primary etiology, presents with "cape-like" symmetric loss of pain and temperature in the upper extremities and upper thorax, sparing the abdomen, lumbosacral areas, and the lower extremities [15, 35, 36]. Loss of hot or cold sensation, along with asymmetric deep tendon reflexes, can also be noted in the upper extremities [15, 37, 38].

Differential Diagnosis

CA shoulder has a broad differential diagnosis, including septic arthritis, tabes dorsalis (neurosyphilis), diabetes, syringomyelia, trauma to the cervical spinal cord, soft tissue sarcoma, tuberculosis, synovial chondromatosis, inflammatory arthropathy, and Gorham disease (vanishing bone disease) [8, 34, 37, 39, 40].

Work-Up

CA shoulder is often a diagnosis of exclusion. So, it is prudent to systematically evaluate and exclude other more prevalent pathological conditions such as septic joint, inflammatory arthropathy, tumor, tabes dorsalis, diabetes, and tuberculosis (TB).

Lab Tests

Given the similarity, the initial stages of CA shoulder may be confused with septic arthritis, a condition that could exist concurrently, as seen in case 1. Routine labs, therefore, start with checking the standard inflammatory markers, including complete blood count (CBC), white blood cell (WBC) count, C-reactive protein (CRP), and erythrocyte sedimentation rate (ESR). These parameters are usually within the normal range in an isolated CA shoulder [3, 10, 41]. The other relevant serologic evaluation includes hemoglobin A1c, rapid plasma reagin, anti-cyclic citrullinated peptide antibody, rheumatoid factor, and antinuclear antibody, as a work-up for the differential diagnosis. The rest include skin testing and a quantiFERON (QFT-Plus) lab test for evaluating TB arthritis. Notably, the QFT-Plus test, unlike skin test, is unaffected by prior vaccination.

Imaging Studies-Radiographs

CA shoulder can have a varied appearance on radiographic imaging based on the state of the disease and commonly includes two disease patterns: atrophic and hypertrophic [1, 10, 13, 14, 36, 42]. Bone resorption is characteristic of the atrophic stage with superomedial flattening of the humeral head. In contrast, the hypertrophic pattern consists of joint destruction, fragmentation, osseous debris, osteophytes, effusion, and periarticular new bone formation.

Magnetic Resonance Imaging (MRI)

The distinct MRI findings of the CA shoulder include effusion, periarticular inflammation, joint destruction, and rotator cuff tears [34]. When CA shoulder is likely, a cervical spine MRI should be obtained to evaluate for syringomyelia, the most common underlying disease. The size and extent of the syrinx can be determined based on its signal intensity, which is equal to or slightly higher than CSF. A non-contrast-enhanced study is usually sufficient to delineate the characteristics of a syrinx and can also differentiate it from a spinal tumor [43, 44].

Computed Tomography (CT)

Although a CT scan has no definitive role in diagnosing a CA shoulder, it may help evaluate bone destruction, sequestra, intra-articular bone debris, and subluxation/dislocation. To assess the primary etiology, a CT myelogram of the cervical spine can be considered when there is a contraindication for an MRI study [45].

Arthrocentesis

Joint aspiration or arthrocentesis is the critical test to differentiate a CA shoulder from septic arthritis, but as a standard practice, it is held until all other relevant non-invasive imaging investigations have been conducted. It typically yields a large quantity of clear yellow fluid with particulate debris [10]. The aspirate specimens should be sent for total cell count (with differential), gram stain, crystal analysis, and microbiology for aerobic, anaerobic, acid-fast bacilli, and fungal culture. Occasionally, septic arthritis may co-exist with CA pathology [46, 47]. When detected, the standard treatment consists of open/arthroscopic surgical drainage and debridement followed by 4–6 weeks of culture-specific antibiotics. However, the overall shoulder function is likely to be poor in this combined situation considering the preexistent damage to the cartilage as well as rotator cuff.

Classification

The CA shoulder may be classified using the Eichenholtz system, which was originally developed for the assessment of a neuropathic foot (Table 5.1). It has three stages of disease progression based on clinical and radiological findings [49]. Features of inflammation including joint swelling, warmth, and erythema accompanied by ligamentous laxity are seen in the first stage (development stage), and the radiographs demonstrate osteopenia, fragmentation, bone debris, and joint subluxation or dislocation. The second stage (coalescence stage) is characterized by a gradual reduction in the above acute symptoms with radiographic absorption of fragmented debris and the appearance of sclerosis. Finally, the third stage (reconstitution or reconstruction stage) demonstrates a complete absence of inflammation, with the radiographic findings of consolidation of the deformity, rounded margins, subchondral sclerosis, joint arthrosis, and fibrous ankylosis. Later on, in 1990, Shibata et al. included stage 0, the prodromal stage that describes the presence of just clinical findings of early inflammation with no radiographic changes [48]. The classification, however, is largely subjective and therefore prone to bias. In general, conservative modality is recommended up to the second stage, while the operative reconstruction is reserved for the third stage of the disease.

Table 5.1 Modified Eichenholtz classification [47]

Stage	Clinical presentation	Radiographic features
0 (prodromal) [48]	Early inflammation with swelling, redness, and warmth	Normal
1 (Fragmentation)	Continued inflammation with persistent swelling, warmth, instability	Periarticular fragmentation, osteopenia, subluxation
II (Coalescence)	Gradual reduction of inflammation with improvement of swelling, redness, and warmth	Resorption of bone debris and coalescence of large fragments
III (Reconstruction)	Resolved inflammation with no swelling or warmth	Joint arthrosis, fibrous ankylosis, consolidation of bone fragments

Adopted from Rosenbaum AJ, DiPreta JA. Classifications in brief: Eichenholtz classification of Charcot arthropathy. Clin Orthop Relat Res. 2015 Mar;473(3):1168–1171

Treatment

The primary goal of managing a CA shoulder is rapid diagnosis and prompt management of underlying etiology, which in most cases means identification of spinal cord syrinx followed by immediate neurosurgical evaluation [2, 4, 8, 38, 40, 41, 50]. Besides neurological improvement, the neurosurgical decompression performed in a timely fashion could halt the silent destruction of the shoulder joint, allowing for moderate preservation of joint ROM and function. Not uncommonly, the CA shoulder is misdiagnosed, as was the case in the above two patients, resulting in suboptimal shoulder procedures.

Syrinx Management

The treatment of cervical/cervicothoracic syrinx depends on its characteristics identified in the MRI scan and the pattern of neurological symptoms. Once a patient is referred to the neurosurgical clinic with symptomatic Charcot arthropathy and an MRI diagnosis of cervical syrinx, the posterior fossa is evaluated for cerebellar tonsillar ectopia. An MRI of the brain is then obtained to rule out hydrocephalus and a supratentorial cause for the tonsillar ectopia. Management of cerebellar ectopia does not necessarily require posterior fossa decompression. If there is a cervical syrinx demonstrating an alteration in CSF flow at the cervicomedullary junction; however, posterior fossa decompression is indicated.

Nonoperative modality with serial MRI spine follow-up is an accepted treatment when the syrinx remains stable and asymptomatic [51, 52]. The presence of sensory/motor deficits in the extremities, cranial nerve involvement, cerebellar manifestations, and the MRI evidence of expansile syrinx are the common indications for surgical decompression [51, 53, 54]. Excellent prognosis is expected with timely surgical intervention in appropriately selected patients. Besides, studies have demonstrated that a neuropathic shoulder can experience a marked improvement in its functioning, solely from neurosurgical treatment, without any orthopaedic surgical intervention for the affected shoulder [3, 4, 37, 50].

Shoulder Management

Initial Treatment

A conservative approach is usually the preferred orthopaedic treatment method for the CA shoulder. Short-term sling immobilization and weightbearing limitations are instructed to protect the joint, and oral anti-inflammatory medicines are prescribed to reduce synovial inflammation. Physical therapy/occupational therapy is essential to maintain shoulder ROM, regain strength, and improve activities of daily living. Serial arthrocentesis is often necessary for symptomatic relief of gross effusions. Further, the aspirate specimens should be tested to detect coexistent septic arthritis. Patient education is critical to prevent direct or indirect trauma to the insensate joint. Awareness of joint protection tactics prevents further cartilage damage from overuse and optimizes shoulder function by keeping it within the safe ROM [3, 8]. The efficacy of bisphosphonates in controlling the disease progression is debatable, though they are often used in neuropathic foot and ankle arthropathy [26, 55, 56]. The other pharmacological agents, such as osteoprotegerin, denosumab, and other TNF-alpha inhibitors, are considered investigational at this point [26, 27, 57].

Operative

Given the high risk of infection, implant-related complications, and poor outcomes, operative management is usually not the primary treatment modality [9, 12, 41]. Shoulder surgical options may need to be considered if patients have persistent or worsening shoulder symptoms despite maximizing all the available conservative methods. As a general rule, the underlying etiology must be addressed adequately before any shoulder surgery is performed. Attempted shoulder reconstructive procedures prior to stabilization of syrinx frequently result in unfavorable outcomes, as seen in one of our cases. Even though incomplete, the improvement in neurological status following a neurosurgical intervention offers enough protective sensations to contemplate shoulder reconstructions in the select population [3, 4, 50]. Other surgical prerequisites include a quiescent shoulder (little or no signs of progressive joint damage) over a minimum of 1 year, absence of persistent neurological deficits, and an infection-free joint [4, 9, 12, 58, 59]. Essentially, the surgical options are composed of arthroscopic debridement, arthrodesis, and arthroplasty.

Arthroscopic Surgery

Arthroscopic shoulder debridement may be indicated to alleviate symptoms of tense effusion, although is generally not necessary if the underlying problem is adequately managed. Alternatively, a simple office-based aspiration using a wide-bore needle, followed by an intra-articular injection of cortisone performed in the office in most patients.

Arthrodesis

In the past, arthrodesis was the only salvage modality for a CA shoulder, due to the high risk of complications from arthroplasty. An arthrodesis in a functional position was considered for a grossly unstable shoulder, yet achieving successful osseous bridging across the glenohumeral joint is not easy due to significant bone resorption [10]. In the literature, there is a scarcity of studies that reported the outcomes of arthrodesis [60]. Currently, shoulder arthrodesis has become obsolete in the surgical armamentarium of Charcot shoulder due to the availability of newer arthroplasty implant options.

Arthroplasty

Various arthroplasty procedures have been explored in the surgical reconstruction of a CA shoulder, including resurfacing arthroplasty, hemiarthroplasty (HA), anatomic total shoulder arthroplasty (ASA), and reverse total shoulder arthroplasty (RSA). Resurfacing arthroplasty is an appropriate procedure in the select younger patient cohort with no significant bone resorption. This procedure preserves the bone stock and allows future reconstructions, if necessary. Crowther and Bell [12] presented a case report of resurfacing arthroplasty using an uncemented humeral head implant and a soft tissue biological interposition graft for the glenoid. At the 2-year follow-up, the patient had no shoulder pain and demonstrated 140° of active elevation and 50° of external rotation. Matsuhashi et al. [58] reported the outcomes of HA with rotator cuff repair for three CA shoulders that had a preserved greater tubercle. At a mean 8-year follow-up, all showed improvement in shoulder pain and ROM. Except for slight central migration of the humeral head, there were no radiographic signs of dislocation, prosthetic loosening, or bone erosions. Ueblacker et al. [59] performed a staged bilateral RSA on a woman with neuropathic destruction of both shoulders accompanied by massive cuff tears secondary to post-traumatic syringomyelia. At the 2-year follow-up, the patient attained satisfactory improvement in function with no pain in either shoulder along with stable radiographic appearance of arthroplasty components. Schoch et al. [61] presented a series of 10 CA shoulders between 2000 and 2011, being managed by HA for six patients and ASA for one patient, while the remaining three patients underwent RSA. At a mean 4-year follow-up, there was an improvement in shoulder pain, but the overall gain in ROM was moderate. The single ASA and one of the three RSA patients needed revision surgery an average of 5 months after the index procedure. Two RSA patients developed postoperative stress fractures of the acromion. Radiographic signs of glenoid erosion were seen in five HA patients. As per recent study by Wawrzyniak et al. [41] the RSA group of two patients showed better ROM and pain relief than the eight nonsurgical patients. Overall, a trend can be seen toward RSA for symptomatic CA shoulder patients who failed all the conservative measures. Undoubtedly, the primary etiology of the CA shoulder must be promptly identified and adequately managed before any surgical procedures are attempted.

Conclusions

CA shoulder is a rare yet critical condition that mandates early diagnosis to minimize irreversible joint destruction and disability. Every orthopaedist must be wary of its characteristic clinical and radiological findings to avoid missed or late diagnosis. The first step in management is identifying and effectively managing the underlying cause. There is currently a paucity of evidence on the nonoperative versus operative management of a neuropathic shoulder. Nonetheless, the conservative approach seems to be a reasonable first-line modality until the primary neurological process is adequately stabilized. With regard to optimal shoulder surgery, given the scarce available data, further studies are necessary to formulate guidelines on operative interventions. In the interim, we recommend effective diagnostic measures to prevent misdiagnosis and allow early treatment for optimal patient outcomes (Fig. 5.11).

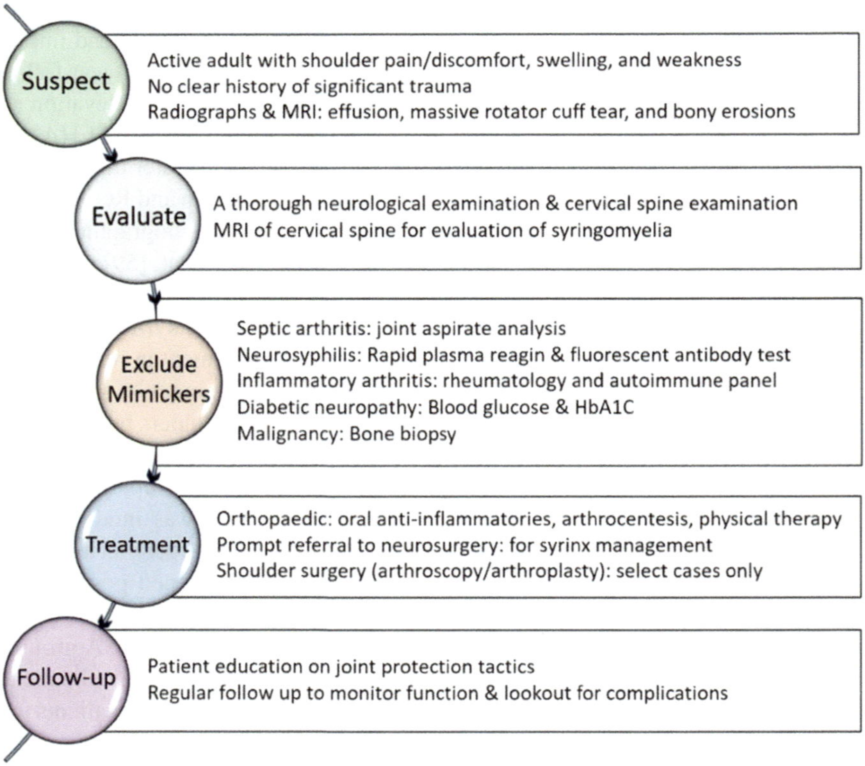

Fig. 5.11 Flowchart for Charcot arthropathy of the shoulder

1. What are the lessons learned?

   Rotator cuff tear in a young, active patient with no clear history of significant trauma should be carefully evaluated for underlying neurological etiology. A high index of suspicion is necessary for early diagnosis of this remarkable pathology. The consequences of a missed diagnosis of cervical spine syringomyelia can be devastating because of its potential for the emergence of a neuropathic shoulder.
2. What could have been done differently (in retrospect)?

   Since early diagnosis and management of the underlying pathology is the goal, emphasis must be placed on taking a comprehensive medical history and performing a thorough clinical examination of both the musculoskeletal and neurological systems. In the first case, the history of neurosurgical procedure for a cervical syrinx was evident only in hindsight. The second one was characterized by acute presentation that closely resembled a septic joint. Nonetheless, a timely MRI of the cervical spine would have brought the underlying syrinx into the limelight in both cases. A prompt referral to the neurosurgery department would have allowed a timely cranial decompression with the possibility of preventing a Charcot shoulder, rather than multiple arthroscopic surgical interventions.
3. What would be the preferred treatment for rotator cuff tear in an established Charcot shoulder?

   A conservative approach is the initial treatment until the neurosurgical team evaluates and addresses the syrinx. It should include (1) temporary immobilization in a sling and weightbearing restrictions to protect the joint, (2) oral anti-inflammatory medications to address synovial inflammation, (3) following resolution of acute symptoms, begin physical therapy/occupational therapy to maintain shoulder ROM, regain strength in the major periarticular muscles, and optimize shoulder function and finally, (4) patient education about this neuropathic nature of the joint and awareness of joint protection techniques as the repetitive trauma from exceeding safe limits of ROM could cause additional cartilage damage.

References

1. Hatzis N, Kaar TK, Wirth MA, Toro F, Rockwood CA. Neuropathic arthropathy of the shoulder. J Bone Jt Surg Am. 1998;80(9):1314–9. https://doi.org/10.2106/00004623-199809000-00010.
2. Rickert MM, Cannon JG, Kirkpatrick JS. Neuropathic arthropathy of the shoulder: a systematic review of classifications and treatments. JBJS Rev. 2019;7(10):e1. https://doi.org/10.2106/JBJS.RVW.18.00155.
3. Snoddy MC, Lee DH, Kuhn JE. Charcot shoulder and elbow: a review of the literature and update on treatment. J Shoulder Elb Surg. 2017;26(3):544–52. https://doi.org/10.1016/j.jse.2016.10.015.
4. Atalar AC. Neuropathic arthropathy of the shoulder associated with syringomyelia: a report of six cases. Acta Orthop Traumatol Turc. 2010;44(4):328–36. https://doi.org/10.3944/AOTT.2010.2216.

5. Guille JT, Forlin E, Bowen JR. Charcot joint disease of the shoulders in a patient who had familial sensory neuropathy with anhidrosis. A case report. J Bone Jt Surg Am. 1992;74(9):1415–7.
6. Parikh JR, Houpt JB, Jacobs S, Fernandes BJ. Charcot's arthropathy of the shoulder following intraarticular corticosteroid injections. J Rheumatol. 1993;20(5):885–7.
7. Kenan S, Lewis MM, Main WK, Hermann G, Abdelwahab IF. Neuropathic arthropathy of the shoulder mimicking soft tissue sarcoma. Orthopedics. 1993;16(10):1133–6. https://doi.org/10.3928/0147-7447-19931001-09.
8. Santiesteban L, Mollon B, Zuckerman JD. Neuropathic arthropathy of the glenohumeral joint a review of the literature. Bull Hosp Jt Dis. 2018;76(2):88–99.
9. Alai A, Reddy CG, Amrami KK, Spinner RJ. Charcot arthropathy of the shoulder associated with typical and atypical findings. Clin Anat. 2013;26(8):1017–23. https://doi.org/10.1002/ca.22110.
10. Alpert SW, Koval KJ, Zuckerman JD. Neuropathic arthropathy: review of current knowledge. J Am Acad Orthop Surg. 1996;4(2):100–8. https://doi.org/10.5435/00124635-199603000-00005.
11. Kelly M. "De arthritide symptomatica" of William Musgrave (1657–1721): his description of neuropathic arthritis. Bull Hist Med. 1963;37:372–7.
12. Crowther MAA, Bell SN. Neuropathic shoulder in syringomyelia treated with resurfacing arthroplasty of humeral head and soft-tissue lining of glenoid: a case report. J Shoulder Elb Surg. 2007;16(6):e38–40. https://doi.org/10.1016/j.jse.2006.11.006.
13. Kumar S, Sharma V, Kumar S, Jain S. Imaging findings in Chiari I malformation with syringomyelia in a case of Charcot shoulder. J Clin Imaging Sci. 2011;1:46. https://doi.org/10.4103/2156-7514.85173.
14. Richards RR, Delaney J. Syringomyelia presenting as shoulder instability. J Shoulder Elb Surg. 1992;1(3):155–61. https://doi.org/10.1016/1058-2746(92)90094-J.
15. Yanik B, Tuncer S, Seçkin B. Neuropathic arthropathy caused by Arnold-Chiari malformation with syringomyelia. Rheumatol Int. 2004;24(4):238–41. https://doi.org/10.1007/s00296-003-0389-x.
16. Archer AG, Roberts VC, Watkins PJ. Blood flow patterns in painful diabetic neuropathy. Diabetologia. 1984;27(6):563–7. https://doi.org/10.1007/BF00276968.
17. Brower AC, Allman RM. Pathogenesis of the neurotrophic joint: neurotraumatic vs. neurovascular. Radiology. 1981;139(2):349–54. https://doi.org/10.1148/radiology.139.2.7220879.
18. Childs M, Armstrong DG, Edelson GW. Is Charcot arthropathy a late sequela of osteoporosis in patients with diabetes mellitus? J Foot Ankle Surg. 1998;37(5):437–9. https://doi.org/10.1016/s1067-2516(98)80054-9.
19. Chisholm KA, Gilchrist JM. The Charcot joint: a modern neurologic perspective. J Clin Neuromuscul Dis. 2011;13(1):1–13. https://doi.org/10.1097/CND.0b013e3181c6f55b.
20. Pinzur MS, Shields N, Trepman E, Dawson P, Evans A. Current practice patterns in the treatment of Charcot foot. Foot Ankle Int. 2000;21(11):916–20. https://doi.org/10.1177/107110070002101105.
21. Chappel R, Willems J, Martin JJ. Charcot joint in idiopathic sensorimotor neuropathy. Clin Rheumatol. 2000;19(2):153–5. https://doi.org/10.1007/s100670050036.
22. Eloesser L. On the nature of neuropathic affections of the joints. Ann Surg. 1917;66(2):201–7. https://doi.org/10.1097/00000658-191708000-00011.
23. Trepman E, Nihal A, Pinzur MS. Current topics review: Charcot neuroarthropathy of the foot and ankle. Foot Ankle Int. 2005;26(1):46–63. https://doi.org/10.1177/107110070502600109.
24. Nacir B, Arslan Cebeci S, Cetinkaya E, Karagoz A, Erdem HR. Neuropathic arthropathy progressing with multiple joint involvement in the upper extremity due to syringomyelia and type I Arnold-Chiari malformation. Rheumatol Int. 2010;30(7):979–83. https://doi.org/10.1007/s00296-009-1013-5.
25. Connors JC, Hardy MA, Kishman LL, Botek GG, Verdin CJ, Rao NM, et al. Charcot pathogenesis: a study of in vivo gene expression. J Foot Ankle Surg. 2018;57(6):1067–72. https://doi.org/10.1053/j.jfas.2018.03.023.

26. Rastogi A, Bhansali A, Jude EB. Efficacy of medical treatment for Charcot neuroarthropathy: a systematic review and meta-analysis of randomized controlled trials. Acta Diabetol. 2021;58(6):687–96. https://doi.org/10.1007/s00592-020-01664-9.
27. Shofler D, Hamedani E, Seun J, Sathananthan A, Katsaros E, Liggan L, et al. Investigating the use of denosumab in the treatment of acute Charcot neuroarthropathy. J Foot Ankle Surg. 2021;60(2):354–7. https://doi.org/10.1053/j.jfas.2020.09.018.
28. Bruhn-Olszewska B, Korzon-Burakowska A, Węgrzyn G, Jakóbkiewicz-Banecka J. Prevalence of polymorphisms in OPG, RANKL and RANK as potential markers for Charcot arthropathy development. Sci Rep. 2017;7:501. https://doi.org/10.1038/s41598-017-00563-4.
29. Dardari D. An overview of Charcot's neuroarthropathy. J Clin Transl Endocrinol. 2020;22:100239. https://doi.org/10.1016/j.jcte.2020.100239.
30. Folestad A, Ålund M, Asteberg S, Fowelin J, Aurell Y, Göthlin J, et al. Role of Wnt/β-catenin and RANKL/OPG in bone healing of diabetic Charcot arthropathy patients. Acta Orthop. 2015;86(4):415–25. https://doi.org/10.3109/17453674.2015.1033606.
31. Kloska A, Korzon-Burakowska A, Malinowska M, Bruhn-Olszewska B, Gabig-Cimińska M, Jakóbkiewicz-Banecka J. The role of genetic factors and monocyte-to-osteoclast differentiation in the pathogenesis of Charcot neuroarthropathy. Diabetes Res Clin Pract. 2020;166:108337. https://doi.org/10.1016/j.diabres.2020.108337.
32. Mabilleau G, Petrova N, Edmonds ME, Sabokbar A. Number of circulating CD14-positive cells and the serum levels of TNF-α are raised in acute Charcot foot. Diabetes Care. 2011;34(3):e33. https://doi.org/10.2337/dc10-1695.
33. Adiyeke L, Durakbaşa MO, Duymuş TM. Bilateral neuropathic osteoarthropathy of the shoulder due to syringomyelia. Clin Pract. 2017;7(2):952. https://doi.org/10.4081/cp.2017.952.
34. Panagariya A, Sharma AK. Bilateral Charcot arthropathy of shoulder secondary to syringomyelia: an unusual case report. Ann Indian Acad Neurol. 2012;15(3):202–4. https://doi.org/10.4103/0972-2327.99718.
35. Gaskins RB, Miller BJ, Scarborough MT. Charcot arthropathy of shoulder: a case report. Orthop Surg. 2011;3(4):268–70. https://doi.org/10.1111/j.1757-7861.2011.00152.x.
36. Jones EA, Manaster BJ, May DA, Disler DG. Neuropathic osteoarthropathy: diagnostic dilemmas and differential diagnosis. Radiographics. 2000;20(suppl 1):S279–93. https://doi.org/10.1148/radiographics.20.suppl_1.g00oc22s279.
37. Deng X, Wu L, Yang C, Xu Y. Neuropathic arthropathy caused by syringomyelia. J Neurosurg Spine. 2013;18(3):303–9. https://doi.org/10.3171/2012.11.SPINE12860.
38. Jones J, Wolf S. Neuropathic shoulder arthropathy (Charcot joint) associated with syringomyelia. Neurology. 1998;50(3):825–7. https://doi.org/10.1212/wnl.50.3.825.
39. Butala RR, Arora M, Rao AA, Samant PD, Mukherjee S. A rare case of ipsilateral shoulder and thumb CMC joint neuropathic arthropathy. J Surg Case Rep. 2014;2014(6):rju054. https://doi.org/10.1093/jscr/rju054.
40. Wang X, Li Y, Gao J, Wang T, Li Z. Charcot arthropathy of the shoulder joint as a presenting feature of basilar impression with syringomyelia: a case report and literature review. Medicine (Baltimore). 2018;97(28):e11391. https://doi.org/10.1097/MD.0000000000011391.
41. Wawrzyniak A, Lubiatowski P, Kordasiewicz B, Brzóska R, Laprus H. Shoulder arthropathy secondary to syringomyelia: case series of 10 patients. Eur J Orthop Surg Traumatol. 2021;32(7):1275–81. https://doi.org/10.1007/s00590-021-03102-0.
42. Deirmengian CA, Lee SG, Jupiter JB. Neuropathic arthropathy of the elbow. A report of five cases. J Bone Jt Surg Am. 2001;83(6):839–44. https://doi.org/10.2106/00004623-200106000-00004.
43. Dowling RJ, Tress BM. MRI—the investigation of choice in syringomyelia? Australas Radiol. 1989;33(4):337–43. https://doi.org/10.1111/j.1440-1673.1989.tb03307.x.
44. Timpone VM, Patel SH. MRI of a syrinx: is contrast material always necessary? AJR Am J Roentgenol. 2015;204(5):1082–5. https://doi.org/10.2214/AJR.14.13310.

45. Tashiro K, Fukazawa T, Moriwaka F, Hamada T, Isu T, Iwasaki Y, et al. Syringomyelic syndrome: clinical features in 31 cases confirmed by CT myelography or magnetic resonance imaging. J Neurol. 1987;235(1):26–30. https://doi.org/10.1007/BF00314193.
46. García Rodríguez C, García-Polín López C, del Olmo HT, Moros Marco S, Jacobo Edo O, Ávila Lafuente JL. Distal biceps tendon rupture: diagnostic strength of ultrasonography and magnetic resonance. Revista Espanola de Cirugia Ortop Traumatol. 2020;64(2):77–82. https://doi.org/10.1016/j.recot.2019.11.004.
47. Strike SA, Johnston JC, Farjoodi P. Septic elbow in the setting of neuropathic joint as the initial presentation of a cervical syrinx. Orthopedics. 2011;34(4):22. https://doi.org/10.3928/01477447-20110228-22.
48. Shibata T, Tada K, Hashizume C. The results of arthrodesis of the ankle for leprotic neuroarthropathy. J Bone Jt Surg Am. 1990;72(5):749–56.
49. Rosenbaum AJ, DiPreta JA. Classifications in brief: Eichenholtz classification of Charcot arthropathy. Clin Orthop Relat Res. 2015;473(3):1168–71. https://doi.org/10.1007/s11999-014-4059-y.
50. Makihara T, Onishi S, Wadano Y, Fujii K, Nagata H, Sakane M. Regrowth of the deteriorated glenoid in advanced Charcot shoulder after suboccipital decompression for syringomyelia: a case report. J Shoulder Elb Surg. 2015;24(8):e223–8. https://doi.org/10.1016/j.jse.2015.04.022.
51. Kleindienst A, Laut FM, Roeckelein V, Buchfelder M, Dodoo-Schittko F. Treatment of posttraumatic syringomyelia: evidence from a systematic review. Acta Neurochir. 2020;162(10):2541–56. https://doi.org/10.1007/s00701-020-04529-w.
52. Rossier AB, Foo D, Shillito J, Dyro FM. Posttraumatic cervical syringomyelia. Incidence, clinical presentation, electrophysiological studies, syrinx protein and results of conservative and operative treatment. Brain. 1985;108(Pt 2):439–61. https://doi.org/10.1093/brain/108.2.439.
53. Cao F, Yang X, Liu W, Li G, Zheng X-S, Wen L. Surgery for posttraumatic syringomyelia: a retrospective study of seven patients. Chin J Traumatol. 2007;10(6):366–70.
54. Klekamp J. Treatment of syringomyelia related to nontraumatic arachnoid pathologies of the spinal canal. Neurosurgery. 2013;72(3):376–89. https://doi.org/10.1227/NEU.0b013e31827fcc8f.
55. Durgia H, Sahoo J, Kamalanathan S, Palui R, Sridharan K, Raj H. Role of bisphosphonates in the management of acute Charcot foot. World J Diabetes. 2018;9(7):115–26. https://doi.org/10.4239/wjd.v9.i7.115.
56. Mascarenhas JV, Jude EB. Pathogenesis and medical management of diabetic Charcot neuroarthropathy. Med Clin N Am. 2013;97(5):857–72. https://doi.org/10.1016/j.mcna.2013.05.002.
57. Carvès S, Bourgeon-Ghittori M, Henry J, Belkhir R, Besson FL, Levante S, et al. Denosumab in active Charcot neuro-osteoarthropathy of the foot. Jt Bone Spine. 2021;88(6):105241. https://doi.org/10.1016/j.jbspin.2021.105241.
58. Matsuhashi T, Nagahama K, Suenaga N, Oizumi N, Minami A. Midterm outcomes after humeral head replacement with rotator cuff repair in patients with syringomyelia shoulder neuroarthropathy: a report on three cases. J Shoulder Elb Surg. 2011;20(8):e8–15. https://doi.org/10.1016/j.jse.2011.04.032.
59. Ueblacker P, Ansah P, Vogt S, Imhoff AB. Bilateral reverse shoulder prosthesis in a patient with severe syringomyelia. J Shoulder Elb Surg. 2007;16(6):e48–51. https://doi.org/10.1016/j.jse.2006.12.003.
60. Kuur E. Two cases of Charcot's shoulder arthropathy. Acta Orthop Scand. 1987;58(5):581–3. https://doi.org/10.3109/17453678709146403.
61. Schoch B, Werthel J-D, Sperling JW, Cofield RH, Sanchez-Sotelo J. Is shoulder arthroplasty an option for Charcot arthropathy? Int Orthop. 2016;40(12):2589–95. https://doi.org/10.1007/s00264-016-3309-x.

Chapter 6
Syphilis

Dirk W. Verheul, Brady Ernst, Jacob Farrar, Wilhelm A. Zuelzer, Christopher Doern, Victoria Kuester, and Shaunette Davey

Case 1: Adult

A 58-year-old male with a past medical history of hypertension and chronic alcohol use presented to the Emergency Department (ED) with 3 weeks of stumbling, fatigue, and generalized body aches. He reported a gradual onset of symptoms, without trauma, and tingling in the hands and feet. The patient denied headaches, visual changes, or weakness in the extremities. The patient was admitted for consuming 2–3 glasses of wine along with 2 beers daily. Basic laboratory evaluation was normal, and a head CT was obtained and demonstrated no acute intracranial

D. W. Verheul · B. Ernst · J. Farrar
Department of Orthopaedic Surgery, Virginia Commonwealth University, Richmond, VA, USA
e-mail: dirk.verheul1@vcuhealth.org; brady.ernst@vcuhealth.org; jacob.farrar@vcuhealth.org

W. A. Zuelzer
Orthopaedic Surgery, Virginia Commonwealth University Medical School, Richmond, VA, USA
e-mail: wilhelm.zuelzer@vcuhealth.org

C. Doern
Department of Pathology, Virginia Commonwealth University, Richmond, VA, USA
e-mail: christopher.doern@vcuhealth.org

V. Kuester
Department of Orthopaedic Surgery, Virginia Commonwealth University, Richmond, VA, USA

Departments of Orthopaedic Surgery and Pediatrics, Children's Hospital of Richmond, Virginia Commonwealth University, Richmond, VA, USA
e-mail: victoria.kuester@vcuhealth.org

S. Davey (✉)
Departments of Orthopaedic Surgery and Pediatrics, Children's Hospital of Richmond, Virginia Commonwealth University, Richmond, VA, USA
e-mail: sdavey@psvcare.org

W. A. Zuelzer, S. Metikala (eds.), *Unusual Conditions That Every Orthopaedic Surgeon Should Know*, https://doi.org/10.1007/978-3-031-58946-1_6

abnormality. The patient was given thiamine in the ED, and an appointment with neurology was scheduled.

Three weeks after his initial presentation, the patient returned to the ED expressing concerns about worsening tingling in his hands and feet. These sensations now included both numbness and pain in both hands and his right heel. Due to the symptoms in his hands, he was unable to make a fist which impacted his work in the food industry. Following evaluation, the patient was given a prescription for oral steroids and was referred to the Ortho Hand clinic for further treatment.

During his follow-up appointment at the orthopaedic clinic, 10 days after his previous visit to the emergency department, it was observed that the patient had a gait abnormality. Upon examination, he was found to have dorsal synovitis of bilateral fourth dorsal compartments and a positive tuck sign. The tuck sign refers to the soft tissue swelling over the dorsum of the wrist when wrist and fingers are placed at maximal extension, causing the swelling to move toward the forearm and tucks under the extensor retinaculum. His wrist range of motion was limited to approximately 30° of flexion and extension with an exaggerated pain response on palpation. Additionally, swelling was observed in multiple distal interphalangeal (DIP) joints without significant synovitis about his metacarpophalangeal (MCP) joints or wrist. The Tinel's test at the wrist was positive for pain, rather than paresthesias and a Spurling's test was negative. The patient also had Dupuytren's nodules and pitting without cords or contracture. At this stage, the patient was suspected to have inflammatory arthritis and therefore, a course of oral steroids was prescribed.

The patient followed up in the neurology clinic 10 days later, and it was noted that he was still having difficulty with ambulation in the setting of diffuse pain symptoms. It was believed that he was experiencing diffuse arthralgias although there was also concern for potential small fiber neuropathic symptoms in hands and feet. The examination did not reveal any proprioceptive deficits. On physical examination, it was found that the patient had limited strength in his wrists and fingers, as well as in the lower extremities, due to pain. He also had a wide-based antalgic gait. The patient's sensory examination showed no abnormalities except for diffuse hyperalgesia with exquisite tenderness to slight stimulation. His reflexes were normal. He also endorsed a 15–20 lbs. unintentional weight loss in the past few months. Further tests showed slightly elevated CRP levels, positive treponemal antibodies, and a positive RPR test at a 256x dilution, indicating an active syphilis infection. An urgent referral to infectious disease was placed and considering the extent of disease activity, indicated by high RPR, a lumbar puncture was recommended to identify the presence of CSF-positive VDRL which would help guide an appropriate treatment regimen. The patient presented to the Public Health Department, where he reportedly received intramuscular penicillin treatment. However, despite being informed about the risks of CNS involvement and the limitations of intramuscular penicillin in treating it, the patient refused to undergo the lumbar puncture. Unfortunately, the patient was lost to follow up.

Case 2: Pediatric

A 2-month-old female without significant past medical history was brought into our emergency room due to 4 days of irritability and 1 day of decreased right arm use without known history of trauma or recent illness. On examination, the patient was noted to have tenderness over the lateral elbow and wrist.

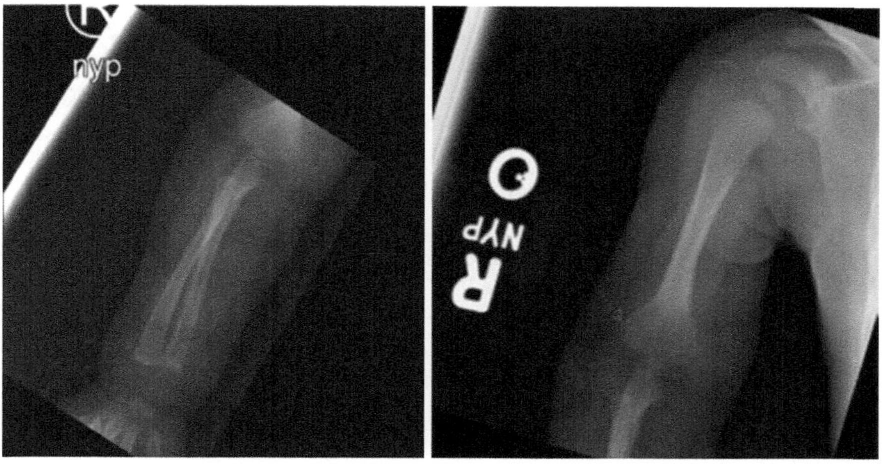

Fig. 6.1 Radiographs from initial presentation reported as fracture of the lateral distal humerus and lateral distal radius

Laboratory workup was notable for a WBC of 14.8, and hemoglobin of 8.6 ESR and CRP were elevated at 73 (mm/h) and 6.1 (mg/dL), respectively. Radiographs of the right upper extremity were obtained and interpreted by our radiologists as fractures of the lateral aspect of the distal humerus and possibly the distal radius (see Fig. 6.1). Ophthalmologic screening, bone survey, and head CT were all negative. However, the combination of heightened irritability with movement of the arm, accompanied by swelling, along with abnormal laboratory results, led to the decision to order an MRI with and without contrast. The MRI findings were not conclusive but raised concerns regarding the possibility of osteomyelitis or bone edema resulting from a fracture.

The decision was made to proceed to the operating room to perform joint and bone marrow aspiration of the affected wrist and elbow. Despite the low suspicion of infection due to the absence of purulent discharge, aspirates were collected and sent for pathological examination and culture. The results came back negative on the first day after the surgery. The patient's overall condition was satisfactory, so she was discharged home with a scheduled outpatient follow-up appointment.

A repeat bone survey was conducted 5 days after the initial presentation, during which it was observed that there were lytic lesions in the same area where fractures were previously a concern. Additionally, lytic lesions were found in the metaphysis of both the proximal and distal tibiae as well as in the distal radius of the left arm. Furthermore, there was evidence of periosteal reaction in both femoral shafts (see Fig. 6.2). Further laboratory tests were carried out, including an RPR and treponemal antibody test, both of which were positive. To investigate the possibility of neurosyphilis, a lumbar puncture was performed, and the results were indicative of neurosyphilis. Subsequently, the patient underwent treatment consisting of a 10-day course of penicillin G and a single dose of intramuscular penicillin G.

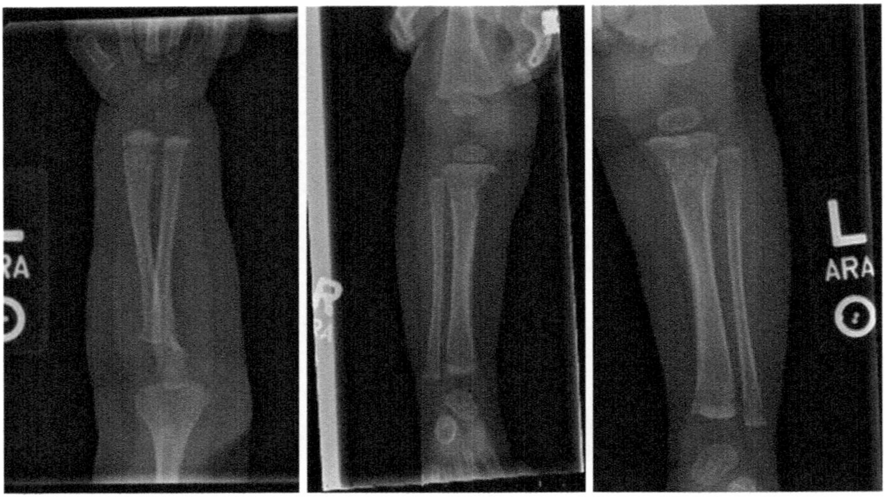

Fig. 6.2 Radiographs obtained 5 days after initial presentation showing Wimberger's sign: lytic lesions in the distal radius as well as in the bilateral tibia

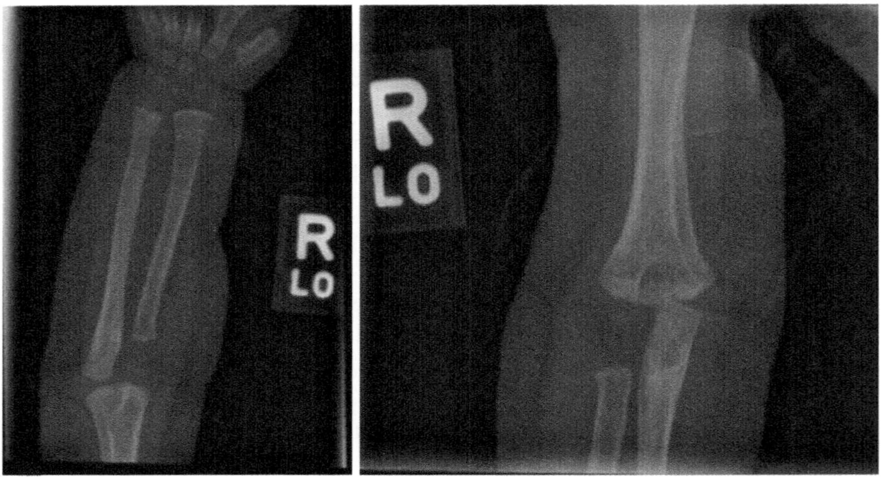

Fig. 6.3 Radiographs obtained at the 4-week follow-up demonstrating resolution of lytic lesions in the right upper extremity

At follow-up 1 month later, repeat radiographs demonstrated complete resolution of bony lesions (see Fig. 6.3). At 19 months, the patient had no symptoms or obvious long-term sequelae of the infection.

Case 3: Pediatric

A 3-month-old male without significant past medical history presented to our clinic as follow up after evaluation at an outside emergency room for fussiness and left wrist pain. The patient had been diagnosed with a left distal ulna fracture and presented in a splint. However, upon examination, he had no discomfort with palpation at the wrist, but rather pain with elbow extension.

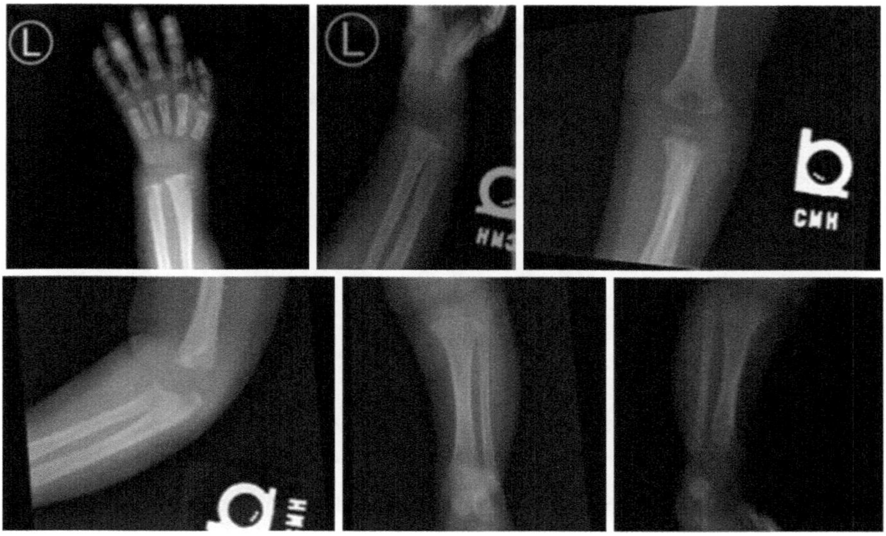

Fig. 6.4 Radiographs from initial presentation with lesions on the left upper extremity and evidence of metaphyseal cortical resorption of the bilateral tibia seen on skeletal survey

Upon review of the images taken at an outside hospital, there were abnormalities in the proximal and distal ulna (see Fig. 6.4). This raised suspicions of hyperparathyroidism, prompting an endocrine evaluation. Laboratory findings of calcium and phosphorus levels were within normal limits, but there was an elevated ESR and CRP of 37 (mm/h) and 4.4 (mg/dL), respectively. A lumbar puncture was performed with no growth at 48 h. Due to these findings, the patient was referred to our hospital for admission, as there were concerns for an infectious etiology.

MRI of the left upper extremity was obtained and resulted with concern for septic elbow and osteomyelitis with indeterminate findings in the wrist. Based on these findings, the decision was made to proceed to the operating room for irrigation and debridement of the wrist and elbow. Fluid samples from both joints were collected and sent for culture analysis, while tissue samples were obtained from the affected bones. To further assess the nature of the lesions, frozen sections were sent to the pathology department.

The patient was started on broad spectrum antibiotics, and on post-operative day 1, an RPR was obtained and was positive. Subsequently, treponemal antibody testing was conducted to confirm the diagnosis. A repeat bone survey was carried out, revealing the presence of additional bone lesions in both tibiae (see Fig. 6.4). The intraoperative cultures remained negative, and the specimens were also negative for Langerhans cell histiocytosis. Spirochetes were noted on spirochete immunostain. A lumbar puncture was later performed with no growth on CSF culture. Once the patient completed the course of Penicillin G, he was discharged. At the 4-month follow-up, the osseous lesions in the patient's left upper extremity completely resolved, and the patient regained full use of their left arm without pain, demonstrating symmetry with the contralateral side (see Fig. 6.5). At the 6-month follow-up, he remained asymptomatic, and his RPR levels showed a downward trend.

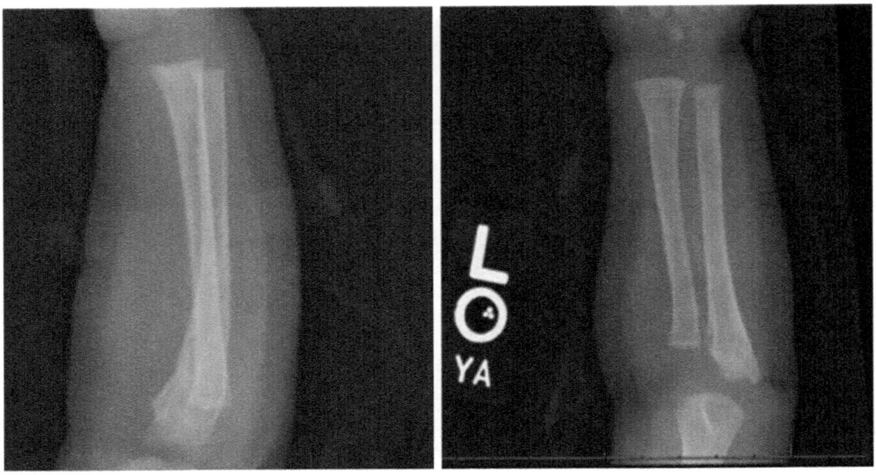

Fig. 6.5 Radiographs obtained at the 4-month follow-up demonstrating complete resolution of distal and proximal ulnar lesions

Questions

1. A patient has serum confirmation for syphilis and has ataxia. What additional workup is required?
2. What are the highest risk groups for acquiring syphilis?
3. What are the classic musculoskeletal signs and symptoms that an orthopaedist will see on presentation of a patient with syphilis?

Background

Syphilis is a sexually transmitted disease caused by the spirochete *Treponema pallidum*. This disease can affect nearly every organ system in the body. There has been a significant increase in syphilis infections over the past decade. Syphilis can present initially to an orthopaedist as a musculoskeletal issue. Musculoskeletal presentations of secondary, tertiary, and congenital syphilis were well known prior to the introduction of penicillin when the prevalence of syphilis was much higher. We need to rediscover these signs and symptoms.

In 1905, Fritz Schaudinn, Erich Hoffmann, and Fred Neufelt were the first to identify the causative agent of syphilis, *Treponema pallidum* (see Fig. 6.6) [1, 2]. This bacterium was described as rotating about the long axis, gliding movements forwards and backwards, with movements of flexion of the whole body, with pointed ends and without evidence of flagella on the surface [1, 2]. The organism was derived from a variety of sites including a genital ulcer and lymph node. It was

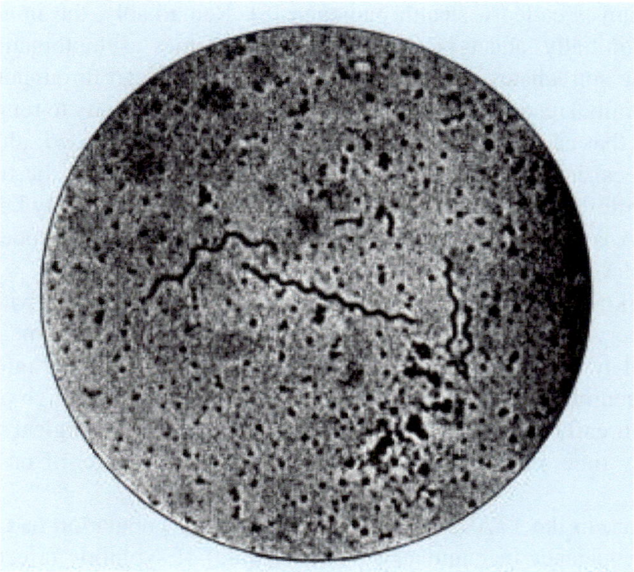

Fig. 6.6 Reproduced with permission a photograph from "3 Spirochetes with Giemesa stained smear from a syphilitic lymph node" [3]

labeled "spirochaete" because of spiral morphology and twisting movements and subcategorized as *Treponema pallidum* (TPA), because of the pale appearance under the microscope.

Syphilis is a sexually transmitted disease; however, very rarely, blood transfusions can be the source of TPA infection [4]. TPA readily disseminates through the blood stream, lymphatics, and CSF fluid and crosses the endothelial, blood–brain, and placental barriers—thus placing all organs and fetus at risk. The TPA outer membrane has a paucity of integral membrane proteins and lipid composition which may explain the often-limited response to invasion. The outer wall may be a barrier to antibody binding with the preponderance of spirochete immunogenic lipoprotein appearing to be in the inner membrane. The fragility and low protein content of the outer membrane have made it very difficult to study these organisms as they are unable to be grown in vitro [5–8].

TPA has a double cell wall like gram-negative bacteria but has a different outer membrane phospholipid composition than the outer membrane of a typical gram-negative bacteria—for example, the density of outer membrane protein in TPA is 100-fold less than *E. coli* [7]. The spirochete reproduces by undergoing asexual transverse binary fission. The current best estimate is that it multiplies at a rate of once every 30–33 h [9, 10]. The average time between acquisition of syphilis on the surface area and the start of the first symptom is 21 days but can range from 10 to 90 days [11]. The spirochaete appears to avoid a significant host response—thus, this bacterium is called a stealth pathogen [8]. Remarkably, the immune system clears TPA initially, and typically the patient becomes asymptomatic. However, clearly some spirochetes may survive, multiply, and spread throughout the body, despite this initial response. Infection does not provide immunity to reinfection. The mechanism that causes the tissue damage is not well understood, although most likely the local inflammatory response from the spirochaetes is the root cause of clinical manifestations. TPA appears to lack potent toxins. The only known natural host for TPA is human beings. However, more recently, a rabbit model has shown promise to develop a vaccine for this remarkable pathogen [12].

It is well known that syphilis can have devastating consequences with damage to the brain, nerves, eyes, cardiovascular system, and fetal development. Although neurological symptoms may not become apparent until years after infection, invasion of the central nervous system occurs relatively early, with a high proportion of patients with early syphilis having CSF abnormalities. Neurological changes can occur at any time and stage of infection—even within weeks of onset of infection [13].

In London, in the 1770s, it was estimated that the population had over a 20% cumulative incidence (accumulated risk over time) of syphilitic infection [14]. In the early 1900s, syphilis affected between 5 and 10% of the adult European population and was the cause of insanity in a third of cases confined to mental asylums and a quarter of stillbirths [15]. By the 1930s, approximately 1 in 10 Americans suffered from syphilis, up to 20% of all mental institution patients suffered from tertiary syphilis, and 60,000 children were born each year with congenital syphilis [16].

In 1937, Thomas Parran, Surgeon General of the USA, recommended five components for syphilis control. They included: (1) Case finding through serological screening, (2) prompt, effective therapy for infected persons, (3) identification of people exposed to infectious syphilis, (4) mandatory serological evaluation of people who might transmit infection to others, and (5) public education with community partnership of the manifestations and consequences of this disease [17]. However, after reaching record lows in 2000, over the past decade, there has been a 700% increase in cases of congenital syphilis (syphilis infecting a child before birth) in the United States, which is a preventable disease that may have devastating consequences for the newborn. The United States, in the past 20 years, had a 2140% increase in reported cases of syphilis, which is the highest level in more than 70 years [18]. There is also a corresponding increase in syphilis throughout the world. Currently, those at increased risk are patients living with HIV infection, those with methamphetamine or opioid use disorder, patients who are gay, bisexual, men who have sex with men, patients with history of incarceration, transactional sex, or military service, and those who have challenges to access to health care coverage and care [19, 20]. Since community prevalence may vary, it is recommended that clinicians monitor the CDC and state and local health departments' data [18].

An untreated syphilis patient remains potentially contagious during the initial years following the incubation period, except for congenital infections [21]. Thereafter, a patient is very unlikely to infect another person, but repeated inoculation remains a concern.

Syphilis Disease Overview and Natural History

The natural history of syphilis is complex (see Fig. 6.7). Syphilis is classified into several stages: primary, secondary, latent (positive test with no symptoms or signs), and tertiary phases. The primary stage occurs after an initial infection and is characterized by a typically painless sore called a chancre, at the entrance site and regional lymphadenopathy (see Fig. 6.8). This predominantly mucocutaneous disorder appears within 9–90 days after incubation. If untreated, the chancre and lymphadenopathy usually resolve in 3–10 weeks [22]. Occasionally, TPA manages to overcome the immunological response, with mechanisms that are not yet fully understood [23].

Thus, if left untreated, a secondary stage may occur within 1–6 months after exposure to TPA, characterized by a maculopapular rash that may appear on the palms and soles of the feet (see Fig. 6.9). Other symptoms include weight loss, malaise, and anogenital papules, known as condyloma lata. In less than 10% of

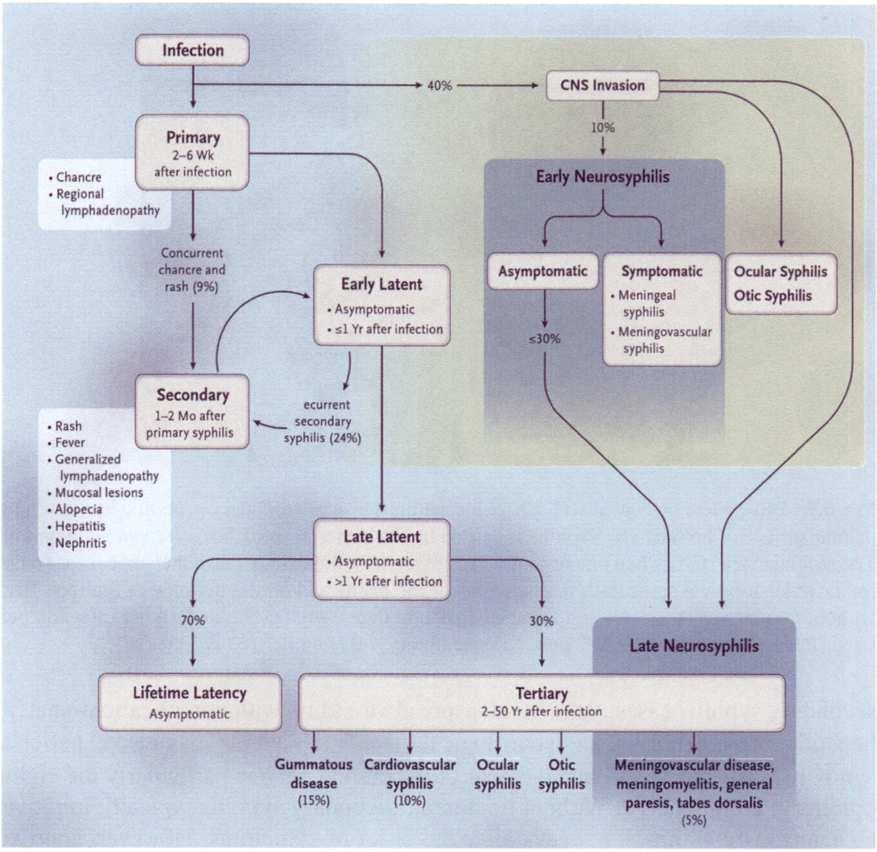

Fig. 6.7 The natural history of syphilis reproduced with permission from The Modern Epidemic of Syphilis [13]

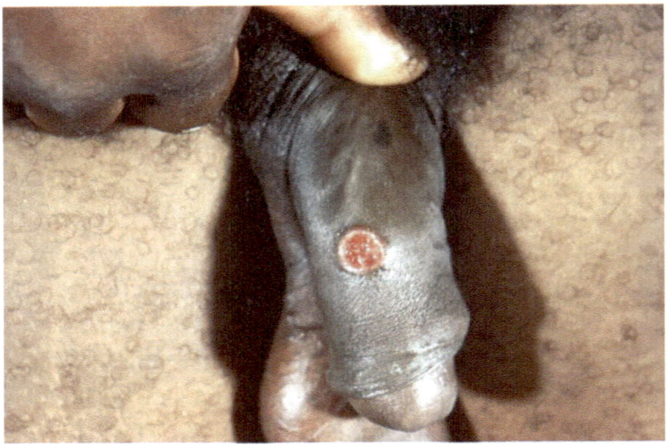

Fig. 6.8 This image depicts a close view of a male patient's penis, revealing a primary syphilitic lesion on the penile shaft. From this view, the chancre appeared to exhibit a raw surface, similar to an open wound, while being ringed by a raised border. Syphilis is caused by the bacterial spirochete, *Treponema pallidum*. (Image obtained from CDC public image library—ID number 17040 [24])

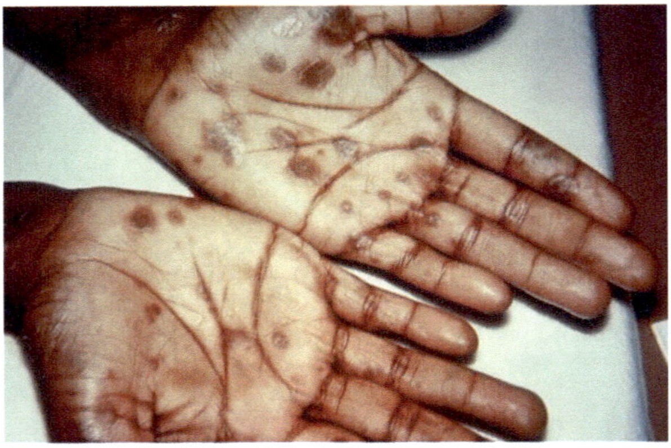

Fig. 6.9 This patient presented with a papulosquamous rash of secondary syphilitic lesions on the palmar surface of both hands. Syphilis is caused by the bacterial spirochete, *Treponema pallidum*. The second stage starts when one or more areas of the skin break into a rash that appears as rough, red or reddish-brown spots both on the palms of the hands and on the bottoms of the feet. Even without treatment, rashes clear up spontaneously, on their own, but the underlying infection persists. (Image obtained from CDC public image library—ID number 16749 [25])

secondary syphilis cases, there is widespread vasculitis with complications such as hepatitis, iritis, nephritis, and neurological disorders. Patients may also experience synovitis, headaches, and involvement of the cranial nerves, particularly the eighth (auditory) cranial nerve. Without treatment, secondary syphilis typically improves spontaneously within 3–6 weeks after the onset of symptoms. However, approximately a quarter of these patients experience relapsing episodes of secondary syphilis with the reappearance of the rash, mucosal ulcerations, and fever. Eventually, almost all patients with untreated secondary syphilis become asymptomatic (latent

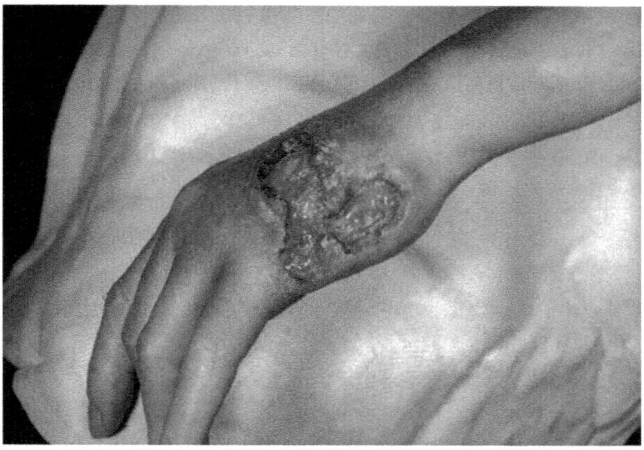

Fig. 6.10 This photograph depicts a dorsomedial view of a patient's left hand, revealing the presence of a gummatous lesion, due to a tertiary syphilitic infection, caused by the bacterium, *Treponema pallidum*. Gummatous lesions due to tertiary syphilis occur many years after initial untreated primary syphilis. The lesions are benign, and if properly treated, the gummas will heal and the patient will recover in most cases. (Image obtained from CDC public image library—ID number 2381 [27])

phase) about 1–2 years after initial presentation of the secondary phase. To be considered in the latent phase, there should be no evidence of syphilis on a thorough history and physical exam.

After more than 2 years in the latent phase, around 35% of individuals may progress to tertiary syphilis. Tertiary syphilis may present as neurosyphilis even after an incubation of almost 20 years. It is important to note that the subset of meningovascular syphilis can occur in both the secondary and tertiary phases of the disease. Symptoms include stroke, intermittent headaches, vertigo, insomnia, and behavioral changes [26]. A patient who presents in the tertiary phase may have cardiovascular involvement, including the large vessels, such as the aorta, up to 30 years after syphilis incubation. Additionally, after an incubation of 3–12 years following primary syphilis, the patient may develop gummatous masses, which typically affect skin or bone (see Fig. 6.10). The orthopaedist will commonly encounter these patients in the secondary or tertiary phase. It is crucial to recognize that syphilis can present with a wide range of symptoms even after even prolonged asymptomatic period, leading to diagnostic confusion. It truly earns its reputation as a "great simulator."

Musculoskeletal Presentation

Secondary Phase: It must be emphasized that an orthopaedist in order to identify this condition would need to identify many issues including sexual history, skin abnormalities or lesions, sore throat, headaches, weight loss, hair loss, or ataxia. There is no other option [28, 29].

Hematogenous and lymphatic spread of TPA can lead to musculoskeletal involvement, affecting various areas such as muscles, tendons, bursa, bones, and joints. This is well described by Hajjaj-Hassounit et al. [30]. It is estimated that up to one-third of patients with secondary syphilis may develop musculoskeletal complaints [31–34]. Below are some of the more common patient findings that may present to an orthopaedic surgeon:

1. Skin lesions: The orthopaedist may be the first to see a patient presenting with multiple macular (flat lesions less than 1 cm size not raised) and maculopapular (macular with small, raised skin lesions). In some cases, the lesions may form rings, known as annular lesions, on the palms and soles (see Fig. 6.9). A characteristic skin lesion of syphilis is this maculopapular lesion, symmetrically distributed especially over the palms and soles. They have a central clearing with a rim of collarette scales with surrounding erythema—this is also called Biett's collarette. Biett's sign is considered a pathognomonic sign of the second phase of syphilis (see Fig. 6.11) [35].
2. Arthralgia (joint aching without any findings on physical exam): In 1927, Todd, in an excellent review, noted that in patients with syphilis, arthralgias may appear even before skin lesions [36]. He reported that joint pain was never severe, but rather described as a dull ache, often occurring at night. Passive range of motion of the involved joint did not increase the discomfort; there were no restrictions of movement and there was no effusion. Todd stressed the importance of ruling out syphilis in patients presenting with arthralgia.
3. Joint synovitis with effusion: Todd felt there were two forms of joint pain associated with this condition. The early form, which primarily affects the knees, but it may be also polyarticular having significant effusion, and a more chronic form of joint pain with effusion. He noted that the pain is typically moderate, without erythema, and fatigue. Additionally, patients may experience fever, but this is not always present. Todd also reported that with more chronic effusions, the condition may appear symmetrical, but that the symptoms may be more severe in one joint compared to the other [36]. Although the effusion may resolve on its own, relapses are common. Classically, symmetrical polyarthritis, rather than migratory arthritis, is the most reported complaint among patients. The knee, ankle, sternoclavicular, wrist metacarpophalangeal, and proximal interphalangeal joints are the most frequently affected areas. However, the resulting disability is typically mild. Reginato et al. reported a more painful joint presentation with an inflammatory arthritis, associated with morning stiffness, limited range of motion, and involvement of one or multiple joints, typically large joints, and primarily the knee joint. Analyzing joint aspirate samples, the white blood cell count usually ranges from 4000 to 13,000 cells/mm^3, with 46–83% polymorphonuclear cells (PMNs). Lymphadenopathy and skin lesions are commonly associated with this presentation. Radiographs of the involved joint usually demonstrate normal joint structures; however, there is often soft tissue and joint swelling [37, 38].

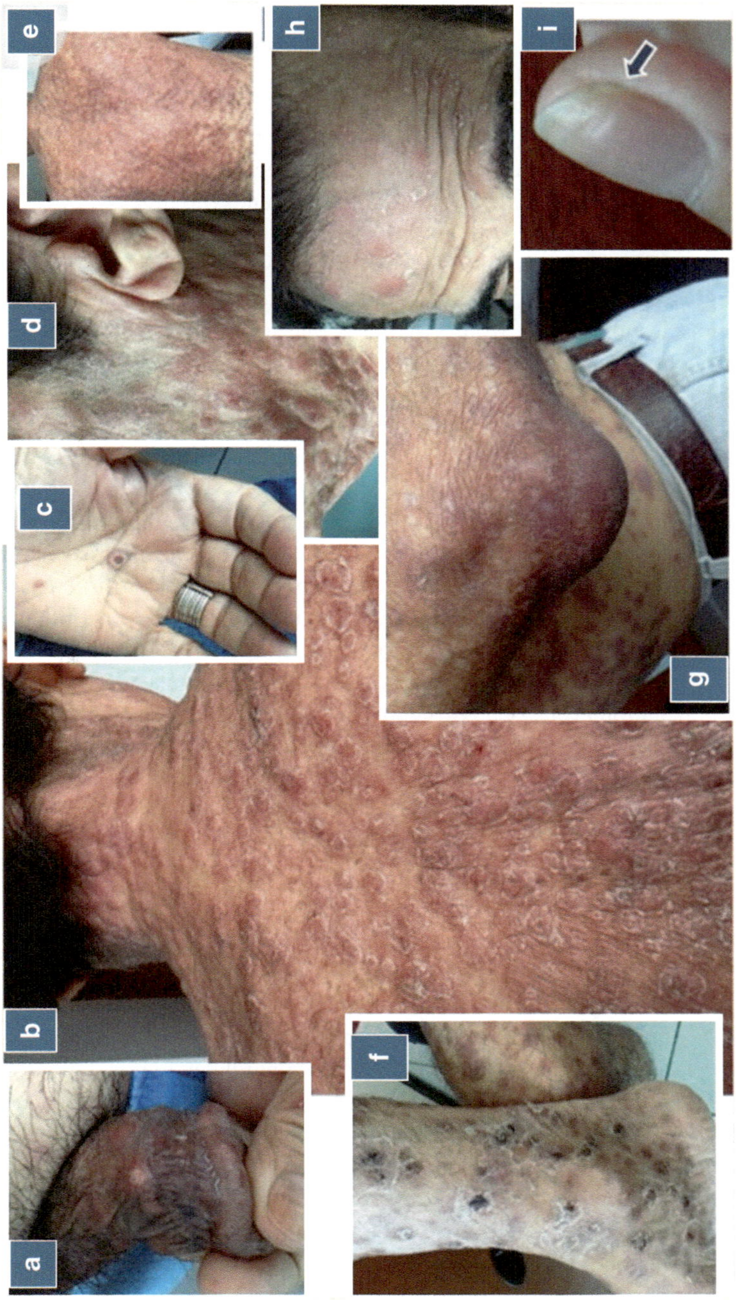

Fig. 6.11 **(a)** A painless healing chancre on penis shaft; **(b, d, e)** generalized papulosquamous and nodular rash leaving no spared area on the back; **(c)** “collarette of Biett” as a feature of the palmar rash: papules surrounded by a ring of scale; **(f)** ulcero-necrotic lesions with a scale-crust, resembling malignant syphilis; **(g)** olecranon bursitis presenting as an asymptomatic, unilateral, fluctuant swelling at the tip of the right elbow; **(h)** “crown of Venus” (corona veneris) bordering the scalp: scaling papular lesions around the hairline; **(i)** transverse depression (Beau’s line) approaches the distal edge of a thumb nail (arrow). Images were taken on the 18th (**a–f**), 25th (**h**), 34th (**g**), and 70th (**i**) day after the rash was first noted. (Reproduced with permission [40])

4. Joint fibrosis (periarticular thickening and swelling without significant effusion): Can be described as a “plastic” form of arthritis, according to Todd. This is typically monoarticular and most commonly occurs in the knee, elbow, midtarsal, shoulder, and wrists. There is loss of motion and resultant disability [36].
5. Tenosynovitis: Classically characterized by painless swelling of the tendon sheaths in the hands or ankles, without erythema [37]. In cases of subacute tenosynovitis involving wrists and ankles, there may be tendon sheath effusions without erythema, heat, or tenderness. Gonococcal infection must be considered in the differential diagnosis. However, gonococcal tenosynovitis is typically much more painful and inflamed.
6. Myositis: Although myositis is a rare occurrence, it is associated with muscle pain and progressive weakness. Myalgia is commonly seen in secondary syphilis. By far, muscle impairment from syphilis is due to brain, spinal cord, and nerve involvement. In patients with syphilis and HIV and/or hepatitis C, the etiology of myositis is more complex and may include the side effects of medications [39].
7. Bursitis: Syphilitic bursitis predominantly affects the olecranon bursa in males, but almost any bursa may be involved (see Fig. 6.11) [40].
8. Dactylitis/nail changes: Characterized by swelling of the entire digit and commonly referred to as sausage fingers and toes. Dactylitis is classically associated with trauma, sickle cell disease, gout, spondyloarthritis, psoriatic arthritis, sarcoidosis, tuberculosis, and syphilis. The swelling is related to enthesitis (inflammation at the attachment of tendon), tenosynovitis, subperiosteal new bone growth, and joint synovial changes. In patients with syphilis related dactylitis, the initial manifestation is classically osteomyelitis primarily in the hands, characterized by bilateral and symmetric exuberant periostitis [41]. The nailbed may be swollen, and the nail could show a pattern of symmetrical transverse depressions of the nail that moves distally, known as Beau’s lines. This commonly affects the thumb nail (see Fig. 6.11). Beau’s lines are felt to be a temporary arrest of proximal nail matrix proliferation. Among the potential causes, psoriasis should be considered in the differential diagnosis [42].
9. Bone involvement: Bony involvement in secondary syphilis is generally considered to be less frequent than in tertiary syphilis [31]. However, it is possible that bone lesions are more prevalent than currently recognized due to their often-asymptomatic nature and limited use of modern technology in studies reporting these in the literature [43]. The most common complaint related to bone involvement is bone pain, which worsens at night and is frequently accompanied by syphilitic skin lesions. Bone lesions become evident as early as 4–6 weeks after primary chancre presentation, and radiographic changes may include periosteal reaction, sclerosis, and lytic lesions, either localized or diffuse. Bone involvement is usually multifocal. It is important to consider syphilis as a potential cause of widespread bone pain in the absence of trauma. However, it should be noted that these patients usually also present with skin lesions and lymphadenopathy [44]. Common sites of involvement include the skull (frontal bone), the shoulder

girdle (distal clavicle), and the long bones (anterior tibia). The long bones are most often affected [32, 33]. Bone involvement in the skull is well described. Thompson and Preston obtained skull radiographs in 80 consecutive patients with syphilis, with clinically recognizable secondary lesions, and identified skull lesions with osteolytic changes on radiographs in seven patients [45]. Diagnostic workup for these patients includes radiographs, MRIs, CT scans, and bone scintigraphy [46]. Finally, it is important to consider the possibility of syphilis when a patient presents with skin ulceration and a lytic defect in the adjacent bone [47].

Tertiary Syphilis

The patients with tertiary syphilis that typically present to an orthopaedic surgeon, are those with Charcot joints and masses in the extremities. Tertiary syphilis is also associated with aortic aneurysm, aortic regurgitation, headaches, confusion, vertigo, personality changes, dementia, fatigue, intention tremors, ataxia, loss of proprioception, and cranial nerve palsies. These symptoms can manifest in varying combinations. While conditions like tabes dorsalis, general paresis, and meningovascular syphilis were more common in the past, seizures, vision problems, strokes, confusion, and personality changes are now more frequently observed instead [48].

1. Tabes dorsalis: Tabes dorsalis, also known as locomotor ataxia, is characterized by loss of sensation associated with demyelination of the dorsal roots and posterior spinal column. This appears to be related to inflammation of the dorsal roots and ganglia, with ascending neuritis from the damaged dorsal roots. Consequently, there is a loss of proprioception, while retaining intact pain sensation. One commonly associated feature of this condition is the development of Charcot joints [28].
2. Charcot joint: Also known as neuropathic arthropathy is observed in approximately 6–10% of patients diagnosed with tabes dorsalis. The loss of protective neurosensory feedback results in repetitive trauma with painless joint swelling, deformity, fragmentation and joint destruction, and eventual functional deficits. When differentiating between potential diagnoses, it is important to consider syringomyelia (which more commonly affects the upper extremities) and diabetes-related complications affecting the feet, leprosy, demyelinating peripheral neuropathies, congenital insensitivity to pain, alcoholism, and repeated corticosteroid injections [49]. The surgical treatment of a Charcot joint is controversial due to the challenges encountered in both joint arthrodesis and the long-term success of arthroplasty in this patient population. The predictability of these procedures remains uncertain.
3. Gumma: The gumma is a type of granuloma that is characterized by the presence of macrophages arranged around a central necrotic zone. Its natural history is variable as it may result in the formation of a scar, necrosis, enlargement, or ulceration. These masses can appear in any part of the body and are often mistaken for tuberculosis [28].

Congenital Syphilis

Congenital syphilis is on the rise, with the number of cases tripling over recent years. In 2020, more than 2000 cases were identified, making this the highest number of cases reported since 1994 [50]. This preventable disease can result in immediate complications, such as low birth weight, anemia, failure to thrive, and stillbirth. There is nothing that more emphasizes the horror of congenital syphilis than reviewing autopsy findings. A review conducted by Oppenheimer and Hardy, which analyzed 16 autopsies of infants with congenital syphilis, unveiled abnormalities in every organ system. These findings revealed that nearly all viscera were infected, with a significant percentage exhibiting lesions of the bone, liver, kidney, pancreas, spleen, eyes, skin, mucous membrane, and intestinal tract [51]. Failure to diagnose and treat early disease can lead to severe and permanent neurological sequelae [52, 53]. The transmission of the disease from mother to fetus usually occurs by transmission of TPA across the placenta before birth, but transmission can also occur during the delivery itself. Newborns may exhibit subtle and nonspecific signs and symptoms, making it crucial to promptly recognize and diagnose congenital syphilis. However, over 50% of infants may not show any symptoms at birth. These asymptomatic infants typically begin to display clinical signs within 3 months of life. Suspicion should be heightened in the presence of bullous skin lesions, maculopapular rash, rhinitis, jaundice, splenomegaly, lymphadenopathy, hepatosplenomegaly, and neurologic impairment. Premature birth or low birth weight can also be possible clues [54]. It is essential for pediatricians and various subspecialties such as orthopaedic surgeons, ophthalmologists, infectious disease specialists, and others to evaluate patients with congenital syphilis early. The late manifestations of congenital syphilis such as bone deformities, i.e., saber shins and frontal bossing, Hutchinson's triad (eighth cranial nerve deafness, interstitial keratitis, Hutchinson's teeth), neurological complications and intellectual disabilities, can be prevented with early treatment, ideally within the first 3 months of life [55].

Early (Before 2 Years)

Bone/cartilage: Bone and cartilage abnormalities are frequently seen in early stages of congenital syphilis. These include periostitis, osteochondritis, osteitis, or chondritis. Orthopaedic manifestations of congenital syphilis occur in 60–80% of patients and in some cases, skeletal findings are the only changes noted on presentation at its onset [56–61]. An early series of congenital syphilis, such as those by McClean, Engeset, Cremin, and Sachdev, highlights the prevalence of skeletal changes [62–66]. In their series of 197 cases of congenital syphilis, Rasool et al. found periosteal reaction along with metaphyseal changes as the most observed radiological abnormality [67]. They reported sparing of the articular cartilage in all but four cases, although joint distension was possible with involvement of a nearby metaphysis, as was the finding in our cases. Radiographs of the long bones often demonstrate the classic pattern of polyostotic periostitis and osteitis, often with a moth-eaten appearance. These findings, along with metaphysitis, often allude to the diagnosis. Specifically, erosions about the medial tibia metaphysis, known as Wimberger's sign, are common (see Fig. 6.2). The presence of these characteristic skeletal features is dependent on the age of the patient at the time of disease manifestation and is typically seen if within the first 2 years of life [68].

Two types of bone involvement in the metaphysis have been described: bone reaction and formation, as well as bone destruction. The metaphyseal involvement in bone reaction and formation includes alterations of mineralization at the zone of provisional calcification [69]. It is common for pathological fractures to occur in the metaphysis due to the destruction of the cancellous and cortical bone by syphilitic granulation tissue [67].

In 1871, Parrot described several children who experienced pain in one or more extremities and lack of movement which he called "pseudoparalysis" [70]. The pseudoparalysis is believed to be a result of intense pain due to chondritis and periostitis. In syphilitic infants under 1 year old, a pathognomonic lesion on radiographs is osteochondritis, which is typically accompanied by symmetric periostitis and can progress to bone destruction and metaphyseal fractures in severe cases [71].

In infants, there is a specific type of osteochondritis known as Parrot's syphilitic osteochondritis, which typically affects the juxta-epiphyseal region of bone, primarily of the proximal humerus. This manifests within the first 3 weeks of life involving upper more than lower extremities. Radiographic findings include irregular epiphyseal line, widened articular space, periosteal changes, and possible fracture. Joint swelling is significant, but pain is usually minimal. This presentation should prompt testing for syphilis.

In our patients, the presenting findings were pseudoparalysis of the involved extremity along with osteitis on radiographs. When assessing these cases, it is important to consider various potential conditions such as Langerhans cell histiocytosis, Caffey disease, scurvy, neuroblastoma, and non-accidental trauma. Non-accidental trauma evaluation is often completed upon presentation. If found to be negative, other etiologies are sought to include infection. In cases where the diagnosis is unclear, it may be worth considering endocrinopathies. This was the scenario for one of our patients who underwent an evaluation for suspected hyperparathyroidism. The diagnosis of congenital syphilis is often made after the exclusion of other potential diagnoses. The skeletal survey demonstrated the characteristic bilateral symmetrical diffuse involvement in one of our patients although several asymmetrical lesions were found in the other patient.

Late: (After 2 Years)

Synovitis: In 1886, Clutton described a presentation in children aged 8–15 with fever and where both knees experienced painless swelling due to presumed congenital syphilis [72]. This specific presentation has been considered pathognomonic for syphilis. The patient typically presents with stiffness in one knee, and upon physical examination, it is discovered that the other knee has an effusion. However, the effusion in the second knee may not become apparent until months or even up to 2 years later. The synovial membrane may be found to be thickened during physical examination. Occasionally, lymphadenopathy can also be observed, and the effusion can persist for several months. Almost all patients in his paper with synovitis exhibited signs of interstitial keratitis, and five of them also had anomalies in their teeth. Further studies have shown that this presentation can occur in individuals aged 5–35 years. Additionally, it is possible for other joints such as the ankle, elbow, wrist, and fingers to be affected.

Borella et al. reported eight children, aged 8–16, who presented with fever up to 102 °F, accompanied by joint effusion (6 bilateral). These patients experienced a delayed onset of symptoms ranging from 15 to 60 days [73]. They noted that the affected joints exhibited more signs of inflammation, including moderate pain and reduced range of motion, which differed from the descriptions provided by Clutton [72]. While these patients did not have any bone changes in the affected joints, periosteal reaction in adjacent areas was observed. The presentation could be unilateral, but bilateral involvement was more common. In cases of bilateral involvement, the second joint could present symptoms months or even years after the initial joint [74].

Comprehensive prenatal screenings and thorough assessment during delivery are critical in minimizing the occurrence of congenital syphilis. It is of utmost importance to correctly identify and complete the treatment of maternal syphilis no later than 30 days prior to delivery, as this prevents up to 98% of cases involving the transmission of syphilis from mother to child [56]. In instances, where the diagnosis is made after childbirth, providing appropriate treatment to the infant proves effective in reversing symptoms and early-stage radiological abnormalities, as supported by several series [55, 62–67, 69].

In a 2014 study, the Centers for Disease Control and Prevention (CDC) found that in 458 mothers with infants diagnosed with congenital syphilis, approximately 20% received no prenatal care. Information on prenatal care was unavailable for another 10% of mothers. Among the mothers who did receive prenatal care, 30% received inadequate treatment for syphilis, while 43% received no treatment at all. This lack of treatment occurred due to various reasons, such as (1) not being tested during pregnancy, (2) testing negative in early pregnancy but acquiring syphilis later, or (3) testing positive but not receiving treatment. It is also important to note that transgender men, that is people whose sex assigned at birth was female, but whose gender identity is male, can also become pregnant and give birth [75]. Another study highlights the association between late or insufficient prenatal care, psychiatric illness, recent substance abuse, and the occurrence of congenital syphilis in newborns. Factors such as disconnected phone numbers and transportation issues contributed to delays in treatment [76].

Laboratory Diagnosis of Syphilis Infections (Not Including Congenital)

Serology is the preferred methodology for the laboratory diagnosis of syphilis infections. In contrast, other conventional methods, such as culture and polymerase chain reaction (PCR), are not routinely used due to their poor performance. In 1906, Landsteiner introduced the utilization of dark-field microscopy to identify this spirochete [77]. Dark-field microscopy blocks direct light and allows light to pass through oblique angles, providing more contrast to distinguish these thin bacteria. The sensitivity of dark-field microscopy for detecting this organism ranges from 86 to 97%, and its specificity is close to 100%. However, this technique has subjectivity as it requires expertise, necessitates immediate examination after sample collection, and may yield false positive results for oral lesions due to the presence of different treponemes in the oral cavity. Additionally, it may result in false-negative outcomes if the patient has undergone treatment [78]. Thus, dark-field microscopy has fallen out of favor and would not be a useful diagnostic for most bone and joint manifestations of syphilis infection.

Due to the poor specificity of serologic methods, tests employing non-treponemal (such as VDRL and RPR) or treponemal tests are considered the gold standard for diagnosing syphilis [12]. As the names suggest, a treponemal test detects antibodies against the protein components of TPA itself, while non-treponemal tests detect antibodies which are produced in response to the infection but are not specific to the organism, particularly cardiolipin. Non-treponemal test titers are highest during secondary syphilis and decrease after infection, including subclinical infection, whereas treponemal tests typically yield positive results throughout an individual's life [79].

While both tests have high sensitivity, they often produce false positives, necessitating confirmatory testing. The recommended order in which testing is performed has changed, with the current practice being to initially perform a treponemal test [like the *Treponema pallidum* particle agglutination assay (TP-PA)] as a screening test. If this is positive, it is then confirmed using a quantitative, non-treponemal test such as RPR. Negative treponemal tests do not require confirmatory testing. This is referred to as the "reverse algorithm." In the "traditional" algorithm, a non-treponemal screening test is performed and then confirmed by a treponemal test. As with the reverse algorithm, negative results from the non-treponemal test do not require confirmatory testing. Syphilis testing is one of the most performed tests in clinical laboratories, and the workflow of automated treponemal tests is preferred over labor-intensive non-treponemal tests such as the RPR. The reason for the reversal in test order is primarily one of convenience, rather than performance. The traditional algorithm, however, is preferred when investigating congenital syphilis, which will be discussed further in this chapter.

Test Performance in Musculoskeletal Manifestations of Syphilis

When syphilis infection results in musculoskeletal manifestations of disease, both treponemal and non-treponemal tests almost always yield positive results. Non-treponemal tests, like RPR, often yield titers above 1:32. While serology is usually reliable in confirming secondary infection, certain clinical conditions, such as HIV, can lead to confusing results such as abnormally high or low titers. In cases where serology is inconclusive, biopsy and microscopy can be performed. Direct observation can be an effective and high yield diagnostic method in cases of typical secondary syphilis infections, with characteristic skin lesions. However, diagnosing osteoarticular syphilis through direct observation may be more difficult, and there is limited published data on the diagnostic accuracy of these methods. Secondary syphilis characteristically resolves after 3–12 weeks and patients become symptom-free, but they remain seropositive [80].

Despite the availability of detailed descriptions of musculoskeletal presentations, limited research has been conducted to assess the effectiveness of laboratory methods in these scenarios. Consequently, our current knowledge in this area is largely derived from the study of non-musculoskeletal manifestations in secondary and tertiary syphilis infections, as well as from case reports. Although systematic evaluations of diagnostic testing for bone and joint manifestations of syphilis have not been performed, several case reports have been published, providing insight into test performance. The table below summarizes select case reports and the results of laboratory testing (Table 6.1).

Table 6.1 Various test results from recent case reports [44, 47, 81–90]

Clinical condition	Patient age	Patient gender	Underlying disease	Treponemal testing	Non-treponemal testing	Other syphilis testing
Tenosynovitis metacarpophalangeal	52 years	Male	None	Not performed	Positive RPR (high titer not specified)	None
Bilateral knee arthralgia and swelling	56 years	Male	None	Positive	Positive RPR (1:64)	Positive PCR—knee effusion
DFE ossification center absent	Infant	Male	None	Positive	Not performed	None
Osteomyelitis foot	73 years	Male	None	Positive	Positive RPR (1:64)	None
Degenerative disk disease	53 years	Male	Hepatitis B	Positive (1:1280)	Positive RPR (1:32)	None
Osteitis	36 years	Male	HIV	Positive	Positive VDRL (1:64)	None

Table 6.1 (continued)

Clinical condition	Patient age	Patient gender	Underlying disease	Treponemal testing	Non-treponemal testing	Other syphilis testing
Swollen joint deformities	50 years	Male	None	Positive	Negative VDRL	None
Osteolytic changes in hyoid bone	58 years	Male	None	Positive	Not performed	None
Osteolysis of tibia, sternal manubrium, ribs, radius, and ulna	61 years	Male	None	Positive (1:20,480)	Positive VDRL (1:16)	None
Charcot knee	67 years	Male	None	Positive	Positive RPR (high titer not specified)	None
Coxofemoral joint degeneration	69 years	Male	HIV, hepatitis C	Positive (1:20,480)	Not performed	Biopsy and Warthin-starry stain negative for organisms
Osteolytic lesions (multiple regions)	48 years	Male	HIV	Positive (1:20,480)	Positive RPR (1:32)	None

Laboratory Diagnosis of Congenital Syphilis

The clinical diagnosis of congenital syphilis is challenging as most infants may be asymptomatic or present with subtle and nonspecific symptoms. Therefore, laboratory testing plays an important role in confirming the diagnosis. Like other forms of syphilis, the clinical presentation of congenital syphilis varies, but can often impact the bones and joints of the child. However, there is limited data regarding the specific performance of laboratory methods in these cases, and it is therefore presumed that the data discussed herein can be extrapolated to children presenting with musculoskeletal symptoms.

The most used diagnostic methods for congenital syphilis are serologic. Dark-field microscopy of amniotic fluid can detect the presence of the organism and may indicate poor outcomes for the infant [91]. However, failure to detect spirochetes does not rule out infection, and dark-field microscopy, as discussed earlier, is no longer performed in most laboratories. PCR from amniotic fluid can also be performed but it is not widely available.

Serologic methods are a mainstay of diagnosis but can be challenging. In infants less than 30 days old, the transfer of maternal treponemal and non-treponemal IgG antibodies across the placenta can complicate the interpretation of test results. Therefore, according to the CDC, it is recommended to perform non-treponemal testing for both the mother and infant and compare titers. A fourfold higher titer in the infant than the mother is indicative of congenital syphilis [92]. It is important to conduct these tests at the same time and in the same laboratory for accurate comparison. Additionally, cord blood should not be used as it may contain maternal blood, leading to confusion in interpreting the results. Unfortunately, comparing the serologic results between mother and infant is rarely useful, with an estimated sensitivity of less than 15% [92].

In cases where both the mother and infant have positive non-treponemal titers, but the infant does not have a fourfold higher titer, close follow-up and additional testing are recommended. This may include a lumbar puncture and CSF VDRL testing, cell count and differential, as well as long-bone radiographs. Treponemal testing is not recommended as the results can be affected by maternal antibodies that are passively transferred and may persist for up to 15 months. Understanding the transmission rates of congenital syphilis from the mother based on her stage of disease can provide valuable information, given the complexities of diagnosing congenital syphilis. Mothers in the primary, secondary, or early latent stages of the disease have a very high rate of transmission, ranging from 40 to 100% [92]. In contrast, mothers with late latent and tertiary infections have a far lower rate of transmission at approximately 10% [92].

Treatment

Penicillin G (benzyl penicillin) should be administered parenterally since it is degraded by gastric acid. It is the preferred drug for treating patients in all stages of syphilis, demonstrating remarkable efficacy in the treatment of TPA infections. Penicillin G's mechanism of action involves interfering with the assembly and/or function of the cell envelope [93]. Due to its short half-life, penicillin G should be given in divided doses 4–6 h apart. Adjustments in the dosage may be needed in specific populations such as breastfeeding women, children, and individuals with severe renal impairment [94]. It is important to emphasize that according to the CDC, alternatives to penicillin have not been extensively studied in patients with syphilis, irrespective of their HIV status. Consequently, it is important to thoroughly evaluate penicillin allergies. Fortunately, penicillin is safe for use during pregnancy and nursing, as the drug appears in breast milk at low concentrations. Caution must be exercised when combining penicillin with tetracycline, as it has an antagonistic effect and may increase the risk of mortality by approximately 2.6 times. Likewise, sulfonamides, erythromycin, and chloramphenicol should be avoided due to their antagonistic effects. Additionally, tubular secretion of penicillin G can be blocked by probenecid resulting in higher and longer lasting plasma concentrations. Other medications such as aspirin, phenylbutazone, sulfonamides, indomethacin, thiazide, furosemide, and ethacrynic acid increase the half-life of penicillin by competing with tubular secretion [95].

In the United States, testing for HIV infection is recommended for all individuals with syphilis. Furthermore, it is recommended to examine the cerebrospinal fluid if there is serological evidence of syphilis, and a clinical syndrome consistent with neurosyphilis. The CDC recommends that patients who are diagnosed with latent syphilis phase, tertiary syphilis phase, neurosyphilis, ocular syphilis, and/or otosyphilis, should receive multiple doses of penicillin G (see Table 6.2). TPA

Table 6.2 With permission from the CDC: sexually transmitted infections treatment guidelines [96]

CDC recommendation for treatment syphilis		
	Infants and children	Adults
Primary and secondary syphilis with or without HIV positivity	Benzathine penicillin G 50,000 units/kg body weight IM, up to the adult dose of 2.4 million units in a single dose	Benzathine penicillin G 2.4 million units IM in a single dose
Latent syphilis early (asymptomatic less than 12 months at risk) with or without HIV positivity		Benzathine penicillin G 2.4 million units IM in a single dose
Latent syphilis late (asymptomatic with unknown or more than 1 year duration) with or without HIV positivity		Benzathine penicillin G 7.2 million units total, administered as 3 doses of 2.4 million units IM each at 1-week intervals
Tertiary syphilis (normal CSF fluid)		Benzathine penicillin G 7.2 million units total, administered as 3 doses of 2.4 million units IM each at 1-week intervals
Neurosyphilis, ocular syphilis, or otosyphilis		Aqueous crystalline penicillin G 18–24 million units per day, administered as 3–4 million units IV every 4 h or continuous infusion for 10–14 days

undergoes slower division than most bacteria. Consequently, it is necessary to maintain penicillin concentrations in the blood above minimum inhibitory concentration (MIC) for at least a 10-day duration.

The goal of follow-up is to confirm the resolution of any symptoms and to ensure serological response. There is a need for additional clinical research to identify the optimal alternative antibiotic management for the truly penicillin allergic patient. Additionally, further studies should be conducted on the subset of patients who do not appear to have adequate serological response to the appropriate treatment. Presently, only 79% of individuals with early syphilis who are HIV-negative, and receive appropriate treatment, achieve serological cure at 6 months posttreatment [97]. Finally, the complexity of syphilis highlights the urgent necessity for the development of a vaccine.

Summary

The incidence of syphilis is on the rise and, if detected early, can be effectively treated. Syphilis can affect any organ system and may present with minimal pain. The increase in congenital syphilis cases can be attributed to the significant rise in syphilis incidence and prevalence among adults. This issue requires attention. The time from infection to the recurrence of symptoms can vary from days to weeks, months, or even years. We must consider syphilis because early diagnosis can greatly benefit both newborns and adult patients. There remains a significant challenge in managing this disease and thus the orthopaedic surgeon must remain vigilant.

Learning Questions, Answered

1. A patient has serum confirmation for syphilis and has ataxia. What additional workup is required?
   This is a finding concerning for tertiary syphilis. Further workup, including echocardiogram and aortic ultrasound can confirm the presence of aortic aneurysm and/or aortic regurgitation. Additionally, the commonly observed manifestations of tabes dorsalis, seizures, vision deficits, strokes, confusion, and personality changes necessitate the pursuit of ophthalmic examination and formal neurologic evaluation, including lumbar puncture. CSF analysis positive for neurosyphilis warrants IV antibiotics rather than IM.
2. What are the highest risk groups for acquiring syphilis?
   Those at highest risk for acquiring syphilis include those with HIV infection, methamphetamine, or opioid use disorder, those who are gay, bisexual, men who have sex with men, patients with a history of incarceration, transactional sex, military service, and those who have limited access to health care coverage and care.
3. What are the classic musculoskeletal signs and symptoms that an orthopaedist will see on presentation of a patient with syphilis?

The patient will typically present in the secondary or tertiary phase of the disease, exhibiting skin lesions (macular, maculopapular, or annular lesions on palms and soles), arthralgia, joint synovitis with effusion, joint fibrosis, tenosynovitis, myositis, bursitis, dactylitis, and/or bone involvement (bone pain, periosteal reaction, sclerosis, and/or lytic lesions).

References

1. Schaudinn F, Hoffman E. Vorlaufiger Bericht uber das Vorkommen von Spirochaeten in syphilitischen Krankheitsprodukten and bei Papillomen. Arb Gesund. 1905;22:527–34.
2. Longo L. Classic pages in obstetrics and gynecology. Vorläufiger Bericht über das Vorkommen von Spirochaeten in syphilitischen Krankheitsprodukten und bei Papillomen. Fritz Richard Schaudinn and Erich Hoffmann. Arbeiten aus dem kaiserlichen Gesundheitsamtes (Berlin), vol. 22, pp. 527–534, 1905. Am J Obstet Gynecol. 1978;12(5):571–2.
3. Kohl PK, Winzer I. 100 Jahre Entdeckung der *Spirochaeta pallida*. Hautarzt. 2005;56(2):112–5. https://doi.org/10.1007/s00105-004-0892-3.
4. Mandelbaum H, Saperstein A. Transmission of syphilis by blood transfusion: a case of acute gummatous osteomyelitis. J Am Med Assoc. 1936;106(13):1061–3. https://doi.org/10.1001/jama.1936.02770130011004.
5. Peeling R, Hook E. The pathogenesis of syphilis: the Great Mimicker, revisited. J Pathol. 2006;208(2):224–32. https://doi.org/10.1002/path.1903.

6. Ávila-Nieto C, Pedreño-López N, Mitjà O, Clotet B, Blanco J, Carrillo J. Syphilis vaccine: challenges, controversies and opportunities. Front Immunol. 2023;14:1126170. https://doi.org/10.3389/fimmu.2023.1126170.
7. Radolf J, Kumar S. *The Treponema pallidum* outer membrane. Curr Top Microbiol Immunol. 2018;415:1–38. https://doi.org/10.1007/82_2017_44.
8. Peeling R, Mabey D, Kamb ML, Chen XS, Radolf JD, Benzaken AS. Syphilis. Nat Rev Dis Prim. 2017;3(1):1–21. https://doi.org/10.1038/nrdp.2017.73.
9. Magnuson H, Eagle H, Fleischman R. The minimal infectious inoculum of *Spirochaeta pallida* (Nichols strain) and a consideration of its rate of multiplication in vivo. Am J Syph Gonorrhea Vener Dis. 1948;32(1):1–18.
10. Cumberland M, Turner T. The rate of multiplication of *Treponema pallidum* in normal and immune rabbits. Am J Syph Gonorrhea Vener Dis. 1949;33(3):201–12.
11. Thompson J. Syphilis: a synopsis, vol. 1. 1st ed. Atlanta: U.S. Department of Health, Education, and Welfare; 1968.
12. Luo Y, Xie Y, Xiao Y. Laboratory diagnostic tools for syphilis: current status and future prospects. Front Cell Infect Microbiol. 2021;10:574806. https://doi.org/10.3389/fcimb.2020.574806.
13. Ghanem KG, Ram S, Rice PA. The modern epidemic of syphilis. N Engl J Med. 2020;382(9):845–54. https://doi.org/10.1056/NEJMra1901593.
14. Szreter S, Siena K. The pox in Boswell's London: an estimate of the extent of syphilis infection in the metropolis in the 1770s. Econ Hist Rev. 2021;74(2):372–99. https://doi.org/10.1111/ehr.13000.
15. Zbar A. Syphilis: a short biography. Springer International Publishing; 2022. https://doi.org/10.1007/978-3-031-08968-8.
16. Englund K. Syphilis 100 years later: another lost opportunity? CCJM. 2017;84(7):514–6. https://doi.org/10.3949/ccjm.84a.16124.
17. Hook E. Is elimination of endemic syphilis transmission a realistic goal for the USA? Lancet. 1998;351:S19–21. https://doi.org/10.1016/S0140-6736(98)90006-X.
18. Lab Recommendations for Syphilis Testing in the United States. 2023. https://www.cdc.gov/std/syphilis/lab/testing/lab-recs-for-testing.htm. Accessed 18 Aug 2023.
19. US Preventive Services Task Force, Mangione CM, Barry MJ, et al. Screening for syphilis infection in nonpregnant adolescents and adults: US Preventive Services Task Force Reaffirmation Recommendation Statement. JAMA. 2022;328(12):1243–9. https://doi.org/10.1001/jama.2022.15322.
20. Kidd S. Increased methamphetamine, injection drug, and heroin use among women and heterosexual men with primary and secondary syphilis—United States, 2013–2017. MMWR Morb Mortal Wkly Rep. 2019;68:6806a4. https://doi.org/10.15585/mmwr.mm6806a4.
21. Hook E. Syphilis. Lancet. 2017;389(10078):1550–7. https://doi.org/10.1016/S0140-6736(16)32411-4.
22. French P. Syphilis. BMJ. 2007;334(7585):143–7. https://doi.org/10.1136/bmj.39085.518148.BE.
23. Drago F, Javor S, Parodi A. Relevance in biology and mechanisms of immune and treatment evasion of *Treponema pallidum*. G Ital Dermatol Venereol. 2019;154(5):573–80. https://doi.org/10.23736/S0392-0488.17.05830-8.
24. Image Number 17040. 1973. https://phil.cdc.gov/Details.aspx?pid=17040. Accessed 25 Aug 2023.
25. Image Number 16749. 1970. https://phil.cdc.gov/Details.aspx?pid=16749. Accessed 25 Aug 2023.
26. Munshi S, Raghunathan SK, Lindeman I, Shetty AK. Meningovascular syphilis causing recurrent stroke and diagnostic difficulties: a scourge from the past. BMJ Case Rep. 2018;2018:bcr2018225255. https://doi.org/10.1136/bcr-2018-225255.
27. Image Number 2381. 1971. https://phil.cdc.gov/Details.aspx?pid=2381. Accessed 25 Aug 2023.
28. Carlson J, Dabiri G, Cribier B, Sell S. The immunopathobiology of syphilis: the manifestations and course of syphilis are determined by the level of delayed-type hypersensitivity. Am J Dermatopathol. 2011;33(5):433–60. https://doi.org/10.1097/DAD.0b013e3181e8b587.

29. Gerster J, Weintraub A, Vischer T, Fallet G. Secondary syphilis revealed by rheumatic complaints. J Rheumatol. 1977;4(2):197–200.
30. Hajjaj-Hassouni N, Rkain H. Syphilis-related musculoskeletal manifestations. In: Espinoza LR, editor. Infections and the rheumatic diseases. Springer International Publishing; 2019. p. 265–75. https://doi.org/10.1007/978-3-030-23311-2_25.
31. McPhee S. Secondary syphilis: uncommon manifestations a common disease. West J Med. 1984;140(1):35–42.
32. Roy R, Laird S. Acute periostitis in early acquired syphilis. Br J Vener Dis. 1973;49(6):555.
33. Tight R, Warner J. Skeletal involvement in secondary syphilis detected by bone scanning. JAMA. 1976;235(21):2326. https://doi.org/10.1001/jama.1976.03260470044027.
34. Wile U, Senear F. A study of the involvement of the bone and joints in early syphilis. Am J Med Sci (1827–1924). 1916;152(5):689.
35. Zampetti A, Rotoli M, Tiberi S. Clinical diagnostic skill in dermatology: how to read palms: learning points from a routine clinical case. Austin J Dermatol. 2015;2(2):1039.
36. Todd A. Syphilitic arthritis. Br J Surg. 1926;14(54):260–79. https://doi.org/10.1002/bjs.1800145410.
37. Reginato A, Schumacher H, Jimenez S, Maurer K. Synovitis in secondary syphilis. Clinical, light, and electron microscopic studies. Arthritis Rheum. 1979;22(2):170–6. https://doi.org/10.1002/art.1780220210.
38. Traczuk A, Chetrit DA, Balasubramanya R, et al. Musculoskeletal manifestations of syphilis in adults: secondary syphilis presenting with ankle inflammatory arthritis and bone involvement with calvarial and sternal lesions. What the rheumatologist needs to know. Clin Rheumatol. 2023;42(4):1195–203. https://doi.org/10.1007/s10067-022-06458-8.
39. Yacyshyn E, Chiowchanwisawakit P, Emery D, Jhamandas J, Resch L, Taylor G. Syphilitic myositis: a case-based review. Clin Rheumatol. 2011;30(5):729–33. https://doi.org/10.1007/s10067-010-1668-z.
40. Eyer-Silva W, da Silva G, Ferry F. Olecranon bursitis, Beau's lines, Biett's collarettes, and crown of Venus. Am J Trop Med Hyg. 2017;96(2):261–2. https://doi.org/10.4269/ajtmh.16-0386.
41. Kaeley G, Eder L, Aydin S, Gutierrez M, Bakewell C. Dactylitis: a hallmark of psoriatic arthritis. Semin Arthritis Rheum. 2018;48(2):263–73. https://doi.org/10.1016/j.semarthrit.2018.02.002.
42. Cormia F. Syphilitic onychia: report of case in which ungual changes helped to establish the diagnosis and the time of syphilitic infection. Arch Dermatol Syphilol. 1938;38(3):432–3. https://doi.org/10.1001/archderm.1938.01480150106017.
43. Bezalely S, Jacob G, Flusser G, Ablin J. Syphilis: an unusual manifestation? BMJ Case Rep. 2014;2014:bcr2014204871. https://doi.org/10.1136/bcr-2014-204871.
44. Colquhoun M, Kirresh O, Keikha M, Haddow L. Osteolytic lesions as the sole presenting feature of secondary syphilis. BMJ Case Rep. 2021;14(6):e242814. https://doi.org/10.1136/bcr-2021-242814.
45. Thompson R, Preston R. Lesions of the skull in secondary syphilis. Am J Syph Gonorrhea Vener Dis. 1952;36(4):332–41.
46. Park K, Lee M, Hong I, et al. Bone involvement in secondary syphilis: a case report and systematic review of the literature. Sex Transm Dis. 2014;41(9):532–7. https://doi.org/10.1097/OLQ.0000000000000164.
47. Gaspari V, Mazza L, Pinto D, Raone B, Calogero P, Patrizi A. Syphilis as osteomyelitis of the fifth metatarsal of the left foot: the great imitator hits once again. Int J Infect Dis. 2020;96:10–1. https://doi.org/10.1016/j.ijid.2020.04.015.
48. Kofman O. The changing pattern of neurosyphilis. Can Med Assoc J. 1956;74(10):807–12.
49. Alpert S, Koval K, Zuckerman J. Neuropathic arthropathy: review of current knowledge. J Am Acad Orthop Surg. 1996;4(2):100–8. https://doi.org/10.5435/00124635-199603000-00005.
50. STD Facts—Congenital Syphilis. 2023. https://www.cdc.gov/std/syphilis/stdfact-congenital-syphilis.htm. Accessed 12 Apr 2023.
51. Oppenheimer E, Hardy J. Congenital syphilis in the newborn infant: clinical and pathological observations in recent cases. Johns Hopkins Med J. 1971;129(2):63–82.

52. Cooper J, Sánchez P. Congenital syphilis. Semin Perinatol. 2018;42(3):176–84. https://doi.org/10.1053/j.semperi.2018.02.005.
53. Lancet T. Congenital syphilis in the USA. Lancet. 2018;392(10154):1168. https://doi.org/10.1016/S0140-6736(18)32360-2.
54. Rothner A, Klein N. Parrot's pseudoparalysis, revisited. Pediatrics. 1975;56(4):604–5.
55. Kimball A, Bowen V, Miele K, et al. Congenital syphilis diagnosed beyond the neonatal period in the United States: 2014–2018. Pediatrics. 2021;148(3):e2020049080. https://doi.org/10.1542/peds.2020-049080.
56. Jacobs K, Vu D, Mony V, Sofos E, Buzi N. Congenital syphilis misdiagnosed as suspected nonaccidental trauma. Pediatrics. 2019;144(4):e20191564. https://doi.org/10.1542/peds.2019-1564.
57. Hussein P, Kew S, Nang K, Kadir F, Teh Y. Skeletal manifestations of congenital syphilis: rare but clinically relevant. Radiol Case Rep. 2021;16(12):3635–7. https://doi.org/10.1016/j.radcr.2021.09.004.
58. Armangil D, Canpolat F, Yiğit S, Demir H, Ceyhan M. Early congenital syphilis with isolated bone involvement: a case report. Turk J Pediatr. 2009;51(2):169–71.
59. Gameiro V, Labronici P, Rosa I, Silva J. Congenital syphilis with bone lesion: case report. Revista Brasileira de Ortopedia (English Edition). 2017;52:740–2. https://doi.org/10.1016/j.rboe.2017.10.002.
60. Hérissé A, Chiaverini C, Hubiche T, et al. Non-accidental injury or congenital infection? Arch Dis Childh. 2017;102(9):852. https://doi.org/10.1136/archdischild-2016-311692.
61. Woods C. Congenital syphilis-persisting pestilence. Pediatr Infect Dis J. 2009;28(6):536–7. https://doi.org/10.1097/INF.0b013e3181ac8a69.
62. Koliou M, Chatzicharalampous E, Charalambous M, Aristeidou K. Congenital syphilis as the cause of multiple bone fractures in a young infant case report. BMC Pediatr. 2022;22(1):728. https://doi.org/10.1186/s12887-022-03789-y.
63. Sachdev M, Bery K, Chawla S. Osseous manifestations in congenital syphilis: a study of 55 cases. Clin Radiol. 1982;33(3):319–23. https://doi.org/10.1016/s0009-9260(82)80278-x.
64. McClean S. The roentgenographic and pathologic aspects of congenital osseous syphilis. Am J Dis Child. 1931;41(1):130–52. https://doi.org/10.1001/archpedi.1931.01940070137018.
65. Cremin BJ, Fisher RM. The lesions of congenital syphilis. Br J Radiol. 1970;43(509):333–41. https://doi.org/10.1259/0007-1285-43-509-333.
66. Engeset A, Eek S, Gilje O. On the significance of growth in the roentgenological skeletal changes in early congenital syphilis. Am J Roentgenol Radium Ther Nucl Med. 1953;69(4):542–56.
67. Rasool MN, Govender S. The skeletal manifestations of congenital syphilis. A review of 197 cases. J Bone Jt Surg Br. 1989;71(5):752–5. https://doi.org/10.1302/0301-620X.71B5.2584243.
68. Zou Y, Marcus MA, Castles C, Kilpatrick S. Congenital syphilis of bone: a potential mimicker of childhood histiocytosis. Am J Surg Pathol. 2017;41(9):1283. https://doi.org/10.1097/PAS.0000000000000893.
69. Toohey J. Skeletal presentation of congenital syphilis: case report and review of the literature. J Pediatr Orthop. 1985;5(1):104–6. https://doi.org/10.1097/01241398-198501000-00021.
70. Parrot M. Sur ene pseudo-paralysie. Arch Physiol. 1871;4:*319*.
71. Pereira A, Castro S, Venturini R, César F, Fortes P, Costa PS. Pseudoparalysis of parrot: a diagnostic aid in congenital syphilis. J Pediatr. 2017;190:282. https://doi.org/10.1016/j.jpeds.2017.07.048.
72. Clutton HH. Symmetrical synovitis of the knee in hereditary syphilis. Lancet. 1886;127(3261):391–3. https://doi.org/10.1016/S0140-6736(00)59101-6.
73. Borella L, Goobar JE, Clark GM. Synovitis of the knee joints in late congenital syphilis: Clutton's joints. JAMA. 1962;180(3):190–2. https://doi.org/10.1001/jama.1962.03050160006002.
74. Klauder J, Robertson H. Symmetrical serous synovitis (Clutton's joints): congenital syphilis and interstitial keratitis. J Am Med Assoc. 1934;103(4):236–40. https://doi.org/10.1001/jama.1934.02750300010004.

75. Bowen V, Su J, Torrone E, Kidd S, Weinstock H. Increase in incidence of congenital syphilis—United States, 2012–2014. MMWR Morb Mortal Wkly Rep. 2015;64(44):1241–5. https://www.cdc.gov/mmwr/preview/mmwrhtml/mm6444a3.htm.
76. Thornton C, Chaisson L, Bleasdale S. Characteristics of pregnant women with syphilis and factors associated with congenital syphilis at a Chicago Hospital. Open Forum Infect Dis. 2022;9(5):ofac169. https://doi.org/10.1093/ofid/ofac169.
77. Luger A. The significance of Karl Landsteiner's works for syphilis research. Wien Klin Wochenschr. 1991;103(5):146–51.
78. Tsang R, Morshed M, Chernesky M, Jayaraman G, Kadkhoda K. Canadian Public Health Laboratory Network laboratory guidelines for the use of direct tests to detect syphilis in Canada. Can J Infect Dis Med Microbiol. 2015;26(Suppl A):13A–7A. https://doi.org/10.1155/2015/685603.
79. Murray P, Rosenthal K, Kobayashi G, Pfaller M. Chapter 41: Treponema, borrelia, and leptospira. In: Medical microbiology. 4th ed; 2006. p. 382.
80. Baughn R, Musher D. Secondary syphilitic lesions. Clin Microbiol Rev. 2005;18(1):205–16. https://doi.org/10.1128/CMR.18.1.205-216.2005.
81. Ratnaraj F, Brooks D, Walton M, Nagabandi A, Abu HM. Forgotten but not gone! Syphilis induced tenosynovitis. Case Rep Infect Dis. 2016;2016:7420938. https://doi.org/10.1155/2016/7420938.
82. Zhou Z, Yang C, Ye J. Severe knee joint damage from syphilitic arthritis. Arthritis Rheumatol. 2018;70(1):133. https://doi.org/10.1002/art.40333.
83. Aoki R, Nagano N, Hijikata M, Seimiya A, Morioka I. Distal femoral epiphyseal ossification center absence in congenital syphilis: a case series. Pediatr Int. 2022;64(1):e15234. https://doi.org/10.1111/ped.15234.
84. Avenel G, Goëb V, Abboud P, Ait-Abdesselam T, Vittecoq O. Atypical forms of syphilis: two cases. Jt Bone Spine. 2009;76(3):293–5. https://doi.org/10.1016/j.jbspin.2008.10.012.
85. Ali R, Perez-Downes J, Baidoun F, et al. Challenges in treating secondary syphilis osteitis in an immunocompromised patient with a penicillin allergy: case report and review of the literature. Case Rep Infect Dis. 2016;2016:4983504. https://doi.org/10.1155/2016/4983504.
86. Gomez J, Molnar S, Val S, Arnal R. Musculoskeletal involvement of syphilis—a forgotten lesson. BMJ Case Rep. 2012;2012:bcr1120115142. https://doi.org/10.1136/bcr.11.2011.5142.
87. Tahara A, Hattori H, Matsuyama T, et al. Syphilis with multiple pulmonary nodules and bone lesions detected on computed tomography and 18F fluorodeoxyglucose-positron emission tomography/computed tomography. J Thorac Imaging. 2022;37(6):W101–5. https://doi.org/10.1097/RTI.0000000000000671.
88. Crépin J, Blot M, Buisson M, Piroth L. Unexplained bone pain and sexual addiction. BMJ Case Rep. 2018;2018:bcr2018225380. https://doi.org/10.1136/bcr-2018-225380.
89. Cardile C, Cazzaniga C, Manzini B, Bongiovanni M, Marasco R, Ragni P. The Charcot knee arthropathy: the diagnostic and surgical challenge. A case of syphilis arthropaty and a review of literature. Arch Bone Jt Surg. 2021;9(4):461–6. https://doi.org/10.22038/abjs.2020.51828.2557.
90. Drago L, De Vecchi E, Pasqualini M, Moneghini L, Bruno M. Rapid, progressive neuropathic arthropathy of the hip in a patient co-infected with human immunodeficiency virus, hepatitis C virus and tertiary syphilis: case report. BMC Infect Dis. 2011;11:159. https://doi.org/10.1186/1471-2334-11-159.
91. Wendel G, Sánchez P, Peters M, Harstad T, Potter L, Norgard M. Identification of *Treponema pallidum* in amniotic fluid and fetal blood from pregnancies complicated by congenital syphilis. Obstet Gynecol. 1991;78(5 Pt 2):890–5.
92. Satyaputra F, Hendry S, Braddick M, Sivabalan P, Norton R. The laboratory diagnosis of syphilis. J Clin Microbiol. 2021;59(10):e0010021. https://doi.org/10.1128/JCM.00100-21.
93. Fisher J, Mobashery S. Constructing and deconstructing the bacterial cell wall. Protein Sci. 2020;29(3):629–46. https://doi.org/10.1002/pro.3737.

94. Yip D, Gerriets V. Penicillin. In: StatPearls. StatPearls Publishing; 2023. http://www.ncbi.nlm.nih.gov/books/NBK554560/.
95. Sexually Transmitted Diseases Treatment Guidelines. 2015. https://www.cdc.gov/mmwr/preview/mmwrhtml/rr6403a1.htm. Accessed 18 Aug 2023.
96. Workowski K, Bachmann L, Chan P, et al. Sexually transmitted infections treatment guidelines, 2021. MMWR Recomm Rep. 2021;70(4):1–187.
97. Seña A, Zhang X, Li T, et al. A systematic review of syphilis serological treatment outcomes in HIV-infected and HIV-uninfected persons: rethinking the significance of serological nonresponsiveness and the serofast state after therapy. BMC Infect Dis. 2015;15:479. https://doi.org/10.1186/s12879-015-1209-0.

Chapter 7
Polymyalgia Rheumatica

Evan Dombrosky and Christopher Wise

Case

A 65-year-old male presents with subacute aching and stiffness in his neck, shoulders, hips, and thighs, which started without any preceding trauma or unusual activity. He responded well to a short course of methylprednisolone, but symptoms rapidly returned after finishing the prescription. He describes fatigue, poor appetite, and several pounds of weight loss during this time.

Physical exam is unremarkable except for mild pain in shoulders during active and passive movement but seemingly normal range of motion. Workup reveals normal blood counts and basic metabolic panel. Erythrocyte sedimentation rate (ESR) and C-reactive protein (CRP) are both elevated. Prednisone is started at 20 mg daily, with significant improvement over the next few days.

At interval follow-up, his symptoms remain improved and now has normalization of inflammatory markers, so the prednisone dose is reduced. One month later, he experiences loss of vision in his right eye while driving his car. He presents to the emergency room (ER) where he undergoes urgent ophthalmology examination, and he receives high dose intravenous methylprednisolone. His visual deficit persists despite this.

Questions

1. Which clinical clues should raise suspicion for PMR?
2. Which differential diagnoses should be considered when suspecting PMR?
3. How is the diagnosis of PMR established?
4. When should GCA be suspected?
5. What should be done if GCA is suspected?

E. Dombrosky (✉) · C. Wise
Division of Rheumatology, Allergy, and Immunology, Department of Internal Medicine, Virginia Commonwealth University, Richmond, VA, USA
e-mail: Evan.Dombrosky@va.gov; christopher.wise@vcuhealth.org

W. A. Zuelzer, S. Metikala (eds.), *Unusual Conditions That Every Orthopaedic Surgeon Should Know*, https://doi.org/10.1007/978-3-031-58946-1_7

Introduction

Polymyalgia rheumatica (PMR) is an inflammatory condition of elderly individuals most often presenting with significant pain and stiffness in the neck, shoulders, and/or hips. Most patients will have elevated acute phase reactants such as the ESR and CRP. It is classically very responsive to medium or low doses of glucocorticoids such as prednisone. PMR has a well-described association with giant cell arteritis (GCA) which may occur before, during, or after clinically apparent PMR. In retrospective analyses, GCA appears to occur in 5 to 30% of those diagnosed with PMR at some point during their lives, while PMR occurs in up to 50% of those with a diagnosis of GCA [1, 2]. The most feared outcome of GCA is permanent vision loss.

Epidemiology

PMR is a disease of adults over the age of 50 [3]. The diagnosis is overwhelmingly unlikely in younger individuals. Prevalence increases with age with peak incidence between 70 and 80. Women are affected more often than men [1]. Caucasians are more likely to develop PMR compared to other ethnicities.

Pathophysiology

Exact pathogenesis of PMR is unknown. There appears to be some genetic predisposition which is not yet well-defined. It is thought to involve activation of both the innate and adaptive immune response. Immune cells migrate to affected tissues and release cytokines including tumor necrosis factor-alpha (TNF-α) and interleukin-6 (IL-6) [4]. This leads to systemic inflammation which may manifest as constitutional symptoms. In PMR, muscle is expected to be normal on histopathologic analysis while periarticular structures demonstrate bursitis and tendonitis [5]. GCA involves similar cytokines though the catalyst driving the development of GCA in those with pre-existing PMR, or vice versa, remains unclear. Multinucleated giant cells (specialized conglomerate of macrophages) may be found on biopsy of affected tissues in PMR or GCA, though their exact role in the disease process remains unclear [6]. Biopsies of affected arteries in GCA may also reveal granulomatous inflammation as well as disruption of the elastic lamina [7].

Clinical Features

The clinical presentations of PMR and GCA can vary widely. Patients with PMR most often present with acute to subacute symmetric pain and stiffness in the neck, shoulders, hips, and/or thighs, with shoulder involvement being the most common.

Occasionally symptoms begin unilaterally but usually become bilateral. A key historical finding is new morning stiffness, lasting at least 30 minutes but often up to several hours. Some patients refer to this as a feeling of weakness. Many patients with PMR will experience constitutional symptoms such as fatigue, diminished appetite, unexpected weight loss, or even low-grade fevers. One cohort of patients with PMR was found to have the following prevalence of symptoms: fatigue (95%), pain in shoulder (88%), pain in neck (67%), pain in thigh (83%), and pain in buttocks (82%). In patients where PMR is suspected, it is important to ask about the most common symptoms of GCA which includes temporal headache, vision changes, and jaw or tongue claudication while eating [8]. Patients with suspected PMR should be warned to look for these symptoms.

There are no tests or established diagnostic criteria for PMR [9]. Clinical diagnosis can be made when another disease is unable to explain a constellation of findings in an individual over 50 years old. There should be a profound response to low to moderate doses of glucocorticoids such as prednisone, prednisolone, or methylprednisolone. Lack of a significant rapid clinical response strongly suggests an alternative diagnosis.

Physical Examination

Close examination of the shoulders and hips should be done in patients with suspected PMR. There may be globally limited range of motion of the shoulders and hips. Strength should remain intact though may be subjectively limited due to pain. There may be non-specific tenderness over proximal muscle groups and bursae. Shoulder symptoms may be mistaken for rotator cuff pathology, and hip symptoms may be mistaken for greater trochanteric pain syndrome. It is reasonable to also assess for GCA by palpating the temporal arteries to assess for tenderness or diminished pulses, especially if there are symptoms more closely associated with GCA.

Workup

When suspecting PMR, it is appropriate to order a complete blood count, a complete metabolic panel, ESR, and CRP [7]. To rule out other mimics, additional testing may be considered such as thyroid-stimulating hormone (TSH), creatine kinase (CK), rheumatoid factor (RF), and anti-cyclic citrullinated peptide (anti-CCP) antibodies. ESR and CRP are often highly elevated but very rarely may be normal. A mild anemia may be present reflecting anemia of chronic disease if the illness has been present long enough. Leukocytosis and thrombocytosis can occur as part of the acute systemic inflammatory response.

Advanced imaging such as MRI may reveal non-specific bursitis and tenosynovitis but is not widely used [6]. If GCA is suspected, ultrasound of the temporal arteries can be helpful in diagnosis in an attempt to avoid temporal artery biopsy.

Management

As mentioned previously, PMR is very responsive to glucocorticoid therapy. If PMR is suspected, it is appropriate to refer urgently to a rheumatologist while also initiating treatment and recommending close follow-up with their primary care provider. In most patients, oral prednisone at 15–20 mg per day is adequate, though this may be tailored to lower or higher doses depending on factors such as BMI, pre-existing diabetes or osteoporosis, or severity of symptoms. If symptoms are not significantly improved within a few days of initiating therapy, the prednisone dose can be escalated further and it may be beneficial to contact your local rheumatologist to expedite the referral.

When patients with PMR do respond well to initial therapy, the prednisone dose is often weaned typically in 2.5 mg increments every 10–14 days until reaching a dose under 10 mg daily at which time the taper should be slowed. It is more common to have relapse of symptoms at prednisone doses of 7.5 mg or less, so it may be wise to avoid tapering below this dose unless frequent clinical monitoring and close follow-up are planned.

Whether it is during initial evaluation or follow-up, if a patient with PMR develops symptoms of GCA, they should be immediately referred to the emergency room to receive high dose glucocorticoids while further evaluation for GCA or alternative diagnoses takes place.

Prognosis of patients with PMR is usually good [10]. Relapses at lower doses of prednisone are common but can usually be treated with a slower prednisone taper, sometimes requiring weaning by 1 mg every several weeks. Most patients will remain on glucocorticoids for 1–2 years, though some will require much longer. Occasionally, patients with persistent or refractory symptoms may be started on a separate immunosuppressive agent by a rheumatologist in an attempt to more successfully wean off glucocorticoids.

Summary

In patients older than 50 years with new-onset pain in the shoulders or hip girdle, the diagnosis of PMR should be considered. The bilateral nature of the disease alongside stiffness are important clinical clues. It is important to assess for constitutional symptoms and those of GCA: new-onset headaches, visual changes, or jaw claudication. Maintain a low threshold to check systemic markers of inflammation such as ESR and CRP. If any classic GCA symptoms are present or there are severe constitutional symptoms, GCA should be ruled out in an emergent manner before permanent vision loss occurs. For less severe cases of PMR without signs of GCA, glucocorticoids can be prescribed alongside referral back to primary care and rheumatology.

Review Questions

1. Which clinical clues should raise suspicion for PMR?
   Age >50, weeks to months of pain and stiffness in the hips and shoulders, lack of swollen joints, good response to glucocorticoids.
2. Which differential diagnoses should be considered when suspecting PMR?
   Rotator cuff tendinitis, bursitis, adhesive capsulitis, osteoarthritis, rheumatoid arthritis, inflammatory myositis, rarely malignancy.
3. How is the diagnosis of PMR established?
   Clinically, should be 50yo, with prolonged (>45 minutes of) morning stiffness, elevated inflammatory markers without another clear cause, and low suspicion for rheumatoid arthritis.
4. When should GCA be suspected?
   If PMR is present and patient has any of the following: new temporal headache tenderness over the temples, asymmetric temporal pulses, jaw or tongue fatigue with chewing.
5. What should be done if GCA is suspected?
   If unable to consult a Rheumatologist directly, send to the emergency room for rapid evaluation and empiric glucocorticoids to prevent potential blindness.

References

1. Salvarani C, Gabriel SE, O'Fallon WM, Hunder GG. The incidence of giant cell arteritis in Olmsted County, Minnesota: apparent fluctuations in a cyclic pattern. Ann Intern Med. 1995;123(3):192–4. https://doi.org/10.7326/0003-4819-123-3-199508010-00006.
2. Salvarani C, Cantini F, Boiardi L, Hunder GG. Polymyalgia rheumatica and giant-cell arteritis. N Engl J Med. 2002;347(4):261–71. https://doi.org/10.1056/NEJMra011913.
3. Salvarani C, Gabriel SE, O'Fallon WM, Hunder GG. Epidemiology of polymyalgia rheumatica in Olmsted County, Minnesota, 1970-1991. Arthritis Rheum. 1995;38(3):369–73. https://doi.org/10.1002/art.1780380311.
4. Weyand CM, Hicok KC, Hunder GG, Goronzy JJ. Tissue cytokine patterns in patients with polymyalgia rheumatica and giant cell arteritis. Ann Intern Med. 1994;121(7):484–91. https://doi.org/10.7326/0003-4819-121-7-199410010-00003.
5. Salvarani C, Cantini F, Olivieri I, Barozzi L, Macchioni L, Niccoli L, Padula A, De Matteis M, Pavlica P. Proximal bursitis in active polymyalgia rheumatica. Ann Intern Med. 1997;127(1):27–31.
6. Mackie SL, Koduri G, Hill CL, Wakefield RJ, Hutchings A, Loy C, Dasgupta B, Wyatt JC. Accuracy of musculoskeletal imaging for the diagnosis of polymyalgia rheumatica: systematic review. RMD Open. 2015;1(1):e000100. https://doi.org/10.1136/rmdopen-2015-000100.
7. Muratore F, Pazzola G, Pipitone N, Salvarani C. Recent advances in the diagnosis and treatment of polymyalgia rheumatica. Expert Rev Clin Immunol. 2016;12(10):1037–45.
8. Soriano A, Muratore F, Pipitone N, Boiardi L, Cimino L, Salvarani C. Visual loss and other cranial ischaemic complications in giant cell arteritis. Nat Rev Rheumatol. 2017;13(8):476–84. https://doi.org/10.1038/nrrheum.2017.98.
9. Bird HA, Esselinckx W, Dixon AS, Mowat AG, Wood PH. An evaluation of criteria for polymyalgia rheumatica. Ann Rheum Dis. 1979;38(5):434–9. https://doi.org/10.1136/ard.38.5.434.
10. Chuang TY, Hunder GG, Ilstrup DM, Kurland LT. Polymyalgia rheumatica: a 10-year epidemiologic and clinical study. Ann Intern Med. 1982;97(5):672–80. https://doi.org/10.7326/0003-4819-97-5-672.

Chapter 8
Postoperative Hyponatremia in the Orthopaedic Patient

Hannah Ruggles, Sreenivasulu Metikala, Jibanananda Satpathy, and Grace Prince

Clinical Vignette

An elective total hip arthroplasty (THA) was planned for a 76-year-old female suffering from chronic right hip pain due to degenerative arthritis [1]. She had significant cardiac history, including coronary artery disease and atrial fibrillation. Her daily medications included hydrochlorothiazide, atenolol, nitroglycerin, losartan, diltiazem, and aspirin. The serum sodium level before surgery was 140 mmol/L. She underwent an uneventful hybrid THA under spinal anesthesia with an estimated blood loss of 685 mL. She received 2200 mL of intravenous fluids during the surgery, and her urine output was 1400 mL. Subsequently, she was admitted to the hospital for routine postoperative care and physical therapy. She had been doing well until the fourth day after the operation when she started to become disoriented and lethargic. The laboratory tests showed a dramatic decline in serum sodium to 107 mmol/L. The sodium concentration in her urine was 23 mmol/L, and the osmolality was 428 mOsm/kg (428 mmol/kg). The patient was found to have symptomatic hyponatremia and was transferred to the intensive care unit (ICU). After being treated with fluid restriction and the infusion of hypertonic saline, the patient's condition gradually improved over a 3-day period. There were no permanent

H. Ruggles (✉)
Department of Internal Medicine, Virginia Commonwealth University, Richmond, VA, USA
e-mail: Hannah.Ruggles@vcuhealth.org

S. Metikala · J. Satpathy
Department of Orthopaedic Surgery, Virginia Commonwealth University, Richmond, VA, USA
e-mail: Sreenivasulu.Metikala@vcuhealth.org

G. Prince
Division of Endocrinology, Department of Medicine, Virginia Commonwealth University, Richmond, VA, USA
e-mail: Grace.Prince@vcuhealth.org

W. A. Zuelzer, S. Metikala (eds.), *Unusual Conditions That Every Orthopaedic Surgeon Should Know*, https://doi.org/10.1007/978-3-031-58946-1_8

neurological impairments, but hospital discharge was delayed until the 13th day after the operation, with a serum sodium concentration of 137 mmol/L.

Another example of postoperative hyponatremia that was unfortunately complicated by serious outcomes was seen in the case of an elderly woman undergoing routine total knee arthroplasty (TKA) [2]. Her preoperative serum sodium level was 134 mmol/L indicating borderline hyponatremia due to prolonged thiazide diuretic use. Postoperatively, she had frequent vomiting and received an infusion of six liters of 5% dextrose saline. On the second day following her surgery, her serum sodium fell to 115 mmol/L, and she slipped into a coma the day after. After 5 days of medical management, the sodium level was brought back to 134 mmol/L, but the patient ultimately suffered permanent cognitive impairment.

Neurological damage due to severe hyponatremia is a rare postoperative complication after major orthopaedic surgical procedures such as total joint arthroplasties and spine reconstructions. The early clinical manifestations are frequently subtle and typically masquerade as routine opioid medication sequelae and general postoperative lethargy. A high index of suspicion is critical for a rapid diagnosis. Delayed or missed diagnosis increases morbidity, length of hospital stays, cost of care, and permanent neurological sequelae, including fatal complications. This chapter reviews the current knowledge about the pathogenesis and clinical manifestations of hyponatremia in a perioperative setting and emphasizes the fundamental principles of management.

Questions Include

1. What are the lessons learned?
2. What could have been done differently (in retrospect)?
3. What would be the preferred treatment for symptomatic hyponatremia following a major orthopaedic surgery?

Introduction

The advancements in implants, surgical techniques, and perioperative care have resulted in greater safety for orthopaedic patients following various surgical procedures. Yet, it is critical to be cognizant of serious postoperative complications, including body fluid and electrolyte disorders, especially when presenting symptoms can be subtle and insidious. Hyponatremia is a common electrolyte disorder occurring in up to 30% of hospitalized patients [3, 4]. Symptoms of hyponatremia can range from mild to severe and can even be life threatening. Many of the milder symptoms, such as lethargy, impaired attention, headache, nausea, and vomiting, are commonly encountered in the postoperative period making discrimination difficult. As a consequence, the potential for misdiagnosis or delayed diagnosis is high.

Hyponatremia, defined as serum sodium <135 mmol/L, is associated with increased morbidity and mortality across a wide range of disorders [5]. Preoperative and postoperative hyponatremia should be recognized as a prognostic marker for perioperative complications. Preoperative hyponatremia, present in up to 7% of orthopaedic surgery patients, is associated with a higher risk of 30-day mortality, perioperative coronary events, wound infections, pneumonia, and prolonged hospitalization [6]. Similarly, postoperative hyponatremia, present in as many as 30% of patients following general orthopaedic surgery [7], is associated with longer hospital stays, more costly admissions, and an increased likelihood of being discharged to an extended-care facility [4, 7, 8]. Particularly relevant to orthopaedic surgeons is the association of hyponatremia with falls, fractures, and low bone mineral density [9, 10]. Astute surgeons should take note of hyponatremia as a marker of increased fall risk and recognize the need for closer surveillance of these patients.

This review presents the current knowledge on the pathogenesis, risk factors, and clinical presentation of perioperative hyponatremia in orthopaedic patients, along with the general strategies for management. As the trend toward shorter hospitalization and outpatient joint arthroplasty continues, improved clinical awareness of hyponatremia as a serious perioperative complication could contribute to providing cost-effective care while maximizing outcomes.

Definition

Hyponatremia is defined as a serum sodium level <135 mmol/L [5, 11]. The severity of hyponatremia can be described by serum sodium levels or by symptomatology. The definition of the severity of hyponatremia is variable among studies. Generally, mild hyponatremia is considered to be serum sodium of 130–134 mmol/L, with moderate to severe hyponatremia occurring with sodium <130 mmol/L [6]. Perhaps the more clinically relevant way to describe hyponatremia is by symptomatology (see Table 8.1). Asymptomatic hyponatremia is a misnomer, and its use should be avoided, as patients with even mild hyponatremia will likely have subtle clinical findings if properly assessed [12].

Table 8.1 Classification of hyponatremia by symptom severity

Severity	Symptom
Mild	Attention deficit Unstable static posture (Romberg) Tandem gait impairment
Moderate	Nausea without vomiting Confusion Headache Fatigue Blurred vision
Severe	Vomiting Cardiorespiratory distress Abnormal and deep somnolence Seizures Coma

Adapted from "Clinical practice guideline on diagnosis and treatment of hyponatraemia," by Spasovski, G., et al., 2014, *European Journal of Endocrinology*, Volume 170, p. G10; and "Is Asymptomatic Hyponatremia Really Asymptomatic?" by Decaux, G., 2006, *The American Journal of Medicine*, Volume 119, p. S82 [11, 12]

The severity of symptoms outlined in Table 8.1 is caused more by the rapidity of the change in serum sodium rather than the absolute number. Nonetheless, more severe symptoms are often associated with serum sodium <125 mmol/L [13]. Describing the acuity of the development of hyponatremia as either acute (<48 h) or chronic (>48 h) becomes clinically relevant in understanding why a patient with the same absolute serum sodium level may present with very different symptomatology [11].

Pathophysiology

Hyponatremia is fundamentally an imbalance between salt and water caused by a relative excess in water with a relative deficiency of sodium. Most cases of hyponatremia are mediated by antidiuretic hormone (ADH), which is responsible for the regulation of body water [11].

Physiologic release of ADH is triggered by low blood volume or low blood pressure via baroreceptors and by increased plasma tonicity or osmolality via osmoreceptors in the anterior hypothalamus [5]. The action of ADH in the kidney leads to the reabsorption of water from the urine. Both appropriate and inappropriate secretion of ADH can lead to water retention and consequent hyponatremia [11].

The most significant pathophysiologic change of hyponatremia is a result of its osmotic effect on the brain. The commonly encountered scenario of hypotonic hyponatremia is caused by water retention [14]. This dilutional state creates an osmotic gradient between the hypertonic intracellular and hypotonic extracellular compartments. If this gradient develops gradually, e.g., over more than 48 h, as is seen with chronic hyponatremia, the brain can alter its effective osmolality to prevent fluid shifts between compartments. However, when this occurs acutely, e.g., in 24–48 h or less, as is seen with acute hyponatremia, the brain's adaptive mechanisms are unable to respond quickly enough, and fluid shifts from the hypotonic extracellular compartment to the relatively hypertonic intracellular compartment (see Fig. 8.1). The end result is cerebral edema, with manifestations such as seizures, coma, or death [11]. Adding further complexity, the danger of rapid fluid shifts similarly applies to treating patients with chronic hyponatremia. Just as rapid fluid shifts can lead to cerebral edema in patients who develop acute hyponatremia, rapid increases in the serum sodium of patients with chronic hyponatremia can also overwhelm adaptive mechanisms, causing fluid shifts in the opposite direction from the intracellular to extracellular space, leading to osmotic demyelination [11] (see Fig. 8.2).

The causes of hypotonic hyponatremia are numerous, and determining the underlying mechanism can be challenging. However, certain perioperative triggers can lead to both appropriate and inappropriate ADH release, ultimately resulting in the retention of water and hypotonic hyponatremia. While not a comprehensive list (e.g., there are numerous medications that have been implicated as causes of the Syndrome of Inappropriate Antidiuretic Hormone Secretion, [SIADH]), Table 8.2 lists causes that are of particular importance to the orthopaedic surgeon.

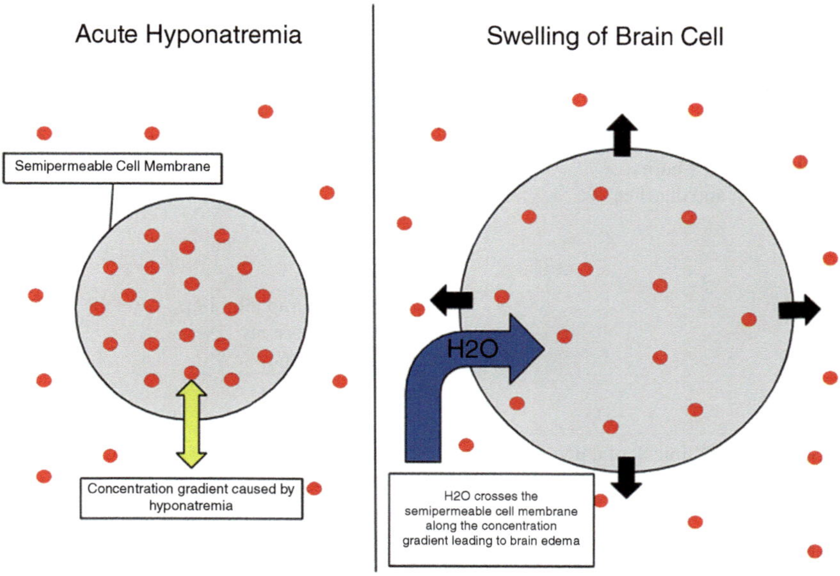

Fig. 8.1 Cellular fluid shifts causing cerebral edema as seen in acute hyponatremia

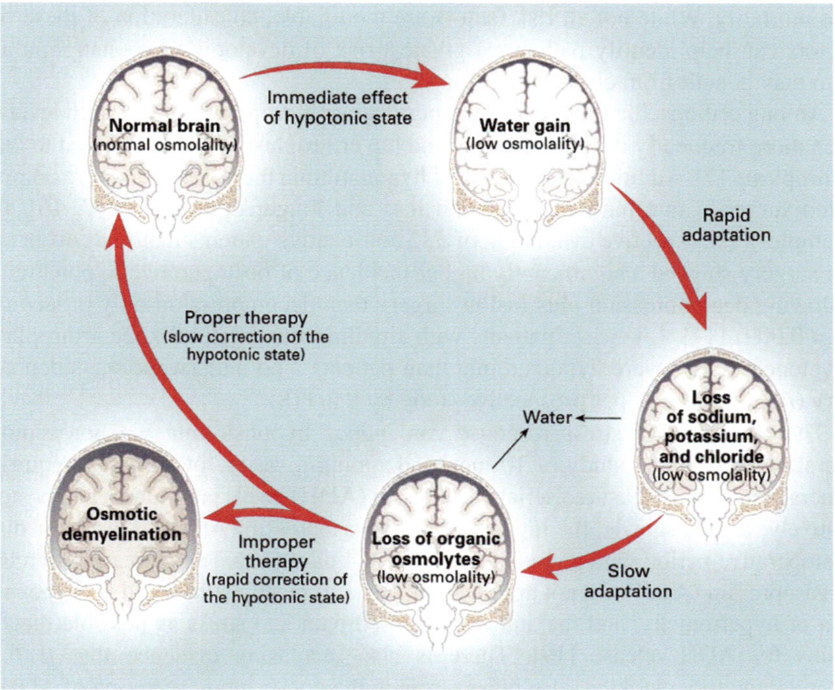

Fig. 8.2 Adaptation of the brain to hypotonicity. (Reproduced with permission from "Hyponatremia," by Adrogue, H.J. & Madias, N.E., *New England Journal of Medicine,* 2000, Volume 342 [15])

Table 8.2 Causes of ADH-mediated hyponatremia commonly encountered in orthopaedic patients

Nature of ADH release	
Appropriate ADH release	Inappropriate ADH release (SIADH)
– Hemorrhage – Hypovolemia or dehydration – Skin losses or burns – Vomiting and diarrhea	Stressors: – Nausea – Pain – Stress
	Medications: – Opiates – NSAIDs – Proton pump inhibitors – Antidepressants – Antiepileptics
	Infections: – Pneumonia

Adapted from "Clinical practice guideline on diagnosis and treatment of hyponatremia," by Spasovski, G., et al., 2014, *European Journal of Endocrinology*, Volume 170. P. G16 [11]

Risk Factors

Hyponatremia in the perioperative period has been associated with a variety of risk factors (see Table 8.3). We have established the clinical importance of hyponatremia as a prognostic marker for perioperative complications with increased morbidity and mortality. While not all risk factors are modifiable, consideration of these risk factors can help identify patients at greatest risk of developing hyponatremia and who may benefit from closer monitoring.

Among orthopaedic procedures, the perioperative drop in serum sodium levels is seen more frequently in spinal surgery and hip arthroplasty when compared to knee arthroplasty [7]. Additionally, the risk of hyponatremia increases with more complicated surgeries that have higher blood loss and longer durations [3, 7, 16]. For example, a retrospective evaluation of 582 consecutive patients that underwent spinal surgery showed a significantly higher incidence of postoperative hyponatremia following decompression plus fusion surgery than decompression-only procedures ($p = 0.009$) [17]. Likewise, patients with simultaneous bilateral knee arthroplasty developed more severe hyponatremia than patients who underwent one-sided surgery ($P < 0.0001$), as per prospective study by Sah [18].

The perioperative stress response can induce hyponatremia via non-osmotic secretion of ADH. A study of 10 men undergoing a variety of surgeries requiring general anesthesia measured serial vasopressin (ADH) levels pre-, intra-, and postoperatively; results showed the highest levels of vasopressin (ADH) in the immediate postoperative period with a gradual fall over 3–4 days [19]. The increased secretion of vasopressin (ADH) did not appear to be physiologically stimulated by hypovolemia or hypertonicity, and the authors proposed pain and stress as possible mechanisms for ADH release [19]. There is also increasing evidence that IL-6, a proinflammatory cytokine, also plays a role in the non-osmotic secretion of ADH, a possible mechanism for water retention and hyponatremia in inflammatory states [20].

Table 8.3 Common risk factors associated with postoperative hyponatremia

Risk factors associated with postoperative hyponatremia		
Preoperative	Operative	Postoperative
Chronic hyponatremia [23] Older age [3, 7, 14] Diuretic use (e.g., thiazides) [7, 15] Chronic medical conditions: CHF, cirrhosis, CKD/renal failure, DM [15, 24]	General anesthesia [21] Higher blood loss [7, 15] Longer operating time [7] More complex operations (e.g., spine surgery, Hip arthroplasty) [7]	Pain and stress [15, 25] Nausea and vomiting [25] Hyperglycemia and steroid use [15]
← Hypotonic Fluids [21] →		

CHF congestive heart failure, *CKD* chronic kidney disease, *DM* diabetes mellitus

Another well-recognized risk factor for postoperative hyponatremia is the use of hypotonic fluids, e.g., dextrose 5% in water or hypotonic saline. In a prospective study, 4.4% of 1088 patients developed postoperative hyponatremia, and 94% of these patients received hypotonic fluids at the time of development of hyponatremia [21]. A small case-control trial with 12 adolescent patients undergoing a scoliosis correction procedure showed a statistically significant drop in serum sodium and serum osmolality in patients receiving hypotonic saline compared to isotonic saline [22].

Preventive Measures

1. Optimal correction of preoperative serum sodium.
   (a) If there is a strong suspicion for drug-mediated SIADH (e.g., SSRIs, see Table 8.2), work with other providers to consider discontinuing these drugs prior to surgery.
   (b) Consider suspending diuretic medications prior to surgery to prevent perioperative dehydration and hypovolemia.
2. Replace volume losses from prolonged fasting or blood losses with isotonic fluids, e.g., normal saline or lactated ringers.
3. For patients with chronic steroid use or known adrenal insufficiency, treat appropriately with stress dose steroids for surgery.
4. Avoid hypotonic fluids, e.g., dextrose 5% in water or hypotonic saline.
5. Avoid starting new medications that could induce SIADH in the perioperative period (see Table 8.2).
6. Have a high clinical index of suspicion when mild symptoms of hyponatremia are recognized (see Table 8.1), and correlate with periodic serum sodium measurements in the perioperative period [26].

Evaluation and Management

The primary goals of hyponatremia management are rapid identification and correction of severely symptomatic hyponatremia if present, followed by the diagnosis of the underlying etiology for disease-specific management.

The evaluation and management of hyponatremia are nuanced and often require expert consultation. This chapter does not serve as a comprehensive guide to the management of hyponatremia. Rather, the following guidelines should help with the initial evaluation and management of hyponatremia to determine when escalation of care or specialty consultation is indicated.

A schematic approach to the evaluation and management of hyponatremia is provided in Fig. 8.3. When hyponatremia is identified, the first step is to assess for the presence of acute or severe symptoms, e.g., vomiting, cardiorespiratory distress, abnormal mentation and/or deep somnolence, seizures, or coma. If severe symptoms are present, this should trigger an immediate escalation in care to an ICU setting along with a specialty consult. Emergent treatment typically involves 100 to 150 mL boluses of hypertonic (3%) saline to help decrease cerebral edema and intracranial pressure, with a goal of increasing serum sodium by 4 to 6 mmol/L within 1–2 h [14]. Delayed treatment can result in severe consequences, including cerebral edema [11].

In a non-emergent setting, additional workup can be initiated before proceeding with treatment. A basic initial workup for hyponatremia should include serum osmolality, urine osmolality, and urine sodium. Using these lab values to work through the flow chart (see Fig. 8.3), one can develop a differential diagnosis and initial management plan.

Looking first at the serum osmolality helps distinguish true hypotonic hyponatremia (serum osmolality <275 mOsm/kg) from other etiologies with normal or elevated serum osmolality. Hyperglycemia is a cause of isotonic and hypertonic hyponatremia due to fluid shifts from the intracellular to the extracellular space, diluting the sodium concentration [14]. Treatment, in this case, would be with the management of blood glucose. Pseudohyponatremia is a cause of isotonic hyponatremia due to a laboratory artifact caused by severe hyperlipidemia or hyperproteinemia [14].

Hypotonic IV fluids, e.g., dextrose 5% in water or hypotonic saline, should be stopped as soon as the diagnosis of hypotonic hyponatremia is made.

In cases of true hypotonic hyponatremia, urine osmolality can help distinguish between ADH-mediated and non-ADH-mediated hypotonic hyponatremia. Physiologically, ADH works in the kidneys to reabsorb water from the urine. Therefore, high levels of ADH lead to concentrated urine (urine osmolality >100 mOsm/kg). In general, higher urine osmolality indicates higher activity of ADH. If the urine osmolality is low (<100 mOsm/kg), this indicates that the kidneys are appropriately excreting water in the setting of hyponatremia (sodium dilution), and ADH secretion is appropriately suppressed. Non-ADH mediated hypotonic hyponatremia is caused by excessive water intake, e.g., primary polydipsia, or by low solute intake, e.g., tea & toast diet or beer potomania [14].

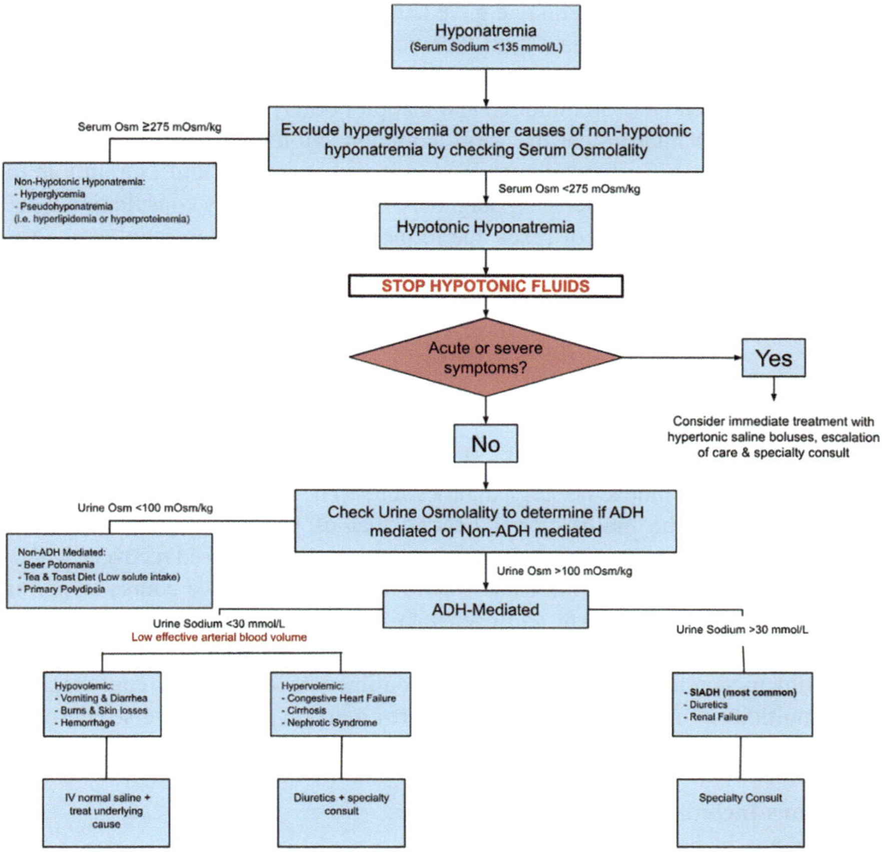

Fig. 8.3 Algorithm for the evaluation and initial management of perioperative hyponatremia. (Adopted from "Clinical practice guideline on diagnosis and treatment of hyponatraemia," by Spasovski, G., et al., 2014, *European Journal of Endocrinology*, Volume 170; and from "The relevance of hyponatraemia to perioperative care of surgical patients," by Cuesta, M., and Thompson, C., 2015. *The Surgeon: Journal of the Royal Colleges of Surgeons of Edinburgh and Ireland.* Volume 13 [11, 26].)

In cases of ADH-mediated hypotonic hyponatremia, urine sodium measurement can help narrow the differential diagnosis. A low urine sodium level (urine sodium <30 mmol/L) indicates that the kidneys are trying to retain salt and water. This occurs when there is low effective arterial blood volume either from true hypovolemia, e.g., vomiting and diarrhea, or from a low flow state, e.g., heart failure. Differentiating between these etiologies is largely based on volume status. In patients with evidence of hypovolemia, e.g., decreased skin turgor, dry mucous membranes, decreased weight, etc., consider treatment with isotonic IV fluids followed by repeat sodium level to look for improvement. To aid in the difficult differentiation between hypovolemia and euvolemia, increased levels of serum urea nitrogen and uric acid are consistent with hypovolemic hyponatremia, whereas low to normal values are more consistent with euvolemic hyponatremia [27]. In patients with evidence of hypervolemia, e.g., edema, elevated JVD, ascites, increased weight, etc., consider treatment with diuretics and specialty consult based on presumed underlying etiology. Finally, in cases of ADH-mediated hyponatremia with elevated urine sodium (>30 mmol/L) and inappropriately concentrated urine (urine osmolality >100 mOsm/kg), the most common etiology is SIADH. However, diuretic use or renal dysfunction can lead to inappropriate sodium excretion in the urine and mask the true underlying diagnosis. Overall, specialty consultation is recommended in the majority of cases due to the difficulty of interpreting diagnostic workup and choosing the next management steps [11, 14].

Conclusion

Clinically significant hyponatremia, though not frequent, is an important occurrence after major orthopaedic surgical procedures. The symptoms can be subtle, and the etiology may be multifactorial beyond that of general surgical stress. The sequelae of the missed or untreated disorder can vary from delayed recovery with an extended hospital stay in an otherwise uneventful postoperative course to permanent neurological impairment and even fatal outcomes. Thus, it is imperative to consider symptomatic hyponatremia for any postoperative orthopaedic patient exhibiting moderate to severe symptoms, as outlined in Table 8.1. Prompt diagnosis and a multidisciplinary treatment approach are crucial to prevent adverse neurological consequences.

Questions Include

1. What are the lessons learned?

   Elderly patients with medical comorbidities and on anti-hypertensive and diuretic medications can be at risk for a rapid decline in serum sodium levels after major orthopaedic surgery. A fall in serum sodium concentration can occur regardless of the preoperative sodium being in the normal range. So, it is important to maintain a high level of suspicion in order to diagnose this remarkable pathology early. A misdiagnosis of hyponatremia can have catastrophic effects due to the possibility of irreversible neurological damage.
2. What could have been done differently (in retrospect)?

   Optimizing the serum sodium during the preoperative visit is the initial step in minimizing the risk of postoperative hyponatremia. Therefore, close attention should have been paid to the list of daily medications to identify the sodium-unfriendly pills and to substitute them with suitable alternatives. Accurate charting of fluid input and output as well as close monitoring of serum electrolytes could have resulted in earlier recognition and management of hyponatremia, thereby preventing a prolonged hospital admission in the first patient. Regarding the second case example, the utilization of isotonic fluids in lieu of large volumes of 5% dextrose saline might have prevented permanent neurological deficits from occurring.

3. What would be the preferred treatment for symptomatic hyponatremia following a major orthopaedic surgery?

   The goal of treatment in patients with acute onset of severe hyponatremia symptoms is rapid diagnosis and prompt electrolyte correction to lower the risk of cerebral edema. This treatment should take place in an ICU setting with an experienced provider. After the initial symptoms have been eased, further treatment is contingent on the additional evaluation (illustrated in Fig. 8.3) to recognize the underlying cause.

References

1. Gluck GS, Lachiewicz PF. Symptomatic hyponatremia in patients undergoing total hip and knee arthroplasty. A report of three cases. J Bone Joint Surg Am. 2008;90(3):634–6.
2. Lane N, Allen K. Hyponatraemia after orthopaedic surgery. BMJ. 1999;318(7195):1363–4.
3. Upadhyay A, Jaber BL, Madias NE. Incidence and prevalence of hyponatremia. Am J Med. 2006;119(7 Suppl 1):S30–5.
4. Wald R, Jaber BL, Price LL, Upadhyay A, Madias NE. Impact of hospital-associated hyponatremia on selected outcomes. Arch Intern Med. 2010;170(3):294–302.
5. Verbalis JG, Goldsmith SR, Greenberg A, Korzelius C, Schrier RW, Sterns RH, et al. Diagnosis, evaluation, and treatment of hyponatremia: expert panel recommendations. Am J Med. 2013;126(10 Suppl 1):S1–42.
6. Leung AA, McAlister FA, Rogers SO Jr, Pazo V, Wright A, Bates DW. Preoperative hyponatremia and perioperative complications. Arch Intern Med. 2012;172(19):1474–81.
7. Hennrikus E, Ou G, Kinney B, Lehman E, Grunfeld R, Wieler J, et al. Prevalence, timing, causes, and outcomes of hyponatremia in hospitalized Orthopaedic surgery patients. J Bone Joint Surg Am. 2015;97(22):1824–32.
8. Pennington Z, Bomberger TT, Lubelski D, Benzel EC, Steinmetz MP, Mroz TE. Preoperative hyponatremia and perioperative complications in cervical spinal fusion. World Neurosurg. 2020;141:e864–e72.
9. Renneboog B, Musch W, Vandemergel X, Manto MU, Decaux G. Mild chronic hyponatremia is associated with falls, unsteadiness, and attention deficits. Am J Med. 2006;119(1):71.e1–8.
10. Rondon-Berrios H, Berl T. Mild chronic hyponatremia in the ambulatory setting: significance and management. Clin J Am Soc Nephrol. 2015;10(12):2268–78.
11. Spasovski G, Vanholder R, Allolio B, Annane D, Ball S, Bichet D, et al. Clinical practice guideline on diagnosis and treatment of hyponatraemia. Eur J Endocrinol. 2014;170(3):G1–47.
12. Decaux G. Is asymptomatic hyponatremia really asymptomatic? Am J Med. 2006;119(7 Suppl 1):S79–82.
13. Gill G, Huda B, Boyd A, Skagen K, Wile D, Watson I, et al. Characteristics and mortality of severe hyponatraemia--a hospital-based study. Clin Endocrinol. 2006;65(2):246–9.
14. Adrogué HJ, Tucker BM, Madias NE. Diagnosis and Management of Hyponatremia: a review. JAMA. 2022;328(3):280–91.
15. Adrogué HJ, Madias NE. Hyponatremia. N Engl J Med. 2000;342(21):1581–9.
16. Deyo RA, Mirza SK, Martin BI, Kreuter W, Goodman DC, Jarvik JG. Trends, major medical complications, and charges associated with surgery for lumbar spinal stenosis in older adults. JAMA. 2010;303(13):1259–65.
17. Kinoshita Y, Tamai K, Oka M, Habibi H, Terai H, Hoshino M, et al. Prevalence, risk factors, and potential symptoms of hyponatremia after spinal surgery in elderly patients. Sci Rep. 2022;12(1):18622.

18. Sah AP. Hyponatremia after primary hip and knee arthroplasty: incidence and associated risk factors. Am J Orthop (Belle Mead NJ). 2014;43(4):E69–73.
19. Haas M, Glick SM. Radioimmunoassayable plasma vasopressin associated with surgery. Arch Surg. 1978;113(5):597–600.
20. Swart RM, Hoorn EJ, Betjes MG, Zietse R. Hyponatremia and inflammation: the emerging role of interleukin-6 in osmoregulation. Nephron Physiol. 2011;118(2):45–51.
21. Chung HM, Kluge R, Schrier RW, Anderson RJ. Postoperative hyponatremia. A prospective study Arch Intern Med. 1986;146(2):333–6.
22. Brazel PW, McPhee IB. Inappropriate secretion of antidiuretic hormone in postoperative scoliosis patients: the role of fluid management. Spine (Phila Pa 1976). 1996;21(6):724–7.
23. Gu A, Chen FR, Chen AZ, Fassihi SC, Thakkar S, Unger AS, et al. Preoperative hyponatremia is an independent risk factor for postoperative complications in aseptic revision hip and knee arthroplasty. J Orthop. 2020;20:224–7.
24. Verghese SC, Mahajan A, Uppal B. Chronic versus new-onset hyponatremia in geriatric patients undergoing orthopedic surgery. Int J Appl Basic Med Res. 2019;9(1):37–43.
25. Richard H, Sterns SMS, Hix JK. Hyponatremia. In: Alpern OWM RJ, Caplan M, editors. Seldin and Giebisch's the kidney. 5th ed. Academic Press; 2013. p. 1511–39.
26. Cuesta M, Thompson C. The relevance of hyponatraemia to perioperative care of surgical patients. Surgeon. 2015;13(3):163–9.
27. Greenberg A, Verbalis JG, Amin AN, Burst VR, Chiodo JA 3rd, Chiong JR, et al. Current treatment practice and outcomes. Report of the hyponatremia registry. Kidney Int. 2015;88(1):167–77.

Chapter 9
Acute Colonic Pseudo-Obstruction (ACPO)

Milan Patel, Jaharris Collier, Jaime Bohl, Laura Carucci, and Wilhelm A. Zuelzer

Case Presentations

Case 1

A 67-year-old male was admitted to the hospital for an elective total right hip replacement surgery in the context of osteoarthritis. The patient had a body mass index (BMI) of 36 with active smoking, dyslipidemia, and hypertension. Surgery was performed under general anesthesia with an anterior approach without any immediate surgical complications for a total intervention time of 1 h and 15 min. Postoperative pain was managed with opioids and additional postoperative medications included enoxaparin, ibuprofen, oxazepam, and paracetamol. Postoperative day one, the patient developed abdominal pain and tenderness with diminished

M. Patel (✉)
Division of Gastroenterology, Hepatology and Nutrition, Department of Medicine, Virginia Commonwealth University, Richmond, VA, USA
e-mail: milan.patel@vcuhealth.org

J. Collier
Phoeniz, AZ, USA

J. Bohl
Department of Surgery, Virginia Commonwealth University, Richmond, VA, USA
e-mail: jaime.bohl@vcuhealth.org

L. Carucci
Department of Radiology, Virginia Commonwealth University, Richmond, VA, USA
e-mail: laura.carucci@vcuhealth.org

W. A. Zuelzer
Orthopaedic Surgery, Virginia Commonwealth University Medical School, Richmond, VA, USA
e-mail: wilhelm.zuelzer@vcuhealth.org

W. A. Zuelzer, S. Metikala (eds.), *Unusual Conditions That Every Orthopaedic Surgeon Should Know*, https://doi.org/10.1007/978-3-031-58946-1_9

bowel sounds and the inability to pass gas. No bowel movement was recorded since his surgery. Given findings suggestive of paralytic ileus, the patient was treated with rectal enemas and laxatives. Opioid medications were stopped. On postoperative day 3, the patient still was unable to have a bowel movement and developed hypotension and tachycardia. Serum blood work showed a white blood count (WBC) of 18 G/L (normal range 4–11 G/L) with abdominal radiograph imaging showing small intestine dilation and multiple air-fluid levels. The patient further decompensated on postoperative day 4 with hypoxia and tachypnea leading to a cardiac-respiratory arrest and death.

Post-mortem computed tomography (PMCT) revealed a cecal diameter of 9 cm without pneumoperitoneum being noted (Fig. 9.1a). Upon autopsy, the cecal serosa was covered by yellow-brownish deposits suggestive of fibrinoid peritonitis (Fig. 9.1b). Similar deposits were noted on the distal segment of the terminal ileum and appendix. Under those deposits, the cecal surface showed diffuse purple and greenish discoloration and a sharp reddish demarcation with an unremarkable ascending colon. The cecum was noted to be thin with mucosa exhibiting the same discoloration and sharp line of demarcation as seen on the cecal serosa. Histological examination showed acute inflammatory necrosis of the cecum confirming acute

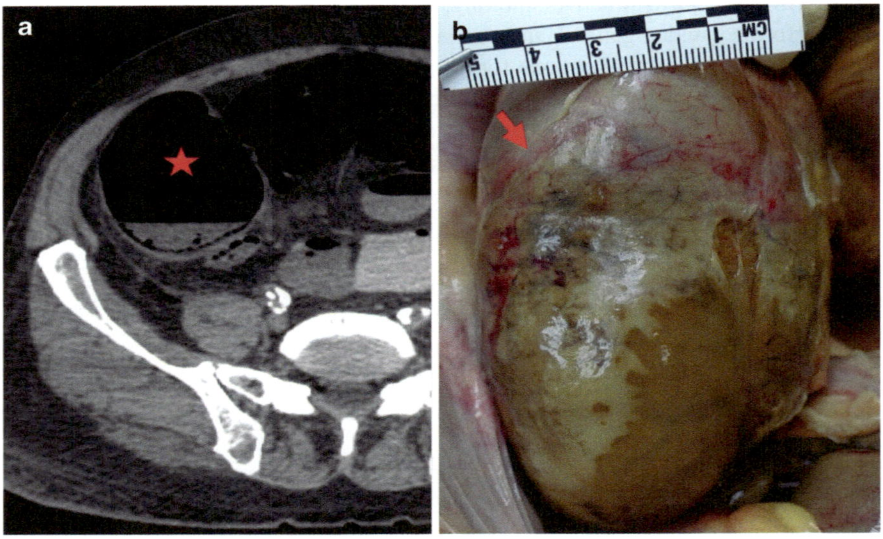

Fig. 9.1 (**a**) Post-mortem CT-scan showing dilation of the cecum (red star). (**b**) Autopsy in situ view of the anterior part of the cecum presenting diffuse green-brownish discoloration with a red–purple well-delineated edge (red arrow). (Reproduced with permission Aguiar, D, Fracasso T and Lardi C, Fatal Ogilvie's syndrome after hip surgery and review of the literature Forensic Science, Medicine and Pathology 18, 170–175 with license http://creativecommons.org/licenses/by/4.0/)

fibrinoid peritonitis. Post-mortem bacteriological analysis revealed the presence of mixed digestive bacterial flora within the peritoneal cavity and blood cultures. The analysis of peritoneal fluid showed various and numerous enteric bacteria such as *Escherichia coli* with blood cultures revealing *Escherichia coli* as well. Cause of death was then attributed to be acute peritonitis in the context of Ogilvie's syndrome with acute cecal necrosis.

Case 2

A 67-year-old male presented with a pathological fracture of the right acetabulum. He had a noted history of multiple myeloma and prostate cancer. On presentation, he was noted to have abdominal distension with an abdominal radiograph as seen in Fig. 9.2. The patient subsequently completed a magnetic resonance imaging (MRI) of the abdomen and pelvis noting a diffusely dilated ascending and transverse colon with maximum diameter of 10 cm in the cecum and a right acetabular mass.

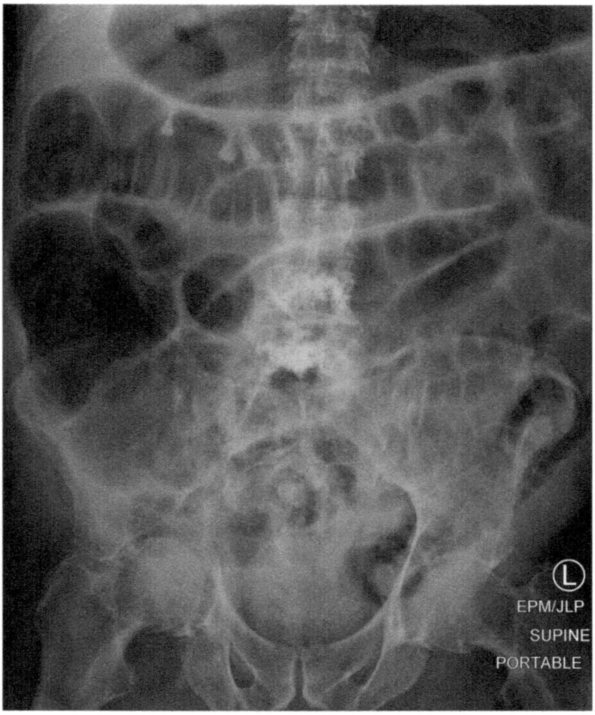

Fig. 9.2 Supine abdominal radiograph shows distension of small and large bowel. Colonic distension is most pronounced in the cecum and ascending colon. Note gastric distension and femoral head protrusion

The following day the patient underwent a soft tissue embolization of the right acetabular mass. Postembolization, the patient was given an aggressive bowel regimen. Post-admission day 2, the patient was prepped for a cemented acetabular cage reconstruction and cemented femoral stem for management of the right acetabular lesion. During intubation, the patient aspirated large volume of coffee ground emesis and the surgery was canceled. He was transferred to the surgical intensive care unit for management of hypoxic respiratory insufficiency, aspiration pneumonia, hypotension, and shock. His follow-up abdominal radiograph showed dilated small and large bowel with a cecal diameter of 13 cm (see Fig. 9.3).

The patient was diagnosed with acute colonic pseudo-obstruction (Ogilvie's syndrome) and underwent exploratory laparotomy with cecostomy tube placement on post-admission day 5. He subsequently underwent right hip reconstruction on post-admission day 13. The patient recovered without any major issues noted on his outpatient visit after discharge.

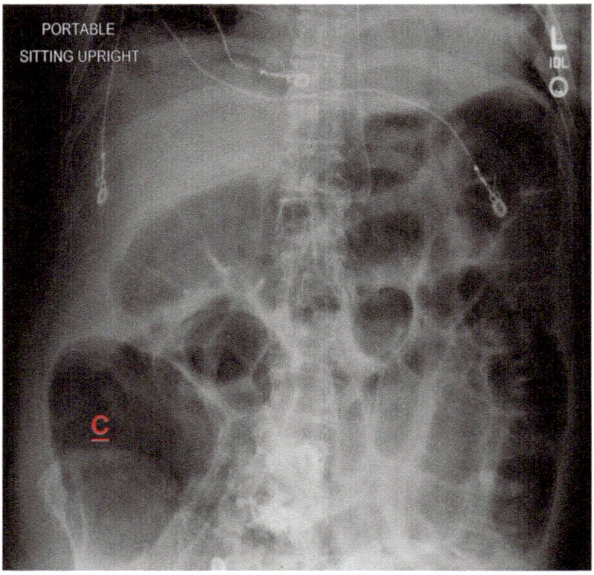

Fig. 9.3 Semi-upright abdominal radiograph with nasogastric (NG) tube in place, gastric distension resolved, and noted colonic distension most pronounced in cecum (C) and ascending colon

Questions

1. What are the main clinical indicators for acute colonic pseudo-obstruction?
2. What are the diagnostic indicators for acute colonic pseudo-obstruction? How do we differentiate it from an ileus?
3. What is the treatment for acute colonic pseudo-obstruction?

Acute Colonic Pseudo-Obstruction (ACPO) (Ogilvie's Syndrome)

Introduction

The colon compromises the distal 1–1.5 m of the gastrointestinal tract and is just distal to the terminal ileum of the small bowel and the ileocecal valve (Fig. 9.4), a muscular sphincter which may prevent reflux of the colonic contents back into the small intestine [1]. The colon's physiologic and mechanical role includes transport of fecal matter, absorption of electrolytes and water, and fermentation of bowel contents. About 1% of orthopaedic injuries and surgeries including joint arthroplasty and spine surgery are associated with acute colonic pseudo-obstruction (ACPO) [2]. Acute colonic pseudo-obstruction is described as functionally impaired transit of colonic contents secondary to uncoordinated, non-peristaltic muscle contractions leading to massive dilatation of the colon in the absence of mechanical obstruction [3]. The physiology and neurological causes of ACPO are not fully understood but suspected to be secondary to dysfunctional colonic neural response to an initial stress. In a paralytic colon, there will be continued buildup of fluid, gas, and stool within the colon. Continued colon dilation can lead to colon ischemia and perforation resulting in sepsis and death. Thus, early recognition and diagnosis of ACPO is key to prevent adverse patient outcomes.

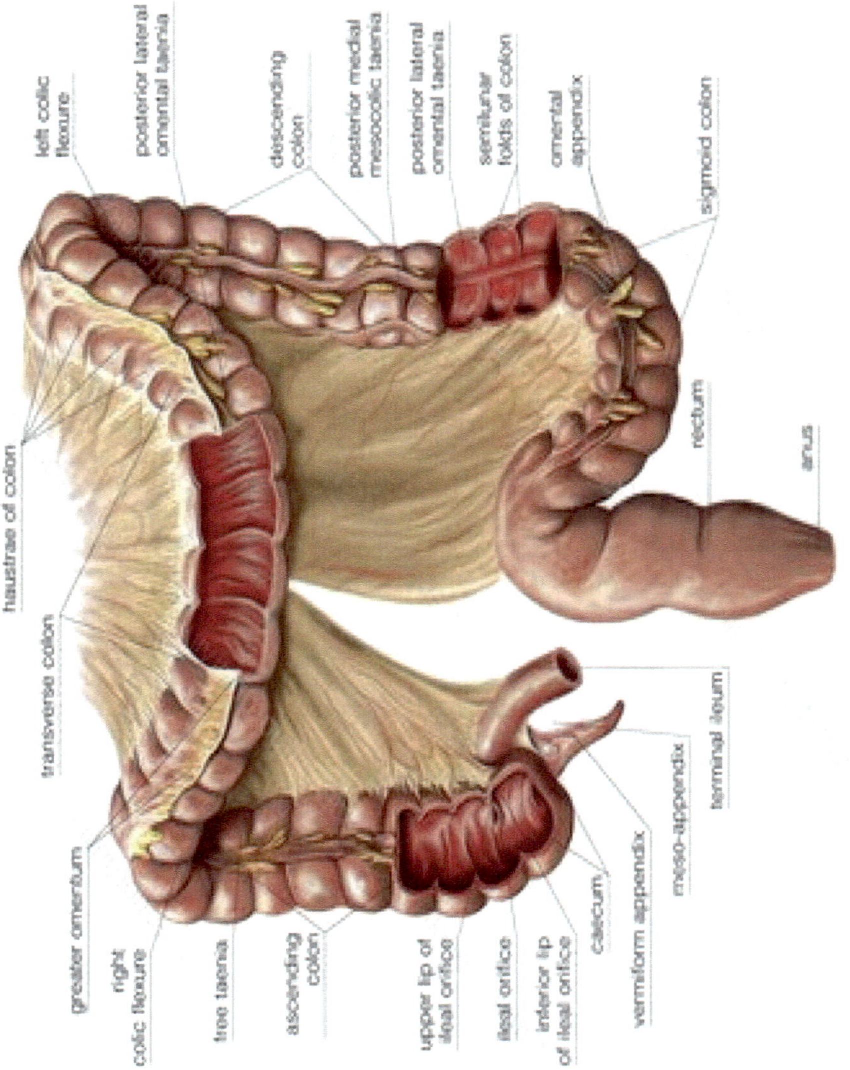

Fig. 9.4 Colon anatomy. (Reproduced with permission: ASKLEPIOS MEDICAL ATLAS/SCIENCE PHOTO LIBRARY)

Overview of Colonic Obstruction

Large-bowel obstruction (LBO) can occur via a mechanical or functional (neurological) mechanism. Mechanical causes includes blockage due to colon malignancy, colon volvulus (twisting), stricture formation (through diverticulitis or inflammatory bowel disease), ischemia, foreign body, intussusception, and external compression (adhesions, ovarian tumor or hernia) [4]. Functional mechanisms include congenital defects in number and locations of neural cells or neural connections or infectious damage leading to impairment of bowel neurological control mechanism. Hirschsprung's disease is a congenital disorder due to absence, maldistribution, or reduced number of neural ganglions in colon at birth, leading to distal colonic obstruction [5]. Depending on the number of neural ganglions missing, presentation of Hirschsprung's can occur in an infant or even in the elderly with varying symptoms [6]. An infectious cause of decreased colonic neural ganglion includes Chaga's disease (*Trypanosoma cruzi* parasitic infection). This infection destroys neural ganglions leading to smooth muscle degeneration with chronic megacolon [7]. Another rare infectious cause is herpes zoster, which can also lead to neural degeneration and functional colon obstruction [8]. The underlying pathophysiology is destruction of neural system in the colon itself.

Mechanical and functional obstruction in the colon can lead to an increase in pressure and proximal colon distention, especially in patients with competent ileocecal valves. Laplace's law states that tension in the walls of colon is proportional to the pressure of colon contents and the colonic radius [9, 10]. When the intraluminal pressure increases with fluid distention in the cecum, it leads to increased wall tension constricting arterial flow and venous congestion within the wall itself. The ensuing bowel ischemia may cause necrosis and perforation. In patients with competent ileocecal valves, ileal contents including stool and gas accumulate in the cecum after passing through the small bowel and cannot decompress retrograde into the small intestines due to the ileocecal valve. The lack of forward flow due to presumed neural pathology places the greatest intraluminal pressure in the cecum, and accordingly, making the cecum the most likely site of perforation [10]. Anatomically the perforation occurs most commonly on the anterior surface of the cecum [11].

Another form of functional paralytic intestinal obstruction is ileus where there is obstruction due to impaired transit of intestinal contents throughout the entire intestine including the stomach, small intestine, and colon. There are many causes of an ileus including recent abdominal surgery [3]. A key distinction between an ileus and other pathologies is that there is no significant cecal dilation. Most commonly, for an ileus, gastrointestinal function returns in the small bowel around 1 to 24 h, gastric function in 24–36 h, and colonic motility around 48–72 h [12]. Colon motility, however, may take up to 6 days to fully recover.

Acute Colonic Pseudo-Obstruction (ACPO)

A functional non-mechanical dilation of the large intestine is acute colonic pseudo-obstruction (ACPO). Commonly known as Ogilvie's syndrome, the condition was first described by Sir W. H. Ogilvie in 1948 [13]. He noted two patients with retroperitoneal malignancy and significant colon dilation without a mechanical obstruction. Sir Ogilvie theorized that there was autonomic dysfunction leading to the dilation. The current prevailing hypothesis for ACPO centers on stressor/s leading to an imbalance between sympathetic and parasympathetic inputs leading to colon atony or uncoordinated peristalsis [14, 15].

Background

The adult colon is a muscular tube between 1 m and 1.5 m [1]. Anatomically, the colonic wall has longitudinal muscular bands that are termed tenia. The tenia are shorter than the intestine itself, thus allowing for the formation of small pouches throughout it length (called haustral sacs) (Fig 9.4). The ascending and descending colon are fixed by visceral peritoneum and are thus retroperitoneal. The transverse colon is fixed at its proximal and distal ends by ligaments at the hepatic and splenic flexure. The omentum arising from the gastrocolic ligament also attaches to the transverse colon. Neural inputs allow for non-propulsive and propulsive forces to move contents from the ileum. This has also been described as haustral contraction and mass movement contraction [16]. Non-propulsive phasic contractions or haustral contractions allow for mixing of chyme, water absorption, and stool formation. Propulsive phasic contractions or mass movement contractions allow for stool passage from the cecum to the rest of the colon.

Function of Colon

The primary digestive and absorptive organ in the gastrointestinal tract is the small intestine [17]. This is the site of absorption of 90% of water as well as nutrients and vitamins. The colon function is to store the contents from the small intestine, secrete antibacterial substances, and allow for further absorption of electrolytes, water, fat-soluble vitamins (including vitamin K), and other bacterial metabolites. The colonic absorption of water leads to stool formation. As noted above, non-propulsive and propulsive forces maximize absorption and move stool from the proximal to distal colon. Overall, approximately 1–1.5 L of liquid contents are presented to the cecum from the small intestine, which eventually forms on average ~0.2 kg stool, per day.

Bacterial Load Colon

The colon microbiota is essential for providing metabolism of vitamins and enhancing the immune system [18, 19]. For an average 70 kg male, the number of bacteria in the colon is estimated at 3.8 x 10^{13} [20]. Bacteria, in the anaerobic, nitrogen-rich environment, specializes in fermentation [21]. In addition to the bacterial population, the colon has fungi, archaea, protozoa, and viral phages [18]. This massive and complex microbiome clearly supports the essential nature of the immune system to protect the colon and organism.

There are four bacterial phyla represented in the colon which comprise 98% of microbes in the gastrointestinal tract: bacteroides (*Bacteroides fragilis*), firmicutes (*Bacillus* and *Staphylococcus*), proteobacteria (*Escherichia Coli, Klebsiella*, and *Enterobacter*) and actinobacteria (*Propionibacterium* and *Corynebacterium*) [18, 21].

Most bacteria reside in the stool itself, but within the colon, certain bacteria reside in the loose outer mucus layer which extends several hundreds of microns into the lumen from the colon inner surface, the mucosa. Those close to the mucosa are oxygen-tolerant bacteria such as proteobacteria and actinobacteria. The intestinal mucosa is covered by an inner mucus layer which limits bacterial colonization of the intestinal mucosa—both physically and biologically [22].

Colon Neural Pathways

The autonomic nervous system has traditionally been described as controlling unconscious activity such as smooth muscle, glands, and heart rate, whereas the somatic nervous system is described as controlling conscious activity such as locomotion through striated muscles, and sensation (Fig. 9.5). The colon is innervated by the autonomic nervous system which includes the enteric nervous system (ENS) which is intrinsic (self-contained) within the colon) and the parasympathetic/sympathetic nervous system which neurally connects the brain and spinal cord to the colon and has a significant presence within the colon including connections to the ENS [23, 24] (Fig 9.6).

The enteric nervous system (ENS) has the largest concentration of neural elements outside of the brain, with over 100 million nerve cell bodies and more than 500 million neurons and supporting glia [25–28]. Initially described by Von Haller in the 1700s, the complexity and redundancy of the ENS allows for an intestinal segment to be removed and still have contracting function [29]. The ENS multidirectionally communicates with the intestinal epithelialium, endocrine cells, immune cells, and the parasympathetic/sympathetic nervous system. The ENS is located between the muscularis propria and epithelium, also called the submucosal plexus or Meissner plexus (see Fig 9.6), which acts in a digestive capacity regulating functions such as absorption, secretion, and local blood flow in response to the presence of contents. The ENS is also located between the longitudinal and circular

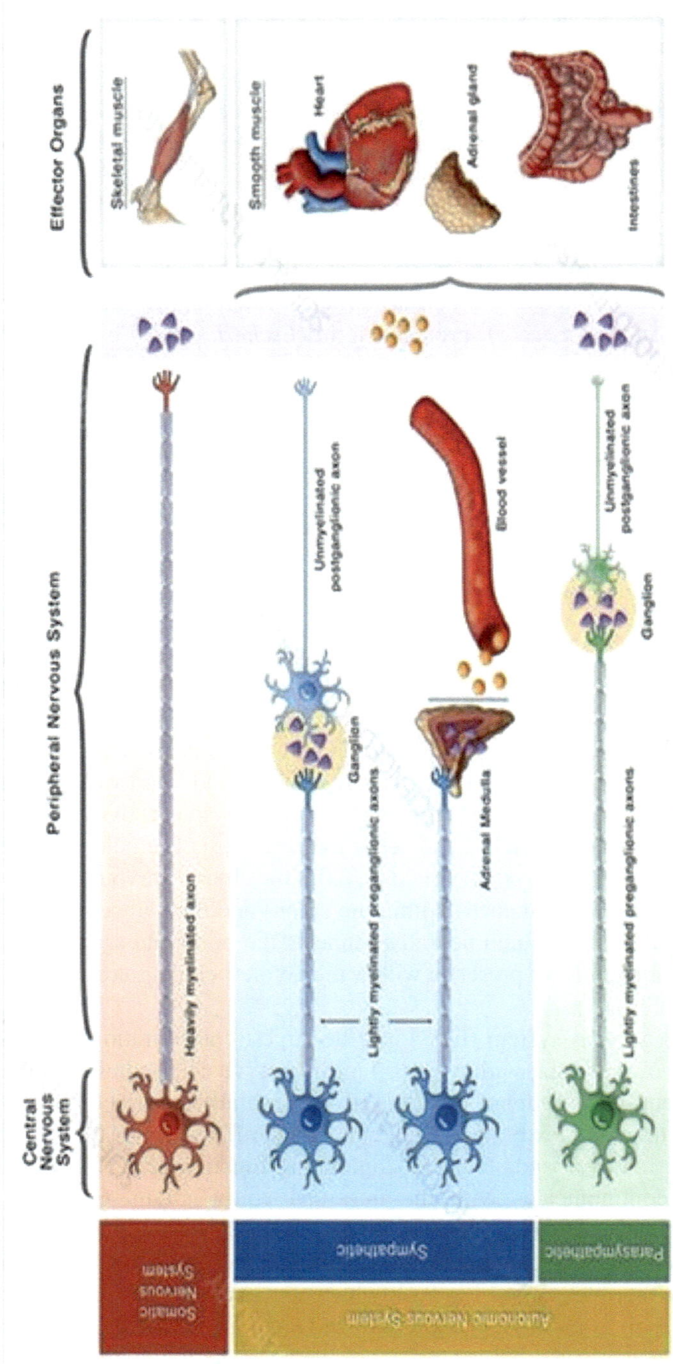

Fig. 9.5 Comparison of autonomic and somatic motor system. (Reproduced with permission OpenStax)

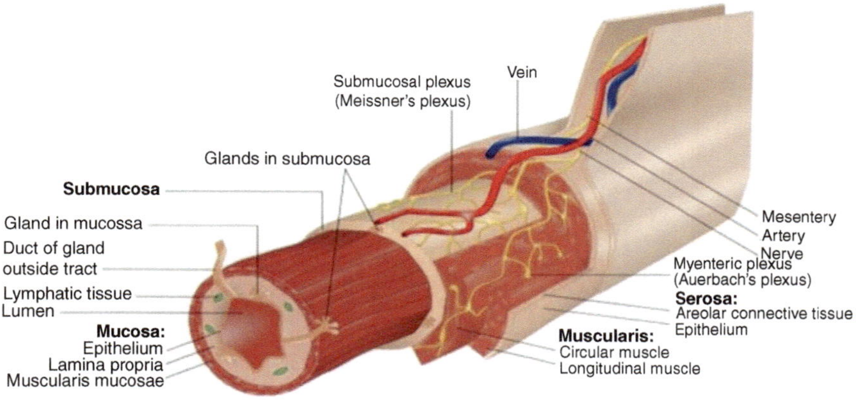

Fig. 9.6 Location of neural component in the colon. (Reproduced with permission OpenStax)

muscle as the myenteric plexus, which regulates peristaltic activity and motility (Fig. 9.5) [25, 28]. The submucosal and myenteric plexus respond to input of both sympathetic and parasympathetic neurons and mucosal enteroendocrine cells [25, 30, 31].

The sympathetic and parasympathetic autonomic nerve system connects the forebrain and brainstem and spine to the ENS system (Figs. 9.5, 9.6, and 9.7). The sympathetic and parasympathetic autonomic nerve system differ in their pathways [31]. Sympathetic innervation to the ascending colon and proximal transverse colon originates in the T7-T12 splanchnic nerve column which travel to celiac and superior mesenteric ganglia (conglomeration of nerve cells). These sympathetic nerves travel along the superior mesenteric artery to the colon. The distal colon (distal transverse), descending and sigmoid receives sympathetic nervous innervation originating from L1 to L3, traveling along the inferior mesenteric blood supply. A major function of the sympathetic nervous system is to inhibit secretory and contractility functions of the colon [23].

The vagus nerve supplies the parasympathetic system from the upper gastrointestinal tract to the splenic flexure and the sacral parasympathetic nerves (S2-S5) supply the left colon, sigmoid, and rectum. Again, sympathetic stimuli result in the inhibition of bowel motility and the contraction of sphincters. T7-T13 supply the sympathetic tone to the right colon, whereas L1-L3 supply the left colon. Parasympathetic input to the proximal colon segments is supplied by the vagus nerve, and distally, colon parasympathetic input is supplied by S2-S4 splanchnic nerves (Fig. 9.7). The parasympathetic system activates gastrointestinal motility and bladder tone. The vast majority of vagal nerve fibers are sensory and thus transmit input from bowel to the central nervous system. In opposition to the parasympathetic input from vagal and sacral outflow, sympathetic pathways inhibit enteric motor circuits through paravertebral ganglia and splanchnic nerves [25].

Notably, there is evidence that bacteria in the microbiome participate in neuronal, endocrine, and immune signaling pathways. ENS pathways respond to microbial signals produced by bacteria which help regulate intestinal secretion, motility,

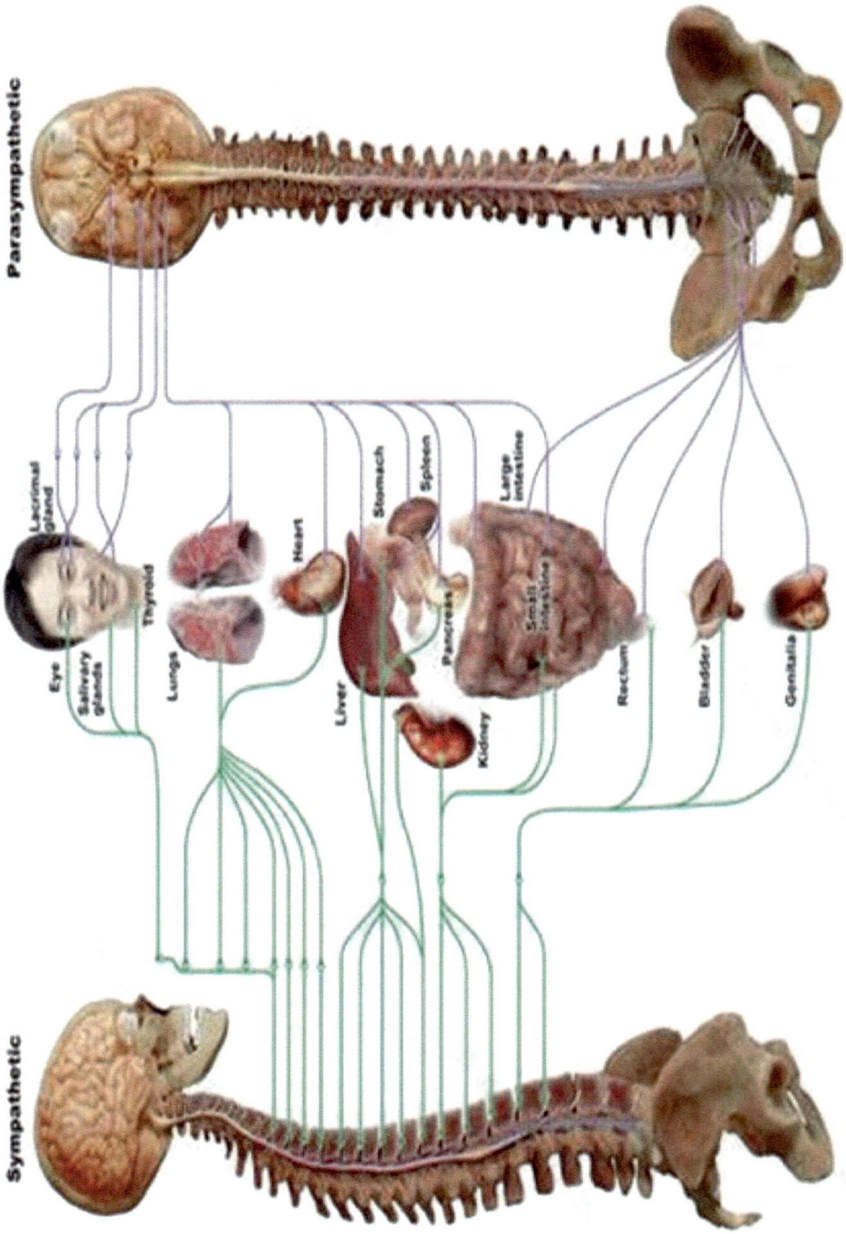

Fig. 9.7 Pathway of Sympathetic and Parasympathetic Branches. (Reproduced with permission from OpenStax)

permeability, and immunity to both control the environment and overall composition of enteric microbiota [28, 32, 33]. Further research is ongoing about the implications on changes to the microbiome and its effect on the brain-gut axis.

Autonomic neuropathy has been noted in patients with chronic idiopathic intestinal pseudo-obstruction [34]. Diabetic and other neurologically afflicted patients have been identified with both abdominal vagal neuropathy and chronic intestinal pseudo-obstruction. Although causal relationship between chronic neurological disorders and ACPO have presumed to be present [35], this is not established. There is some data suggesting a loss of interstitial cells of cajal in the colon, which are "pacemaker" cells (where peristaltic waves originate) is associated with cases of chronic pseudo-obstruction [36].

Parasympathetic Drug Activity

Acetylcholine is a cholinergic neurotransmitter of the parasympathetic nervous system that promotes the digestive and motility functions of the gastrointestinal tract. Anticholinergic medications inhibit the action of acetylcholine both in the central and peripheral nervous system thereby reducing digestion and gut motility. Adverse effects of anticholinergics include flushing, anhidrosis, altered mental status, urinary retention, and gastrointestinal paralysis [37]. These adverse effects are more prevalent in the geriatric population due to a greater exposure to these medications and enhanced sensitivity [38]. There have been associations with polypharmacy and admissions to the hospital for the geriatric population with the use of anticholinergics (particularly antipsychotics) [39, 40]. The use of these medications opposing the natural cholinergic effect on the colon is amplified with anticholinergics as aging per se reduces the cholinergic function of individuals above 65 years of age [41]. Thus constipation is a more significant issue in the elderly. Moreover, anticholinergic medications have been associated with ACPO. Thus, it is important to identify medications that could lead to anticholinergic effects on the gastrointestinal tract. Table 9.1 lists common parasympathetic related anticholinergic medications. Some medications have been noted to have a higher cholinergic load; however, unfortunately, anticholinergic potency is difficult to determine and scale appropriately, given the differences in metabolism, drug interactions, and complexity in measuring cumulative doses and effect [42].

Sympathetic Drug Activity

In opposition to the effect of anticholinergics are the sympathomimetic drugs, which increase the effect of neurotransmitters that inhibit colon motility and function. Sympathetic-stimulating agents (including epinephrine and norepinephrine) can release a "fight or flight" response acting on sympathetic ganglions to indirectly counteract the innate cholinergic activity of the body which has been empirically demonstrated in animal models [45]. Table 9.2 identifies medications that stimulate

Table 9.1 Anticholinergic drugs (inhibit parasympathetic system) [42–44]

Antidepressants	
Clomipramine[a] Desipramine [a] Imipramine [a] Doxepin [a] Fluoxetine Fluvoxamine Mirtazapine	Nortriptyline Paroxetine Sertraline Trazodone Protriptyline Trimipramine
Antiemetics	
Promethazine Prochlorperazine	
Antiepileptics	
Carbamazepine[a] Oxcarbazepine[a] Valproate	
Antihistamines (typically sleep and cold medication over the counter)	
Azelastine nasal spray Brompheniramine Carbinoxamine Clemastine Chlorpheniramine Cyproheptadine Dexbrompheniramine Dexchlorpheniramine	Diphenhydramine[a] Hydroxyzine Loratadine Mepyramine Olopatadine nasal spray Phenyltoloxamine Promethazine Triprolidine
Antihypertensives (including calcium channel blocking agents)	
Verapamil Clonidine	
Anti-Parkinson medications	
Amantadine Benztropine Mesylate Biperiden[a] Bromocriptine	Carbidopa- Levodopa Pramipexol Selegiline Trihexyphenidyl[a]
Antipsychotic medications	
Chlorpromazine [a] Clozapine[a] Fluphenazine[a] Haloperidol Loxapine[a] Molindone	Perphenazine[a] Quetiapine Thioridazine Ziprasidone Olanzapine[a]
Antispasmodics/antidiarrheal	
Atropine[a] Belladonna alkaloids [a] Clidinium Dicyclomine	Hyoscyamine Loperamide Methscopolamine Propantheline
Anti-ulcer	
Cimetidine Glycopyrrolate	Ranitidine

Table 9.1 (continued)

Benzodiazepines	
Alprazolam Chlordiazepoxide Clonazepam Clorazepate Diazepam	Flurazepam Lorazepam Midazolam
Bladder (urological) drugs	
Oxybutynin Tolterodine Darifenacin	Flavoxate Solifenacin Trospium
Bronchodilator medications	
Fluticasone-Salmeterol	
Cardiac medications	
Digoxin Diltiazem Warfarin	
Corticosteroids	
Cortisone Dexamethasone Methylprednisolone	Prednisone Hydrocortisone
Diuretics	
Captopril Chlorthalidone	
Opioids	
Codeine Fentanyl	Morphine Tramadol
Infection	
Ampicillin Cefalotin Cefamandole Cefoxitin Clindamycin	Cycloserine Gentamicin Piperacillin Tobramycin Vancomycin
Movement disorder medications	
Benztropine[a] Trihexyphenidyl[a] Procyclidine	

[a]high anticholinergic load

Table 9.2 Sympathomimetic drugs (promote sympathetic nervous system) [46–48]

Ephedrine (direct agonist)	Cocaine
Dobutamine	Phentolamine
Clonidine	Isoproterenol
Epinephrine	Isoprenaline
Tyramine	Salmeterol
Monoamine oxidase inhibitor	Terbutaline
Phenylephrine	
Amphetamines	
Dopamine	
Methyldopa	

the sympathetic nervous system. Unlike anticholinergics, sympathetic-stimulating medications have not been demonstrated to be associated with ACPO.

Acute Colonic Pseudo-Obstruction (ACPO)

Epidemiology of ACPO

ACPO has an estimated incidence of one case per 1000 inpatient admissions per year in the United States [49]. Orthopaedic admissions for joint arthroplasty have reported ACPO rates of 0.29–5.6% [50–53]. In a large retrospective cohort of 1060 patients, ACPO was diagnosed in 1.6%, 2.7%, and 2.6% for acetabular, pelvic, and combined fractures, respectively [54]. ACPO has also been noted as a complication of post-cardiac surgery at 0.06–5%, post-C-section at 0.1%, and burn surgeries at 0.29% [49, 55, 56]. The elderly are at greater risk for complications involving ACPO post-procedure or surgery [57]. Average age for ACPO was 59.9 for males and 56.5 for females without a difference in the frequency between the genders [58, 59]. ACPO seems to occur (94.5%) after an initial stressor, commonly after surgery or a medical condition [58]. Table 9.3 lists conditions associated with ACPO. In the elderly and in certain postoperative conditions, opioids use is associated with ACPO. Opioids mediate their gastrointestinal effects through mu, kappa, and delta opioid effects affecting areas in the submucosal and myenteric plexus to decrease intestinal secretion, disrupting peristalsis and reducing gut motility [95].

Presentation

Acute Colonic Pseudo-Obstruction (ACPO) is defined as severe functional impairment of transit for colonic contents in the absence of mechanical obstruction (colon volvulus, malignancy, stricture). This results in massive colon dilation with a risk of colonic perforation above 11 cm in diameter [52]. The mechanism behind ACPO, as noted, is suspected to be autonomic dysfunction leading to an imbalance between sympathetic and parasympathetic inputs into the enteric nervous system causing uncoordinated, non-peristaltic muscle contractions [3, 57]. Prolonged recumbency has been postulated to play a role in decreased peristalsis and increasing risk of ACPO.

Although ACPO can occur at any age, ACPO occurs most often in elderly, bedridden patients with severe underlying disease. Patients present with loss of bowel movements and progressive abdominal distension. Surgical patients with ACPO onset of symptoms from 1 to 6 days (typically at day 3–5) postoperatively [58]. Symptoms include abdominal pain, nausea, and vomiting (present in 80% of patients). Other symptoms may include obstipation and fever. Although constipation is the most common symptom, there is a subset of ACPO with profuse diarrhea with hypokalemia, due to colonic hypersecretion of potassium [96]. On physical

Table 9.3 Conditions associated with acute colonic pseudo-obstruction [60–62]

Connective Tissue Disease	
Systemic sclerosis [63] Lupus [64] Vasculitis [65]	
Neurological	
Dementia [66] Alzheimer's disease Spinal cord injury Epilepsy	Ventriculoperitoneal shunt placement [67] Guillain-Barré syndrome [68] Parkinson's disease
Cardiopulmonary	
Myocardial infarction [58]	
Endocrine	
Diabetes [69] Thyroid dysfunction [70] Amyloidosis [71]	Calciphylaxis [72] Pheochromocytoma [73]
Surgery	
Intra-abdominal surgery [3] Joint reconstruction [2, 50, 51, 74] Cervical spine surgery [75] Lumbar spine surgery [76] Appendicitis [77] Cesarean section [78] Burns [79]	Hip or pelvic fractures [80] Renal transplantation [81] Renal calculus [82]
Neoplasm	
Retroperitoneal malignancy [13] Pancreatic malignancy [10]	
Infection	
Chagas [7] CMV [83] Herpetic/varicella zoster [8, 84] SARS-CoV2 [85] Lyme [86] Pneumonia [87]	
Electrolyte abnormalities	
Hypokalemia [88] Hyponatremia [89] Hypercalcemia [89, 90]	
Miscellaneous	
Sickle cell [91] Post-colonoscopy [92] Obesity Acute intermittent porphyria [93] Age > 65 [94]	

exam, patients most often have a tympanitic, distended abdomen with hypoactive or absent bowel sounds (Fig. 9.9). A minority of patients may have bowel sounds, given small bowel function may still be present. There may be an empty rectum on digital exam. The most relevant of these findings is the abdominal distention which is present in 90–100% of patients and can be progressive, in addition to nausea and vomiting [58]. Patient evaluation with thorough history and physical exam is required to identify the urgency of clinical condition. Patients with tachycardia, hypotension, and peritonitis on abdominal exam (rebound pain and guarding to palpation in all quadrants) may require emergent surgical exploration for suspected perforation. Patients with stable vital sign with otherwise benign findings and abdominal distention, require timely workup including review of potassium, sodium, calcium, magnesium, thyroid-stimulating hormone (TSH) and medications (opioids). A rectal exam should be completed to exclude a very distal mechanical obstruction such as impacted stool or tumor. Consultation with a gastroenterologist or general surgeon should be expedited to confirm diagnosis and initiate early treatment management.

Diagnosis

Radiographic imaging is critical to determine the degree and extent of colonic distention, presence of perforation, status of colon wall itself, and identify causes of colon obstruction. Plain films of the abdomen (supine and ideally upright or left side down decubitus) help identify signs of perforation (free air), degree of colonic distention, presence of fecal impaction, and competence of the ileocecal valve (air-fluid levels within the small intestine are consistent with an incompetent valve) (Figs. 9.8, 9.9, 9.10, 9.11, and 9.12). CT is the test of choice since it can better assess presence and cause of obstruction, including evidence for free air, bowel perforation, and ischemia. CT with intravenous contrast is preferrable to non-contrast studies as it allows a more optimal evaluation of the bowel wall and mesenteric vasculature (Fig. 9.13).

Although the entire colon can dilate with ACPO, the cecum has the greatest baseline diameter and receives ileal contents first, thereby typically having the highest

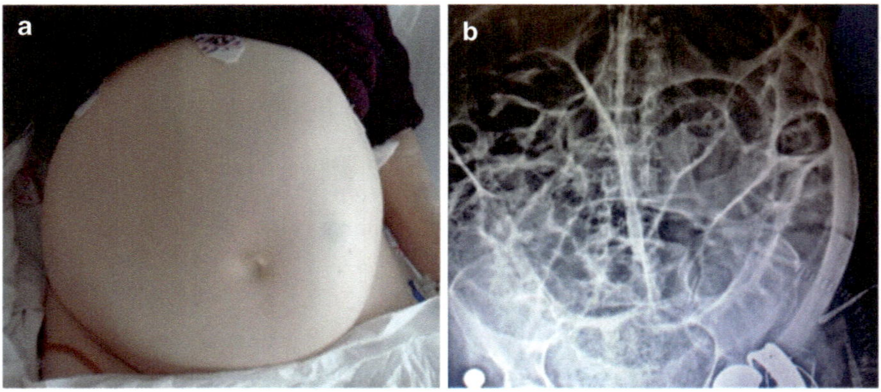

Fig. 9.8 (**a**) Distended abdomen. (**b**) Correlation with radiographs

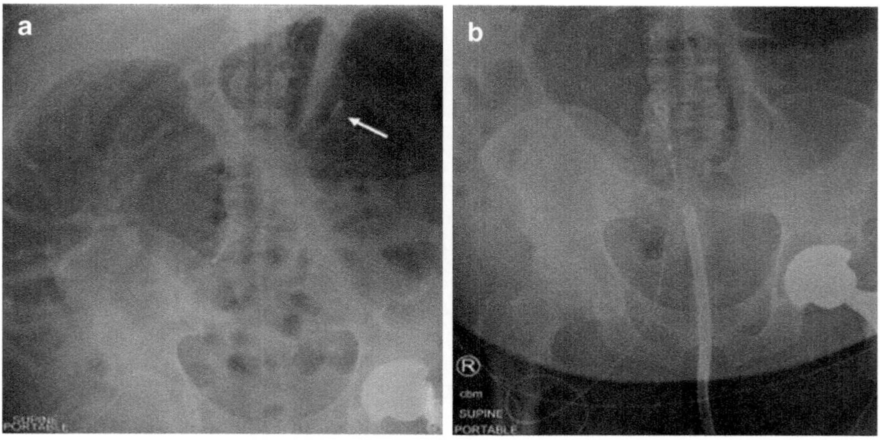

Fig. 9.9 (**a**) KUB with colonic distention with feeding tube terminating in the distal duodenum (white arrow). (**b**) Supine KUB following large bore rectal tube placement

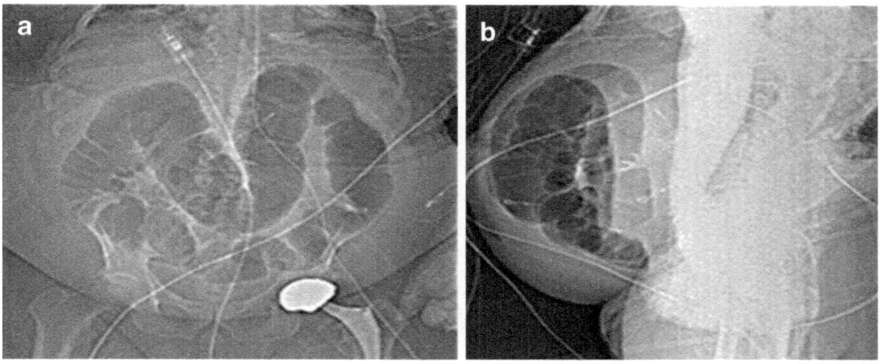

Fig. 9.10 Supine (**a**) and lateral (**b**) scout topograms showing colonic distention

intralumenal pressure. Thus, cecal diameter is used as a measure for risk of colon ischemia and perforation. Cecal diameter of 11 cm or greater has been associated with a greater rate of perforation [58, 97, 98]. Clinical or radiographic signs of perforation or colonic ischemia are indications for urgent surgery.

Non-operative cases should be closely monitored with serial patient evaluations including abdominal exams and radiography to ensure the patient does not progress to signs and symptoms of colonic perforation or ischemia. In addition, continual monitoring of vitals, electrolytes, and medications are important to exclude reversible causes to ACPO.

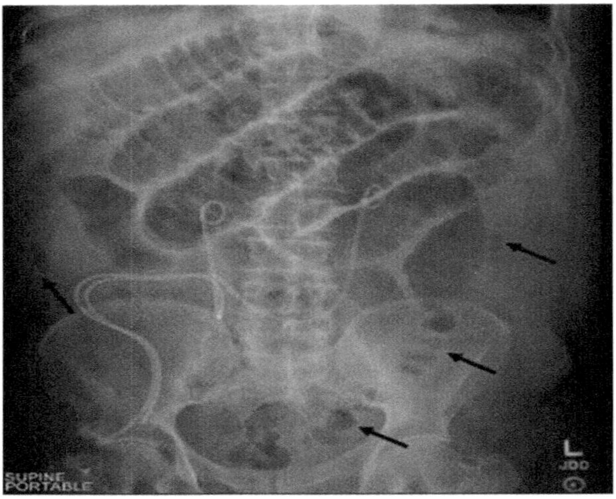

Fig. 9.11 Small bowel distention with supine radiograph of the abdomen showing multiple dilated, gas-filled loops of small bowel centrally located in the abdomen with a small amount of gas in the decompressed distal small bowel and in the colon (black arrows). Findings are consistent with small bowel obstruction. Also note bilateral nephron-ureteral stents in this patient status post-cystectomy with ileal conduit

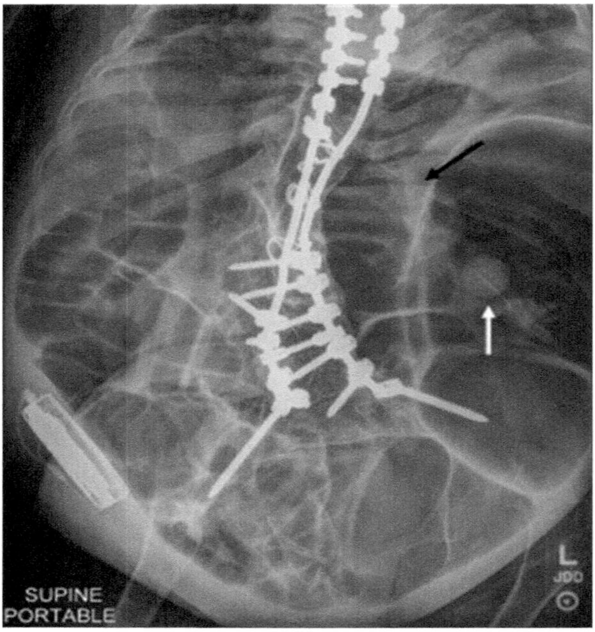

Fig. 9.12 Colonic distention. Supine radiograph of the abdomen shows a diffusely dilated, gas-filled colon. There is a nasogastric tube in pace (black arrow) as well as a gastrostomy tube (white arrow). Also note extensive surgical hardware in the spine and a neurostimulator device in place with mechanical pack in the right lower abdominal wall

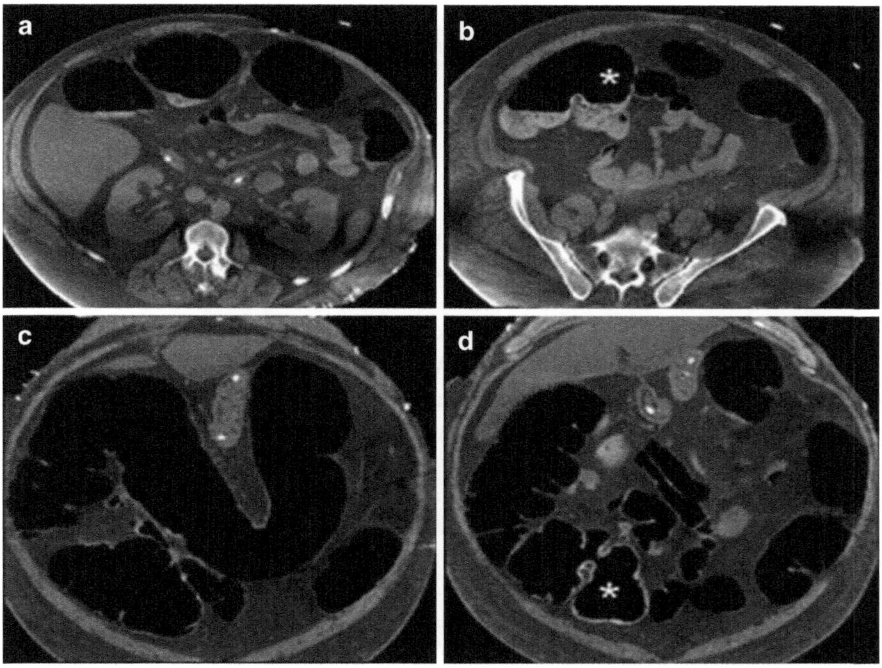

Fig. 9.13 Colonic distention on CT. (**a** and **b**) Axial and (**c** and **d**) coronal non-contrast CT images show a diffusely dilation, gas-filled colon. Small bowel loops are decompressed. No transition point was seen to suggest obstruction. * = Cecum

Treatment

Historically, there has been a strong recommendation for placement of a nasogastric (NG) tube to suction in all patients with ACPO, even in the absence of nausea and vomiting [99]. The nasogastric tube not only drains gastric secretions and decompresses the stomach, but it theoretically limits the amount of swallowed air. However, more recent literature suggests that the NG tube may not be as impactful as previously thought. Case 2 demonstrates a scenario where an NG tube may have had a therapeutic effect.

In patients with less than 11 cm of cecal dilation without perforation or signs of ischemia, initial treatment should be conservative management. This includes bowel rest, consideration of nasogastric tube decompression, and rectal tube placement (red rubber). There should be close surveillance of patients to include serial abdominal examinations, abdominal radiographs, and laboratory studies to monitor for electrolyte disturbances and infection. Specifically, serum potassium, calcium, sodium, phosphate, and magnesium should be monitored. It is important to continually monitor the patients' medications and limit opioids or other anticholinergic medications. Rates of success with conservative management are reported from studies in the 1980s as above 77% [58, 100]. Notably, spontaneous resolution of ACPO was less likely in post-surgical patients and patients with opioid exposure [100, 101].

Medical

Medical treatment can be considered for individuals who fail to improve with conservative measures. Neostigmine is a short-acting anticholinesterase parasympathomimetic that currently has the highest quality of evidence for ACPO but is not currently FDA approved for this indication. Patients given neostigmine should be monitored.

A meta-analysis in 127 patients with ACPO comparing one dose of neostigmine (2.5 mg) versus control group (conservative therapy) showed an effectiveness of 85–94% to resolve ACPO in neostigmine patients compared to 14.8% of control patients. Most common side effects were abdominal pain in 53.1%, hypersalivation in 31.1%, vomiting in 15.6%, and bradycardia in 6.3% [102–105]. Atropine should be available for symptomatic bradycardia and glycopyrrolate for hypersalivation. Absolute contraindications to neostigmine include mechanical bowel or urinary obstruction. Relative contraindications include recent myocardial infarction, acidosis, asthma, bradycardia, peptic ulcer disease, and β-blocker therapy [102, 106]. The initial neostigmine dose in an adult is 2.0–2.5 mg intravenous once over 3–5 min. Neostigmine treatment can be repeated with a second dose for patients with an incomplete response, patients without a response, or those with a recurrence. Repeat neostigmine doses can be given one to two times within 3 h of the initial dose. A study in 2018 also demonstrated efficacy with subcutaneous neostigmine ACPO [107]. Similar to intravenous dosing, atropine and glycopyrrolate should be available in case of bradycardia and hypersalivation. A benefit to subcutaneous dosing is not requiring intensive care unit monitoring; instead, subcutaneous dosing of neostigmine can be given on a regular hospital ward floor.

Recurrence of ACPO after neostigmine treatment may be prevented by administration of polyethylene glycol (PEG). In a group of 30 patients randomized to PEG versus placebo treatment following successful neostigmine treatment for ACPO, patients treated with PEG had a recurrence rate of 0% compared to 33% of controls. PEG treatment also resulted in greater gas and stool evacuation and decreased cecal distension compared to control treatment [108].

Failure of response to neostigmine should then lead to consideration of endoscopic or surgical management. As noted previously, patients should be continually monitored for signs of electrolyte abnormalities and infection. In addition, if there is any opioid exposure, addition of methylnaltrexone can be considered.

Endoscopic Decompression

Endoscopic decompression is reserved for patients who have failed conservative measures, have contraindications to neostigmine, or in whom neostigmine has failed. Endoscopic decompression of the colon is highly variable with highest response rates seen in the 70% of patients in the acute phase of ACPO [109]. However, recurrence rates of cecal distention of 10–65% have been noted after initial success [110, 111].

Additional benefits of endoscopic decompression include definitive assessment of the colon to rule out mechanical obstruction and visualization of the colonic mucosa to rule out early ischemic changes [112]. Colonoscopy for ACPO should be performed with narcotic sparing anesthesia, if possible [113]. If there is concern for aspiration due to small bowel distention, the patient may require rapid sequence intubation. In order to avoid further colonic dilation, carbon dioxide insufflation during colonoscopy is preferred due to its greater solubility compared to air.

Surgical Decompression

Surgical Intervention is reserved for patients with persistent ACPO despite maximal medical treatment and intervention. Traditionally, laparotomy with placement of colostomy has been used in patients without signs of ischemia or perforation on abdominal exploration. More recently, cecostomy placement has been used in patients with refractory ACPO. Cecostomy tube decompression may be performed percutaneously, laparoscopically or with open surgical technique [114–116]. Overall, surgery is the treatment of last resort in ACPO patients, unless there are signs of ischemia or perforation.

Conclusion

Ogilvie's syndrome, although uncommon, can cause significant morbidity and mortality in hospitalized patients. ACPO patients can enjoy a good prognosis and early resolution of symptoms (6–8 days) with prompt diagnosis and medical treatment. Due to its association with major orthopaedic procedures, the orthopaedic surgeon should be knowledgeable about ACPO to initiate early recognition. Most patients will respond to medical optimization (avoidance of exacerbating medications and increased mobility) but some patients will require medical treatment with neostigmine, endoscopic decompression, or surgical decompression. Failure to properly recognize and manage this process can result in perforation and ischemia, which can lead to a 44% surgical mortality rate [58]. With advancing technology, improved medical treatment for ACPO can be anticipated but early provider recognition and patient treatment will remain paramount.

Summary

1. What are the main clinical indicators for acute colonic pseudo-obstruction (ACPO)?
   ACPO or Ogilvie's syndrome should be considered in patients who have abdominal distention, abdominal pain and nausea. Absence of flatus or bowel movements are likely but not required and the patient may still have loose bowel

movements. A patient with ACPO may progress to fever and sepsis and in severe cases colon perforation and death (Case 1).

2. What are the diagnostic indicators for acute colonic pseudo-obstruction? How do we differentiate it from an ileus?
After clinical suspicion of ACPO, radiographic imaging is necessary to rule out mechanical obstruction and assess the colon wall. Computed tomography (CT) imaging with contrast is most often used to assess cecal diameter and determine if there is a perforation. A cecal diameter greater than 11 cm has a higher risk of perforation. CT imaging can also assess for ischemia and necrosis and more sensitive, if completed with contrast. Abdominal plain films can be used to assess interval changes.
An ileus is another form of paralytic intestinal obstruction involving the whole gastrointestinal tract. Radiographically, an ileus will not have cecal dilation typical of ACPO. Bowel motility returns within 72 hrs, most often, and does not lead to complications, such as perforation.
3. What is the treatment for acute colonic pseudo-obstruction (ACPO)?
ACPO may resolve without any medical intervention. For patients with a cecal diameter greater than or equal to 11 cm, neostigmine, an acetylcholinesterase inhibitor, can be administered. Endoscopic decompression of the colon can be considered if patients do not respond to neostigmine. Surgical or interventional radiology placement of a cecostomy tube is reserved for patients who fail to respond to neostigmine treatment and endoscopic decompression.

References

1. Levine DS, Haggitt RC. Normal histology of the colon. Am J Surg Pathol. 1989;13(11):966–84.
2. Norwood MG, Lykostratis H, Garcea G, Berry DP. Acute colonic pseudo-obstruction following major orthopaedic surgery. Color Dis. 2005;7(5):496–9. https://doi.org/10.1111/j.1463-1318.2005.00790.x.
3. Batke M, Cappell MS. Adynamic ileus and acute colonic pseudo-obstruction. Med Clin North Am. 2008;92(3):649–70. https://doi.org/10.1016/j.mcna.2008.01.002.
4. Jaffe T, Thompson WM. Large-bowel obstruction in the adult: classic radiographic and CT findings, etiology, and mimics. Radiology. 2015;275(3):651–63. https://doi.org/10.1148/radiol.2015140916.
5. Doodnath R, Puri P. A systematic review and meta-analysis of Hirschsprung's disease presenting after childhood. Pediatr Surg Int. 2010;26(11):1107–10. https://doi.org/10.1007/s00383-010-2694-2.
6. Ahmad T, Riaz M, Khan A, Khan MM. Hirschsprung's disease: A rare entity in adults. J Coll Physicians Surg Pak. 2019;29(7):674–6. https://doi.org/10.29271/jcpsp.2019.07.674.
7. Jabari S, de Oliveira EC, Brehmer A, da Silveira AB. Chagasic megacolon: enteric neurons and related structures. Histochem Cell Biol. 2014;142(3):235–44. https://doi.org/10.1007/s00418-014-1250-x.
8. Edelman DA, Antaki F, Basson MD, Salwen WA, Gruber SA, Losanoff JE. Ogilvie syndrome and herpes zoster: case report and review of the literature. J Emerg Med. 2010;39(5):696–700.
9. Basford JR. The law of Laplace and its relevance to contemporary medicine and rehabilitation. Arch Phys Med Rehabil. 2002;83(8):1165–70. https://doi.org/10.1053/apmr.2002.33985.

10. Slam KD, Calkins S, Cason FD. LaPlace's law revisited: cecal perforation as an unusual presentation of pancreatic carcinoma. World J Surg Oncol. 2007;5:14. https://doi.org/10.1186/1477-7819-5-14.
11. Novy S, Rogers LF, Kirkpatrick W. Diastatic rupture of the cecum in obstruction carcinoma of the left colon. Radiographic diagnosis and surgical implications. Am J Roentgenol Radium Therapy, Nucl Med. 1975;123(2):281–6. https://doi.org/10.2214/ajr.123.2.281.
12. Condon RE, Cowles VE, Ferraz AA, et al. Human colonic smooth muscle electrical activity during and after recovery from postoperative ileus. Am J Phys. 1995;269(3 Pt 1):G408–17. https://doi.org/10.1152/ajpgi.1995.269.3.G408.
13. Ogilvie H. Large-intestine colic due to sympathetic deprivation; a new clinical syndrome. Br Med J. 1948;2(4579):671–3. https://doi.org/10.1136/bmj.2.4579.671.
14. Dudley HA, Paterson-Brown S. Pseudo-obstruction. Br Med J (Clin Res Ed). 1986;292(6529):1157–8. https://doi.org/10.1136/bmj.292.6529.1157.
15. Stephenson BM, Morgan AR, Drake N, Salaman JR, Wheeler MH. Parasympathomimetic decompression of acute colonic pseudo-obstruction. Lancet. 1993;342(8880):1181–2. https://doi.org/10.1016/0140-6736(93)92167-r.
16. Azzouz LLSS. Physiology, large intestine. In: StatPearls. Treasure Island (FL): StatPearls Publishing; 2023.
17. Biga LM, Bronson S, Dawson S, et al. Anatomy and Physiology. OpenStax/Oregon State University; 2019.
18. Coyne MJ, Comstock LE. Type VI secretion systems and the gut microbiota. Microbiol Spectr. 2019;7(2):10–128.
19. Lai LA, Tong Z, Chen R, Pan S. Metaproteomics study of the gut microbiome. In: Functional Proteomics: methods and protocols; 2019. p. 123–32.
20. Sender R, Fuchs S, Milo R. Revised estimates for the number of human and bacteria cells in the body. PLoS Biol. 2016;14(8):e1002533.
21. Lee J-Y, Tsolis RM, Bäumler AJ. The microbiome and gut homeostasis. Science. 2022;377(6601):eabp9960.
22. Tropini C, Earle KA, Huang KC, Sonnenburg JL. The gut microbiome: connecting spatial organization to function. Cell Host Microbe. 2017;21(4):433–42.
23. Karemaker JM. An introduction into autonomic nervous function. Physiol Meas. 2017;38(5):R89.
24. Horn JP. The sacral autonomic outflow is parasympathetic: Langley got it right. Clin Auton Res. 2018;28(2):181–5.
25. Furness JB, Callaghan BP, Rivera LR, Cho H-J. The enteric nervous system and gastrointestinal innervation: integrated local and central control. In: Microbial endocrinology: The microbiota-gut-brain axis in health and disease; 2014. p. 39–71.
26. Goldstein A, Hofstra R, Burns A. Building a brain in the gut: development of the enteric nervous system. Clin Genet. 2013;83(4):307–16.
27. Schemann M. Control of gastrointestinal motility by the "gut brain"-the enteric nervous system. J Pediatr Gastroenterol Nutr. 2005;41:S4–6.
28. Schneider S, Wright CM, Heuckeroth RO. Unexpected roles for the second brain: enteric nervous system as master regulator of bowel function. Annu Rev Physiol. 2019;81:235–59.
29. Von HA. A dissertation on the sensible and irritable parts of animals. Translated from The Latin. London: J. Nourse, 1755. Reprint, with introduction by Owsei Temkin. Supplemnet to the Bulletin of the History of Medicine; 1755. p. 651–99.
30. Gershon MD. The enteric nervous system: a second brain. Hosp Pract. 1999;34(7):31–52.
31. Benarroch EE. Physiology and pathophysiology of the autonomic nervous system. Continuum (Minneap Minn). 2020;26(1):12–24.
32. Gershon MD, Margolis KG. The gut, its microbiome, and the brain: connections and communications. J Clin Invest. 2021;131(18):e143768.
33. Lyte M. Microbial endocrinology and the microbiota-gut-brain axis. Adv Exp Med Biol. 2014;817:3–24.

34. Mattsson T, Roos R, Sundkvist G, Valind S, Ohlsson B. Sympathetic nerve dysfunction is common in patients with chronic intestinal pseudo-obstruction. J Clin Gastroenterol. 2008;42(2):174–7.
35. Camilleri M, Balm RK, Low PA. Autonomic dysfunction in patients with chronic intestinal pseudo-obstruction. Clin Auton Res. 1993;3:95–100.
36. Jain D, Moussa K, Tandon M, Culpepper-Morgan J, Proctor DD. Role of interstitial cells of Cajal in motility disorders of the bowel. Am J Gastroenterol. 2003;98(3):618–24.
37. Mangoni AA. Assessing the adverse effects of antimuscarinic drugs in older patients: which way forward? Expert Rev Clin Pharmacol. 2011;4(5):531–3.
38. Lozano-Ortega G, Johnston KM, Cheung A, Wagg A, Campbell NL, Dmochowski RR, Ng DB. A review of published anticholinergic scales and measures and their applicability in database analyses. Arch Gerontol Geriatr. 2020;87:103885.
39. Vidal X, Agustí A, Vallano A, Formiga F, Moyano AF, García J, López-Soto A, Ramírez-Duque N, Torres OH, Barbé J, San-José A. Potentially Inappropriate Prescription in Older Patients in Spain (PIPOPS) Investigators' project. Elderly patients treated with psychotropic medicines admitted to hospital: associated characteristics and inappropriate use. Eur J Clin Pharmacol. 2016;72(6):755–64.
40. Akgün Ö, Oudshoorn C, Mattace-Raso FUS, Egberts A. Anticholinergic Drug Use on Admission and the Risk of In-Hospital Falls in Older Hospitalized Patients. Clin Interv Aging. 2022;17:277–28.
41. McCrea GL, Miaskowski C, Stotts NA, Macera L, Varma MG. A review of the literature on gender and age differences in the prevalence and characteristics of constipation in North America. J Pain Symptom Manage. 2009;37(4):737–45.
42. López-Álvarez J, Sevilla-Llewellyn-Jones J, Agüera-Ortiz L. Anticholinergic Drugs in Geriatric Psychopharmacology. Front Neurosci. 2019;13:1309.
43. Lechevallier-Michel N, Molimard M, Dartigues JF, Fabrigoule C, Fourrier-Réglat A. Drugs with anticholinergic properties and cognitive performance in the elderly: results from the PAQUID study. Br J Clin Pharmacol. 2005;59(2):143–51. https://doi.org/10.1111/j.1365-2125.2004.02232.x.
44. Chew ML, Mulsant BH, Pollock BG, et al. Anticholinergic activity of 107 medications commonly used by older adults. J Am Geriatr Soc. 2008;56(7):1333–41. https://doi.org/10.1111/j.1532-5415.2008.01737.x.
45. Gillis RA, Souza JD, Hicks KA, et al. Inhibitory control of proximal colonic motility by the sympathetic nervous system. Am J Physiol. 1987;253(4):G531–9. https://doi.org/10.1152/ajpgi.1987.253.4.G531.
46. Neal MJ. Medical pharmacology at a glance. Wiley; 2020.
47. Burns C, Kidron A. Biochemistry, Tyramine. Treasure Island (FL): StatPearls Publishing; 2022.
48. Bell C. Dopamine release from sympathetic nerve terminals. Prog Neurobiol. 1988;30(2):193–208.
49. Ross SW, Oommen B, Wormer BA, Walters AL, Augenstein VA, Heniford BT, Sing RF, Christmas AB. Acute colonic pseudo-obstruction: defining the epidemiology, treatment, and adverse outcomes of ogilvie's syndrome. Am Surg. 2016;82(2):102–11.
50. Clarke HD, Berry DJ, Larson DR. Acute pseudo-obstruction of the colon as a postoperative complication of hip arthroplasty. J Bone Joint Surg Am. 1997;79(11):1642–7.
51. Hsiue PP, Greig D, Chen CJ, Patel B, Trikha R, Rowan FE, Khoshbin A, Stavrakis AI. Incidence and risk factors for the development of acute colonic pseudo-obstruction (Ogilvie Syndrome) in total joint arthroplasty patients. J Am Acad Orthop Surg. 2021;29(4):159–66.
52. Nelson JD, Urban JA, Salsbury TL, Lowry JK, Garvin KL. Acute colonic pseudo-obstruction (Ogilvie syndrome) after arthroplasty in the lower extremity. J Bone Joint Surg Am. 2006;88(3):604–10.
53. Petrisor BA, Petruccelli DT, Winemaker MJ, de Beer JV. Acute colonic pseudo-obstruction after elective total joint arthroplasty. J Arthroplasty. 2001;16(8):1043–7.

54. Jensen LR, Possfelt-Møller E, Nielsen AE, Singh UM, Svendsen LB, Penninga L. Ogilvie Syndrome in Patients With Traumatic Pelvic and/or Acetabular Fractures: A Retrospective Cohort Study. J Orthop Trauma. 2023;37(3):122–9.
55. Wells CI, O'Grady G, Bissett IP. Acute colonic pseudo-obstruction: A systematic review of aetiology and mechanisms. World J Gastroenterol. 2017;23(30):5634–44.
56. Ford E, Bozin M, Shedda S, McCormick J, Skandarajah A, Cade T. Risk factors for acute colonic pseudo-obstruction after caesarean section: A retrospective case-control study. Aust N Z J Obstet Gynaecol. 2023;63(1):86–92.
57. Tenofsky PL, Beamer L, Smith RS. Ogilvie syndrome as a postoperative complication. Arch Surg. 2000;135(6):682–6; discussion 686-7
58. Vanek VW, Al-Salti M. Acute pseudo-obstruction of the colon (Ogilvie's syndrome). An analysis of 400 cases. Dis Colon Rectum. 1986;29(3):203–10. https://doi.org/10.1007/bf02555027.
59. Haj M, Haj M, Rockey DC. Ogilvie's syndrome: management and outcomes. Medicine. 2018;97(27):e11187.
60. Saunders MD. Acute colonic pseudo-obstruction. Best Pract Res Clin Gastroenterol. 2007;21(4):671–87. https://doi.org/10.1016/j.bpg.2007.03.001.
61. De Giorgio R, Barbara G, Stanghellini V, et al. The pharmacological treatment of acute colonic pseudo-obstruction. Aliment Pharmacol Ther. 2001;15(11):1717–27. https://doi.org/10.1046/j.1365-2036.2001.01088.x.
62. Wells CI, O'Grady G, Bissett IP. Acute colonic pseudo-obstruction: A systematic review of aetiology and mechanisms. World J Gastroenterol. 2017;23(30):5634–44. https://doi.org/10.3748/wjg.v23.i30.5634.
63. Brandler JB, Sweetser S, Khoshbin K, Babameto M, Prokop LJ, Camilleri M. Colonic manifestations and complications are relatively under-reported in systemic sclerosis: A systematic review. Am J Gastroenterol. 2019;114(12):1847–56.
64. Zheng J, Ni R, Liu H. Intestinal pseudo-obstruction in systemic lupus erythematosus: an analysis of nationwide inpatient sample. Clin Rheumatol. 2022;41(11):3331–5.
65. Wright GD, McCullagh CD, Walsh IK, Roberts SD. Digital necrosis with Ogilvie's syndrome. Ann Rheum Dis. 1997;56(4):224–5.
66. Fraisse A, Brosse S, Manckoundia P, Popitéan L, Pfitzenmeyer P. Ogilvie syndrome in the elderly: retrospective study of 40 cases. Presse Med. 2003;32(32):1500–4.
67. Liu C, Smerin D, Comba I, Bhatia L. Acute colonic pseudo-obstruction after Ventriculoperitoneal shunt placement for Normal pressure hydrocephalus. Cureus. 2020;12(5):e8295.
68. Man BL, Fu YP. Intestinal pseudo-obstruction as a presenting symptom of Guillain-Barré syndrome. BMJ Case Rep. 2014;2014:bcr2014205155.
69. Katz LA, Spiro HM. Gastrointestinal manifestations of diabetes. N Engl J Med. 1966;275(24):1350–61. https://doi.org/10.1056/nejm196612152752406.
70. Bastenie PA. Paralytic ileus in severe hypothyroidism. Lancet. 1946;1(6395):413–6. https://doi.org/10.1016/s0140-6736(46)90364-9.
71. Gilat T, Spiro HM. Amyloidosis and the gut. Am J Dig Dis. 1968;13(7):619–33. https://doi.org/10.1007/bf02232969.
72. Mitchell TA, Hoffer ZS, Cancio LC. Extracutaneous manifestations of Calciphylaxis: Ogilvie's syndrome with perforation. Am Surg. 2020;86(5):546–8. https://doi.org/10.1177/0003134820919736.
73. Sweeney AT, Malabanan AO, Blake MA, de Las Morenas A, Cachecho R, Melby JC. Megacolon as the presenting feature in Pheochromocytoma. J Clin Endocrinol Metabol. 2000;85(11):3968–72. https://doi.org/10.1210/jcem.85.11.6947.
74. Aguiar D, Fracasso T, Lardi C. Fatal Ogilvie's syndrome after hip surgery and review of the literature. Forensic Sci Med Pathol. 2022;18(2):170–5. https://doi.org/10.1007/s12024-022-00470-9.

75. Cakir E, Baykal S, Usul H, Kuzeyli K, Cinel A. Ogilvie's syndrome after cervical discectomy. Clin Neurol Neurosurg. 2001;103(4):232–3. https://doi.org/10.1016/s0303-8467(01)00167-6.
76. Feldman RA, Karl RC. Diagnosis and treatment of Ogilvie's syndrome after lumbar spinal surgery. Report of three cases. J Neurosurg. 1992;76(6):1012–6. https://doi.org/10.3171/jns.1992.76.6.1012.
77. Gortani G, Pederiva F, Ammar L, et al. Ogilvie syndrome in a 8 year old girl after laparoscopic appendectomy. BMC Pediatr. 2019;19(1):82. https://doi.org/10.1186/s12887-019-1457-z.
78. Ravo B, Pollane M, Ger R. Pseudo-obstruction of the colon following cesarean section. A review. Dis Colon Rectum. 1983;26(7):440–4. https://doi.org/10.1007/bf02556522.
79. Kadesky K, Purdue GF, Hunt JL. Acute pseudo-obstruction in critically ill patients with burns. J Burn Care Rehabil. 1995;16(2 Pt 1):132–5. https://doi.org/10.1097/00004630-199503000-00007.
80. Jensen LR, Possfelt-Møller E, Nielsen AE, Singh UM, Svendsen LB, Penninga L. Ogilvie syndrome in patients with traumatic pelvic and/or acetabular fractures: a retrospective cohort study. J Orthop Trauma. 2023;37(3):122–9. https://doi.org/10.1097/bot.0000000000002506.
81. O'Malley KJ, Flechner SM, Kapoor A, et al. Acute colonic pseudo-obstruction (Ogilvie's syndrome) after renal transplantation. Am J Surg. 1999;177(6):492–6. https://doi.org/10.1016/s0002-9610(99)00093-8.
82. Gillies M, AlDujaili T. Acute colonic pseudo-obstruction secondary to renal calculus: A case report and review of pathophysiology. Cureus. 2023;15(2):e34756. https://doi.org/10.7759/cureus.34756.
83. Shapiro AM, Bain VG, Preiksaitis JK, Ma MM, Issa S, Kneteman NM. Ogilvie's syndrome associated with acute cytomegaloviral infection after liver transplantation. Transpl Int. 2000;13(1):41–5. https://doi.org/10.1007/s001470050006.
84. Anaya-Prado R, Pérez-Navarro JV, Corona-Nakamura A, Anaya-Fernández MM, Anaya-Fernández R, Izaguirre-Pérez ME. Intestinal pseudo-obstruction caused by herpes zoster: Case report and pathophysiology. World J Clin Cases. 2018;6(6):132–8. https://doi.org/10.12998/wjcc.v6.i6.132.
85. Wang J, Marusca G, Tariq T, Mohamad B. Ogilvie syndrome and COVID-19 infection. J Med Cases. 2021;12(8):328–31. https://doi.org/10.14740/jmc3728.
86. Chatila R, Kapadia CR. Intestinal pseudoobstruction in acute Lyme disease: a case report. Am J Gastroenterol. 1998;93(7):1179–80. https://doi.org/10.1111/j.1572-0241.1998.00361.x.
87. MacColl C, MacCannell KL, Baylis B, Lee SS. Treatment of acute colonic pseudoobstruction (Ogilvie's syndrome) with cisapride. Gastroenterology. 1990;98(3):773–6. https://doi.org/10.1016/0016-5085(90)90301-g.
88. Sunnoqrot N, Reilly RF. Hypokalemia Associated with colonic pseudo-obstruction (Ogilvie's Syndrome). Case Rep Nephrol Dial. 2015;2:118–23.
89. Manappallil RG, Suresh CC, Kadengil D, Thomas P, Jayaraj J. A case of Ogilvie’s syndrome associated with electrolyte imbalance in a healthy individual. Asian J Med Sci. 2023;8(1):101–3.
90. Tsai WC, Chuang TY, Chen MC, Chen JC, Tsao YT. Ogilvie syndrome: a potentially life-threatening phenotype of immobilization hypercalcemia. Am J Emerg Med. 2014;32(7):816.e1–3. https://doi.org/10.1016/j.ajem.2013.12.056.
91. Knox-Macaulay H, Ayyaril M, Nusrat N, Daar A. Colonic pseudo-obstruction in sickle cell disease. South Med J. 2003;96(1):93–5. https://doi.org/10.1097/01.smj.0000047056.99409.0f.
92. Tenofsky PL, Beamer RL, Smith RS. Ogilvie syndrome as a postoperative complication. Arch Surg. 2000;135(6):682–7. https://doi.org/10.1001/archsurg.135.6.682.
93. Pahadiya HR, Lakhotia M, Gandhi R. Acute intermittent porphyria presented with acute intestinal pseudo-obstruction. Indian J Endocrinol Metab. 2018;22(4):573–4. https://doi.org/10.4103/ijem.IJEM_677_17.
94. Schermer CR, Hanosh JJ, Davis M, Pitcher DE. Ogilvie's syndrome in the surgical patient: a new therapeutic modality. J Gastrointest Surg. 1999;3(2):173–7. https://doi.org/10.1016/s1091-255x(99)80029-8.

95. Yan Y, Chen Y, Zhang X. The effect of opioids on gastrointestinal function in the ICU. Crit Care. 2021;25(1):370.
96. Bazerbachi F, Haffar S, Szarka LA, Wang Z, Prokop LJ, Murad MH, Camilleri M. Secretory diarrhea and hypokalemia associated with colonic pseudo-obstruction: A case study and systematic analysis of the literature. Neurogastroenterol Motil. 2017;29(11):e13120. https://doi.org/10.1111/nmo.13120.
97. Joechle K, Guenzle J, Utzolino S, Fichtner-Feigl S, Kousoulas L. Ogilvie's syndrome-is there a cutoff diameter to proceed with upfront surgery? Langenbecks Arch Surg. 2022;407(3):1173–82. https://doi.org/10.1007/s00423-021-02407-2.
98. Schermer CR, Hanosh JJ, Davis M, Pitcher DE. Ogilvie's syndrome in the surgical patient: a new therapeutic modality. J Gastrointest Surg. 1999;3(2):173–7.
99. Pereira P, Djeudji F, Leduc P, Fanget F, Barth X. Ogilvie's syndrome-acute colonic pseudo-obstruction. J Visc Surg. 2015;152(2):99–105.
100. Sloyer AF, Panella VS, Demas BE, Shike M, Lightdale CJ, Winawer SJ, Kurtz RC. Ogilvie's syndrome. Successful management without colonoscopy. Dig Dis Sci. 1988;33(11):1391–6.
101. Loftus CG, Harewood GC, Baron TH. Assessment of predictors of response to neostigmine for acute colonic pseudo-obstruction. Am J Gastroenterol. 2002;97(12):3118–22.
102. Valle RG, Godoy FL. Neostigmine for acute colonic pseudo-obstruction: A meta-analysis. Ann Med Surg (Lond). 2014;3(3):60–4.
103. Ponec RJ, Saunders MD, Kimmey MB. Neostigmine for the treatment of acute colonic pseudo-obstruction. N Engl J Med. 1999;341(3):137–41.
104. van der Spoel JI, Oudemans-van Straaten HM, Stoutenbeek CP, Bosman RJ, Zandstra DF. Neostigmine resolves critical illness-related colonic ileus in intensive care patients with multiple organ failure--a prospective, double-blind, placebo-controlled trial. Intensive Care Med. 2001;27(5):822–7.
105. Amaro R, Rogers AI. Neostigmine infusion: new standard of care for acute colonic pseudo-obstruction? Am J Gastroenterol. 2000;95(1):304–5.
106. Hutchinson R, Griffiths C. Acute colonic pseudo-obstruction: a pharmacological approach. Ann R Coll Surg Engl. 1992;74(5):364–7.
107. Kram B, Greenland M, Grant M, Campbell ME, Wells C, Sommer C. Efficacy and Safety of Subcutaneous Neostigmine for Ileus, Acute Colonic Pseudo-obstruction, or Refractory Constipation. Ann Pharmacother. 2018;52(6):505–12.
108. Sgouros SN, Vlachogiannakos J, Vassiliadis K, Bergele C, Stefanidis G, Nastos H, Avgerinos A, Mantides A. Effect of polyethylene glycol electrolyte balanced solution on patients with acute colonic pseudo obstruction after resolution of colonic dilation: a prospective, randomised, placebo controlled trial. Gut. 2006;55(5):638–42.
109. Rex DK. Acute colonic pseudo-obstruction (Ogilvie's syndrome). Gastroenterologist. 1994;2(3):233–8.
110. Sariego J, Matsumoto T, Kerstein MD. Colonoscopically guided tube decompression in Ogilvie's syndrome. Dis Colon Rectum. 1991;34(8):720–2.
111. Nano D, Prindiville T, Pauly M, Chow H, Ross K, Trudeau W. Colonoscopic therapy of acute pseudoobstruction of the colon. Am J Gastroenterol. 1987;82(2):145–8.
112. Kukora JS, Dent TL. Colonoscopic decompression of massive nonobstructive cecal dilation. Arch Surg. 1977;112(4):512–7.
113. Lee JT, Taylor BM, Singleton BC. Epidural anesthesia for acute pseudo-obstruction of the colon (Ogilvie's syndrome). Dis Colon Rectum. 1988;31(9):686–91.
114. Casola G, Withers C, vanSonnenberg E, Herba MJ, Saba RM, Brown RA. Percutaneous cecostomy for decompression of the massively distended cecum. Radiology. 1986;158(3):793–4.
115. Benacci JC, Wolff BG. Cecostomy. Therapeutic indications and results. Dis Colon Rectum. 1995;38(5):530–4.
116. Ramage JI Jr, Baron TH. Percutaneous endoscopic cecost omy: a case series. Gastrointest Endosc. 2003;57(6):752–5.

Chapter 10
Coagulation Review

Wesley Lemons, Dallas Hampton, Meric Mericliler, and J. Christian Barrett

Clinical Vignette

A 78-year-old female was involved in a motor vehicle crash and subsequently arrived at a level one medical center for the treatment of her injuries. She presented with left thigh pain with obvious deformity and bilateral open ankle fractures. She was subsequently placed in femoral traction and underwent operative fixation the following day. She tolerated her operative course without concern. She received intramedullary nailing of her femur and a plate and screw construct with primary closure of her ankle fractures. She was then transferred to the orthopaedics floor on postoperative day 1. She was restarted on her home medications and unfractionated heparin for deep vein thrombosis prophylaxis. She was kept non-weightbearing due to her ankle injuries. On postoperative day 6, laboratory work demonstrated a platelet count of 55×10^9/L which was a decrease from previous laboratory work-up demonstrating a platelet count of 160×10^9/L. No further work-up was conducted for isolated thrombocytopenia, and no medication changes were made at this time.

W. Lemons (✉)
Department of Orthopaedic Surgery, Virginia Commonwealth University, Richmond, VA, USA
e-mail: wesley.lemons@vcuhealth.org

D. Hampton
Eastern Virginia Medical School, Norfolk, VA, USA
e-mail: hamptoDJ@EVMS.edu

M. Mericliler
Division of Hematology/Oncology, Virginia Commonwealth University, Richmond, VA, USA
e-mail: Meric.Mericliler@vcuhealth.org

J. C. Barrett
Division of Hematology/Oncology, Department of Internal Medicine, Virginia Commonwealth University, Richmond, VA, USA
e-mail: john.barrett@vcuhealth.org

W. A. Zuelzer, S. Metikala (eds.), *Unusual Conditions That Every Orthopaedic Surgeon Should Know*, https://doi.org/10.1007/978-3-031-58946-1_10

On postoperative day 8, the patient called nursing staff with increasing pain attributed to her original injuries. The following day, nursing staff noted that the patient was starting to bleed from her intravenous access sites. On postoperative day 9, the patient experienced crushing chest pain, shortness of breath, and tachycardia. The patient subsequently experienced a cardiopulmonary arrest. Unfortunately, the resuscitation efforts failed, and she was pronounced dead.

Questions

1. What is the cause of death for this patient?
2. What laboratory studies could have confirmed the diagnosis?
3. What medication should the patient be switched to after identifying laboratory changes on postoperative day 6?

Introduction

The nature of orthopaedic injuries put all patients at increased risk for venous thromboembolism (VTE). This inherent risk stems from the idea of Virchow's triad of venous stasis, endothelial injury, and hypercoagulability [1]. In the realm of orthopaedic trauma, patients often fulfill this triad with a long list of injuries including but not limited to spine injuries, pelvic fractures, lower extremity injuries, vent dependency, and a multitude of other orthopaedic and non-orthopaedic injuries [1]. In these patients, the risk of deep vein thrombosis (DVT) without chemical prophylaxis can be as high as 80% in some studies [1–3]. In patients identified as elevated risk for VTE and treated with chemical prophylaxis, the rate of DVTs (Deep Vein Thrombosis) drops to 11%, with many of these being subclinical [1–3]. The prevalence of DVTs has been studied thoroughly. One study, completed in 2009, demonstrating DVT incidence of 2.1% in patients treated with a joint-spanning external fixator who were on chemical prophylaxes [1, 4]. A study conducted by Smith et al. demonstrated that 10% of patients who had ultrasound screenings free of DVTs and underwent operative intervention for acute femur or hip fractures subsequently developed a DVT [1, 5]. In the setting of foot and ankle surgery, a retrospective review, completed in 2011, of 57,000 patients with ankle fractures treated with surgery revealed a readmission rate of 0.05% due to DVTs [1, 6]. Although the risk of readmission was low in the overall population, the risk was higher in patients who are older, those with open fractures, and those with a higher Charlson comorbidity score.

In the United States alone, there is 300,000–600,000 cases of VTE a year with an estimated cost to the healthcare budget of more than seven billion dollars per year [7].

All these studies underscore the high incidence and economic burden of venous thromboembolism in orthopaedic practice. Accordingly, we will review the coagulation cascade as it pertains to orthopaedics and covers common pathologies associated with coagulation errors and their treatments of choice.

Physiology of Coagulation

The coagulation process follows a complex and tightly regulated pathway with coordinated steps to prevent excessive blood loss. In every orthopaedic patient, this pathway comes into play whether the patient is arriving as a trauma alert or undergoing surgery. The imbalance of this pathway can lead to significant morbidity and eventual mortality thus making the understanding of key steps important in a surgeon's daily practice. The clotting cascade can be broken down to two primary stages: Platelet plug formation (primary hemostasis) and stabilization of the platelet plug (secondary hemostasis) [8].

Formation of a Platelet Plug

The process of forming a stable clot begins with an injury to the vessel itself or activation of the endothelium, thus releasing different cellular factors that prompt clot formation. One of the initial responses to vascular injury is vasoconstriction. Vasoconstriction is primarily mediated by release of endothelin-1 from the damaged endothelium of the blood vessel and leads to constriction for up to 4 h [8–10]. Other substances, such as serotonin and thromboxane A2, also contribute to vasoconstriction. Vasoconstriction following vascular injury restricts blood flow and promotes thrombosis. The next step in primary hemostasis involves platelet adhesion, primarily mediated by von Willebrand factor (vWF), synthesized by both megakaryocytes and Weibel-Palade bodies in endothelial cells, and sub-endothelial collagen [10]. Von Willebrand factor is a large multimeric glycoprotein that possesses multiple receptors binding sites, including the GP Ib-IX-V and GP IIb-IIIa receptor complexes. The interaction between vWF and the GP Ib-IX-V receptor complex on the platelet membrane is the primary receptor-ligand binding for platelet adhesion. However, interactions between other membrane glycoproteins, such as GPIa/IIa and GPVI, and collagen have also been shown to play a role in platelet adhesion [11, 12]. The subsequent step in primary homeostasis is the activation of the platelet where the platelets undergo two distinct changes [10–12]. Platelets first increase their surface area by undergoing a permanent change in shape. After the interaction between platelet receptors and collagen, along with subsequent conformational changes, platelets release the contents of their alpha and delta granules, resulting in stronger platelet activation. Platelet granules contain many agonists, coagulation factors such as fibrinogen and factor V, and von Willebrand factor. Specifically, ADP is one of the agonists released from granules that binds two receptors (P2Y1 and P2Y12) on the platelet membranes, both of which play roles in platelet activation and aggregation. Thrombin also plays a direct and indirect role in the platelet activation phase through proteolytic cleavage and platelet granule release [10]. Thromboxane A2 is also synthesized by the platelets which results in further vasoconstriction and plays a key role in the final step in primary homeostasis, platelet aggregation. Platelet aggregation is mediated primarily by the cross-linking of fibrinogen between the activated GP IIb/IIIa receptors expressed on the surfaces of platelets. This interaction additionally intensifies the recruitment of additional platelets.

Stabilization of the Platelet Plug

Secondary homeostasis consists of a cascade of coagulation that results in thrombin cleavage of fibrinogen to fibrin, which is insoluble allowing for a stronger cross-linked mesh [13]. While it may seem as though the two stages of homeostasis occur separately, this cross-linking begins during the platelet aggregation stage of primary homeostasis. The coagulation factors involved in the cascade are known as serine protases as they create a catalytic triad composed of serine, aspartic acid, and histidine [14]. Normally, the surface of an activated platelet allows most of these reactions to take place, but they require calcium. Therefore, the introduction of calcium chelators can prevent this cascades formation. Certain coagulation factors within the cascade (II, VII, IX, and X) along with proteins C and S (inhibitors of coagulation) require Vitamin K to bind the phospholipid surface of platelets. Vitamin K is an important cofactor in the gamma-carboxylation of glutamate which is a necessary step to activate the previously listed coagulation factors and proteins (factors II, VII, IX, and X along with proteins C and S). Importantly, warfarin is a vitamin K antagonist that interferes with the gamma-carboxylation of these coagulation factors [14].

Coagulation Cascade

While still a part of secondary homeostasis, the coagulation cascade can be further broken down into the intrinsic or extrinsic pathway that leads to a common pathway [16]. Normal homeostasis is initiated by the extrinsic pathway with exposure of endothelial tissue following vessel injury. Feedback is then amplified through the intrinsic pathway to lead to sufficient thrombin burst for fibrin clot formation. Activation directly through the extrinsic pathway plays a role in the pathologic process and can lead to thrombosis. Interestingly, factor XII deficiency is not typically associated with an increased risk of bleeding due to the presence of multiple feedback mechanisms in the coagulation cascade [16]. The blood test that is typically performed to measure intrinsic pathway function is partial thromboplastin time (PTT).

The extrinsic pathway is activated by the release of tissue factor from the damaged epithelial cells of the vessel and leads to activation of factor VII which then activates factor X (Fig. 10.1). At this point, the two pathways converge to the common pathway. When clinically measuring the extrinsic pathway, prothrombin time (PT) is used. The two pathways result in an activating complex called Tenase, the components of which depend on which pathway produced the product, which

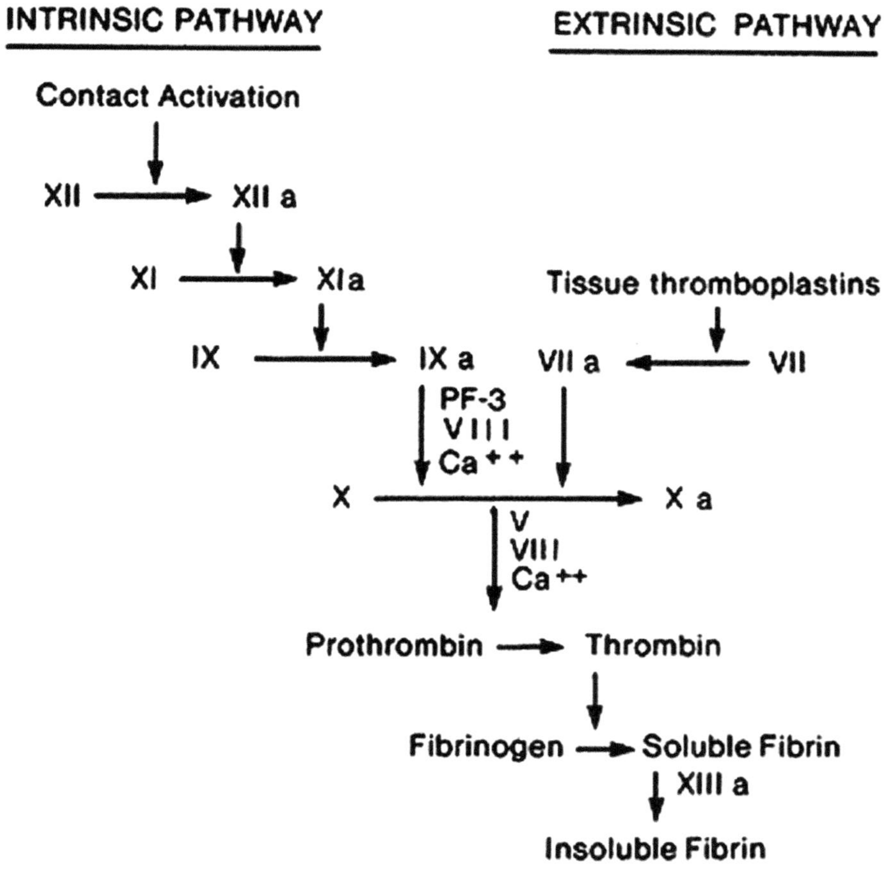

Fig. 10.1 Coagulation Cascade. Adapted from Nacca, Christopher & Shah, Kalpit & Truntzer, Jeremy & Rubin, Lee [15]

activated X to Xa [16]. Prothrombin (II) is then activated into thrombin (IIa), but this reaction relies on the presence of factor V as a cofactor in order to proceed. Thrombin converts fibrinogen to fibrin while also activating other factors within the intrinsic pathway. The platelet plug is stabilized by factor XIII acting on the fibrin strands, composed of fibrin subunits, leading to the improved stabilization of the mesh [16].

VTE Prophylaxis in Orthopaedic Surgery Patients: Introduction

In every orthopaedic patient, as discussed, the risk of venous thromboembolism is exceedingly high. In the context of VTE prophylaxis, the goal is to prevent not only deep vein thrombosis but also pulmonary embolism, with the latter capable of carrying an initial fatality rate as high as 24% [17].

To reduce the risk of thromboembolism and provide better outcomes for patients, several different anticoagulants can be used. This section will review various methods of VTE prophylaxis.

Sequential Compression Devices

Sequential Compression Devices (SCDs) can be used for mechanical DVT prophylaxis in non-ambulatory or bed-bound patients. SCDs function by providing pneumatic compression to the lower extremity thus aiding in blood return to the heart theoretically eliminating one component of Virchow's triad (venous stasis) though physiologic effects on homeostasis may additionally contribute to the reduction in thrombosis seen with SCDs [18, 19]. In the ambulatory patient, this return of blood or prevention of statis is performed by the contraction of the gastrocnemius muscle as the patient walks or moves around. SCDs come in several different forms including foot pumps, calf sleeves (most common), and compression hose, all of which attempt to prevent DVTs through mechanically preventing statis. A randomized prospective study comparing the effectiveness of low-dose warfarin with sequential compression devices for DVT prophylaxis in patients after total hip arthroplasty demonstrated that the use of SCDs significantly outperformed low-dose warfarin, particularly in average-risk patients [20]. Practice guidelines suggest that intermittent pneumatic compression devices are viable options for VTE prophylaxis in patients undergoing total hip arthroplasty or total knee arthroplasty [21]. The data regarding the use of SCD (Sequential Compression Devices) alone for VTE prophylaxis is controversial, and it is considered a beneficial adjunct to chemical prophylaxis [22]. However, in patients who are at significant risk for bleeding and/or place a high value on avoiding bleeding complications, SCDs might be preferred over chemical thromboprophylaxis.

Unfractionated Heparin

Heparin is one of the most used forms of anticoagulation across different specialties in the hospital setting. Heparin itself was first discovered in 1916 by Mclean but was not approved for clinical use until 1935 [23]. Unfractionated Heparin, itself, is a sulfated polysaccharide with a mean molecular weight of 15,000 Daltons. Heparin primarily works by binding to antithrombin III (ATIII) which in turn primarily inactivates Factor IIa (thrombin) and Factor Xa. The inactivation of both thrombin and antithrombin III occurs only with unfractionated heparin as the mean molecular weight must be over roughly 6000 Daltons to bind both molecules [24, 25]. The binding and inactivation of these factors then prevent fibrinogen conversion to fibrin thus preventing clot formation [25]. Heparin can be administrated to the patient either subcutaneously or intravenously depending on the desired effect. In most orthopaedic patients, the subcutaneous route is preferred for DVT prophylaxis which typically takes 1–2 h for full effect [25]. Heparin is also preferred in patients with acute traumatic injuries due to its short half-life of 1.5 h for subcutaneous administration and 30 min for intravenous dosing [26]. When a patient is receiving heparin, the patient's partial thromboplastin time (PTT) as well as hemoglobin, hematocrit, and platelet count should be followed to monitor for any adverse events if the patient is on therapeutic and prophylactic dosing [25, 26]. In the event of a significant drop in hemoglobin or concern for active bleeding, the effects of unfractionated heparin can be reversed with the use of protamine sulfate [26]. The dose required for complete reverse of protamine varies based on total volume of heparin administered and time since the dose [26].

Low-Molecular-Weight Heparin

Low-molecular-weight heparin (LMWH) functions similarly to unfractionated heparin but the mean size of LMWH is 5000 Daltons meaning that its function is through inhibition of factor Xa [27]. LMWH does exert some effect on factor IIa and AT III; however, the effect is normally one-fourth that of its effect on Xa. The advantage of LMWH over the use of heparin is that LMWH usually does not require monitoring; however, if indicated LMWH can be monitored through anti-factor ten levels. Indications for anti-Xa monitoring may include poor renal function, weight above 150 kg (about 330.69 lb.) or less than 50 kg, pregnancy, recurrent thrombosis on prophylaxis, and unexpected bleeding episodes [28]. Enoxaparin is one of the most used low-molecular-weight heparin products (LMWH), but this class also includes drugs such as dalteparin and tinzaparin [27]. The enoxaparin dosing for VTE prophylaxis varies based on practice guidelines; however, the dosing of 0.5 mg/kg twice a day is supported by recent studies [28–30]. LMWH is preferred in a stable patient that does not require urgent surgical intervention or has an elevated risk for reversal of anticoagulation.

Fondaparinux

Fondaparinux is a synthetic sulfated pentasaccharide based on the structure of heparin. Fondaparinux functions similarly to LMWH and unfractionated heparin as it exerts its effects through the enhancement of ATIII thus inhibiting factor Xa [31]. Fondaparinux, like low-molecular-weight heparin, undergoes renal processing and should be used with caution in patients with poor renal function defined as a GFR (Glomerular Filtration Rate) less than 30 mL/min [28]. Fondaparinux does have some advantages and disadvantages when compared to other heparin products. Fondaparinux does not cause heparin-induced thrombocytopenia (to be discussed later in the chapter). However, it is typically more expensive than LMWH and has a half-life of 17–21 h, which can pose a challenge in patients with higher bleeding risk. Practice guidelines recommend that fondaparinux can be an option for antithrombotic prophylaxis for patients undergoing major orthopaedic surgery. Extended-duration fondaparinux has been shown to reduce the rates of VTE compared to placebo although it is associated with an increased risk of bleeding. Fondaparinux effectiveness, compared to other popular anticoagulants such as enoxaparin, has been studied with the double-blinded MATISSE (Mondial Assessment of Thromboembolism treatment Initiated by Synthetic Pentasaccharide with Symptomatic Endpoints-DVT) trial. The incidence of recurrent VTE in patients with DVT was 3.9% in the Fondaparinux group compared to 4.1% in the enoxaparin group [31]. Major bleeding occurred in 1.1% of patients receiving fondaparinux, whereas 1.2% of patients receiving enoxaparin experienced major bleeding [31].

Direct Oral Anticoagulants

Direct oral anticoagulants target specific coagulation factors involved in secondary hemostasis without functioning through antithrombin. They are categorized into two broad groups: (1) selective factor Xa inhibitors (e.g., apixaban, rivaroxaban, and edoxaban); (2) direct thrombin inhibitors (dabigatran) [32]. Additionally, new selective anticoagulants targeting other coagulation factors are currently being investigated [33]. Pharmacological properties such as bioavailability, plasma half-life, and renal excretion vary significantly among different DOACs. Thus, the appropriate DOAC should be chosen based on different patient factors. Dose monitoring is not required, and antidotes have been approved for certain DOACs. Considering these pharmacologic properties and ease of use, as well as their favorable efficacy, DOACs have been increasingly used. DOACs have been approved for different indications including treatment of VTE, primary prevention of stroke in patients with atrial fibrillation, and postoperative VTE thromboprophylaxis. The efficacy and safety of DOACs for postoperative prophylaxis have been assessed in multiple trials. A meta-analysis suggests that factor Xa inhibitors are associated with fewer symptomatic DVTs but an increased risk of bleeding when compared with low-molecular-weight heparin in patients undergoing total hip or knee replacement [34].

The choice and duration of chemical prophylaxis should be individualized in the postoperative setting. Typically, an extended duration of anticoagulation (e.g., up to 35 days) is recommended for patients undergoing THA, whereas a shorter duration (e.g., 10–14 days) is advised for patients undergoing TKA [35]. The EPCAT II trial compared extended-duration prophylaxis with rivaroxaban versus aspirin in patients who underwent total hip or total knee arthroplasty and received initial thromboprophylaxis with the DOAC for 5 days. This trial demonstrated that transitioning to aspirin after the initial 5 days of DOAC treatment resulted in comparable rates of VTE and major bleeding when compared to continuing with rivaroxaban. It is worth noting that most patients in the trial were at low risk for VTE, which limits the generalizability of the results [36].

Aspirin

As one of the most frequently used drugs worldwide, aspirin can be used in both acute management and secondary prevention as it acts to inhibit platelet aggregation [20]. The use of aspirin as primary DVT prophylaxis has been heavily debated in recent years with some data suggesting lower risk for bleeds with a slight increased risk for DVTs which may become clinically significant [37]. Following total joint arthroplasty, aspirin is inexpensive and safe in the prevention of VTE although trials are currently underway to establish more specific guidelines though evidence currently shows a hybrid strategy involving low-dose aspirin after a period of low-dose anticoagulation such as lovenox [37].

Pathologies of the Coagulation Cascade

Deep Vein Thrombosis and Pulmonary Embolism

Prevention of both deep vein thrombosis (DVT) and pulmonary embolism (PE) hinges on an adequate balance among prothrombotic and antithrombotic factors [38]. Virchow's triad composed of venous stasis, vascular injury, and hypercoagulability helps determine the likelihood of experiencing a DVT which is a common postoperative complication in orthopaedic surgery and, while variable depending on the source, occurs within 4 weeks postoperative period [38–40]. Studies of patients undergoing orthopaedic surgeries of the lower extremities found that the site of operation such as knee joint surgery, age greater than 60, female gender, and duration of greater than 120 for the operation were significant factors in the development of a DVT [39, 40]. Interestingly, it was suggested to even try to avoid the use of a tourniquet when performing knee surgery due to the risk for DVT if possible [40]. DVTs can be assessed using ultrasound to help detect the presence of a DVT within the veins prior to embolism of these clots, or spiral CT (Computed Tomography) imagining for PE/DVT detection [40, 41]. Pulmonary embolism is the most dangerous form of venous thromboembolism, resulting in an obstruction in the lungs' arteries, potentially leading to right ventricular dysfunction; if left untreated, it can be fatal. Two different validated assessment tools are available in the assessment of the likelihood of a PE in a patient, but they should only be used once a PE is suspected based on clinical assessment [42]. These two tests are the Revised Geneva Score and the Wells Score whose criteria vary in values and exact criteria but have many overlapping features such as previous PE or DVT, the presence of hemoptysis, heart rate, malignancy, and recent surgery. One study found that patients with low oxygen saturation and those who had a previous DVT or PE were more likely to have a positive spiral CT scan [41]. It has been postulated that the increased sensitivity of spiral CT scans can lead to over-treatment with prolonged anticoagulation that does not actually improve mortality as subsegmental clots not detected on less sensitive VQ scans did not show greater morbidity [41]. In postoperative orthopaedic patients, the cost-benefit analysis for spiral CT in all patients is not recommended and exposes patients to unnecessary radiation though spine and total joint arthroplasty were found to have the highest positive rate in one study. The use of a D-dimer is also not recommended as most postoperative patients will have a positive laboratory result. Larger clinical trials are needed to determine the best algorithm when assessing and testing a PE/DVT after orthopaedic operations. The mainstay treatment for radiologically confirmed VTE is therapeutic anticoagulation (e.g., DOACs, LMWH, or warfarin). In rare cases, thrombolysis may be needed for extensive VTE. Due to the low risk of recurrent VTE after orthopaedic surgery, a limited duration of anticoagulation (3–6 months) is recommended [40–42].

Disseminated Intravascular Coagulation

Commonly associated with live threatening illnesses, disseminated intravascular coagulation (DIC) is associated with multiorgan dysfunction syndrome as widespread activation of the coagulation cascade occurs, with concurrent consumption of clotting factors and platelets that may result in life-threatening hemorrhage [43, 44]. Both microvascular and macrovascular thrombosis can occur due to the hypercoagulable state present and thus compromises blood flow to the effected organs [43]. The main goal in treatment of DIC is to control the underlying disease with the most common cause being severe sepsis [43, 44]. Other causes of DIC include hematologic malignancies, severe trauma, and pregnancy complications such as placental abruption.

Patients may present with a variety of symptoms such as bleeding from multiple sites, through devices such as urinary catheters, hemoptysis if pulmonary hemorrhage or pulmonary embolism are present, and even mental status changes if areas of the brain are affected by thrombi or hemorrhage [43]. There is no single subjective or objective component that can be used when diagnosing DIC, but laboratory findings including increased prothrombin time and partial thromboplastin time, decreased fibrinogen level, or the presence fragmented erythrocytes present on peripheral blood smears can lend support for the diagnosis. There are currently five different diagnostic scoring systems reported for DIC, requiring measurement of platelet count, fibrin markers such as D-dimer, prolonged PT, fibrinogen level, and nonlaboratory findings such as underlying disease and symptoms, depending on the criteria used [43, 44].

In orthopaedic surgery, there is significant morbidity and mortality in patients who experience DIC [45]. Self-limited cases of DIC can also occur during elective orthopaedic surgeries, in which patients can have a negative bleeding history and normal preoperative coagulation laboratory results [46]. Examples of conditions that can lead to DIC in orthopaedic surgery include shock, severe trauma, sepsis, and fat embolism [47]. There has been reports of intraoperative DIC, a recent report of two patients who underwent scoliosis stabilization developed massive bleeding during the procedure, with intraoperative laboratory results showing decreased platelets, plasma coagulation factors, and fibrinogen with elevated fibrin split products. It was suggested that decortication or chipping of the bones could be a trigger for fibrin products leading to intraoperative bleeding that resolves when the operation ends. Heparin should be avoided in these cases with major active hemorrhage therefore, treatment involves blood component replacement. A case report regarding prophylactic intramedullary femoral nailing in a metastatic prostate carcinoma patient describes a patient who developed DIC and became hemodynamically unstable with significant bleeding and subsequent death, despite treatment [45]. This emphasizes the importance of early recognition of DIC in orthopaedic patients, especially in the case of metastatic cancer, or other risk factors for developing DIC. Ideally, patients should be screened for coagulopathies and other potential conditions which could lead to DIC. Patients with increased risk factors such as sepsis, major organ damage (cirrhosis, pancreatitis, burns, poly traumas, transplant patients, pregnancy, and cancer patients) should produce a higher clinical suspicion.

Heparin-Induced Thrombocytopenia (HIT)

Heparin-induced thrombocytopenia is an adverse drug reaction following sensitizing exposure to heparin, resulting in the formation of antibodies directed against platelet factor 4 (PF4) and heparin [48, 49]. These antibodies activate platelets, endothelial cells, monocytes, and neutrophil extracellular traps (NETs), leading to thrombocytopenia and an increased risk for venous and arterial thrombosis [48]. Recent evidence has indicated that thrombotic complications observed in heparin-induced thrombocytopenia might be related to neutrophil activation and NETosis [50, 51]. The mechanisms of thrombocytopenia involve the removal of platelets in the reticuloendothelial space and consumption at the site of thrombosis [48]. This immune-mediated reaction typically occurs over a time range of around 5–10 days after starting the offending drug although the decrease in platelet count can occur at any time [49]. HIT should be suspected in patients experiencing thrombocytopenia following orthopaedic surgery. Clinical decision tools such as 4 T's score can be used to determine the pretest probability, thereby indicating the need for testing. In case of moderate-to-high pretest probability for HIT (e.g., 4 T's score of 4 or above), treatment should be initiated even before confirmatory diagnostic testing is obtained [48]. Immediate cessation of heparin products is of paramount importance, and it is recommended to initiate alternate anticoagulation. The non-heparin anticoagulant options in the context of HIT include DOACs, fondaparinux, danaparoid, argatroban, and bivalirudin [52]. Warfarin should be avoided when platelet count remains low due to the increased risk for thrombosis [48].

It is worth noting that there are reported cases of "spontaneous" HIT which occurs in the absence of drugs from the heparin class but yield positive results for anti-PF4/heparin IgG ELISA and the serotonin release assay [53]. While rare, spontaneous HIT can lead to severe thrombotic complications with most of the reported cases occurring after total knee replacement [53]. Treatment of spontaneous HIT is similar and involves the initiation of non-heparin anticoagulant while severe cases may require vascular interventions [48, 53].

Von Willebrand Disease

Von Willebrand disease (VWD) is an inherited bleeding disorder, though there are also acquired causes, associated with excessive bruising, and prolonged bleeding from mucosal membranes and skin bleeding caused by deficiency of pro-von Willebrand factor [54, 55]. Intraarticular bleeds can also be observed in von Willebrand disease (VWD), particularly in cases associated with more profoundly low Factor VIII activity, which is more commonly found in type 3 and type 2 N VWD. Recurrent intraarticular bleeding can lead to chronic arthropathy necessitating surgery [55]. In addition, these patients are also susceptible to surgical indications seen within the general population. Due to the nature of the disease leading to arthropathies, the need for orthopaedic intervention can arise [56, 57]. Perioperative bleeding complications are also a distinct possibility [56].. This lends to the importance of taking a through history to identify patient with underlying VWD, assess the bleeding phenotype and recognizing the value of close collaboration among interdisciplinary treatment teams for the most effective management of these patients [56]. Often, patients with VWD undergoing major orthopaedic surgery require perioperative von Willebrand factor replacement therapy. Antifibrinolytics can also be considered as adjunctive therapy to minimize excessive bleeding [56, 57].

Hemophilia

The hemophilias are a group of inherited, or rarely acquired, disorders of secondary hemostasis caused by a deficiency or complete absence of a coagulation factor [58, 59]. The classic hemophilias include Factor VIII deficiency (Hemophilia A) and Factor IX deficiency (Hemophilia B). Both congenital Factor VIII and Factor IX deficiencies are X-linked disorders and represent the majority of hemophilia cases, while other coagulation deficiencies are much rarer and mostly autosomal recessive. Hemophilias are characterized by their severity, which is classified as mild, moderate, or severe, based on the baseline factor activity levels. Severe hemophilia is defined as having less than 1% activity, and patients with severe hemophilia typically experience early-onset spontaneous bleeding [59, 60]. Hemophilic arthropathy may warrant surgical management depending on severity and its impact on the patient's quality of life [61, 62]. Surgical management should involve a multidisciplinary approach to ensure surgical success and adequate postoperative hemostasis. Hemophilia can destroy the joints at a young age if left untreated, and it not only leads to a higher risk of bleeding during surgery, but also an increased risk of infection [62]. The use of prophylaxis at a young age significantly reduces the number of intraarticular bleeds and improves preservation of the joints. Therefore, careful attention to hemostasis during and after surgery must be considered including infusion of the deficient factor. A consideration for patients on inhibitors is infusion with activated prothrombin complex concentrates or recombinant-activated FVII [58–62].

Inherited Thrombophilia

Inherited thrombophilia indicates a genetic risk factor that predisposes patients to developing venous thromboembolism.

The most common forms of testing for inherited thrombophilia include Factor V Leiden, the Prothrombin G20210A mutation, and deficiencies in protein S, protein C, and antithrombin. Among inherited thrombophilia, Factor V Leiden is the most prevalent. Factor V Leiden occurs when the cleavage activation site is removed by a point mutation leading to a greater risk for venous thromboembolism, with greater severity in homozygous individuals [63]. The risk for the initial venous thromboembolism (VTE) is modestly increased (four to five-fold) [64]. Although the risk for these patients is increased, many of them will not ever develop a VTE. In addition, the presence of this genetic mutation does not confirm the disorder due to the incomplete penetrance of the autosomal dominant condition. Following any type of orthopaedic surgery, one study found that patients with factor V Leiden, elevated levels of factor VIII, or blood groups other than O were found to have a higher risk of venous thromboembolism [65].

Proteins C and S are vitamin K-dependent glycoproteins that are synthesized in the liver predominantly and can be inherited or acquired [66]. Without these proteins, unchecked thrombin production can lead to thromboembolism due to the disruption of normal hemostasis. The inherited form of protein C deficiency is typically autosomal recessive and can be broken down into types I and II, low protein C antigen and activity level, and normal quantity of protein C but low activity, respectively. There are many causes of acquired protein C deficiency including physiologic low levels in newborns, infectious processes, or low vitamin K levels due to inadequate stores or medication-induced deficit. Also, low protein C activity levels can be seen in acute thrombosis setting. Warfarin is an example of a vitamin K antagonist medication that leads to low protein C concentrations and in patients who already have low protein C due to inherited causes can induce severe skin necrosis

[66, 67]. Protein S is inherited in an autosomal dominant pattern with three distinct types composed of qualitative and quantitative, type II and types I/III, respectively [66]. Like protein C deficiency, newborns may have insufficient levels of protein S. Other causes of deficiency can be caused by chemotherapy, malignancy, acute thrombosis, and combined oral contraceptives. While skin necrosis is most often associated with warfarin usage in protein C-deficient patients, there are rare cases of protein S deficiency with skin necrosis reported. Though various forms of treatment are available in the treatment of protein C deficiency such as APC (antigen-presenting cells) concentrates or fresh frozen plasma, one case report describes the utilization of human zymogen protein C concentrate along with enoxaparin while performing a total hip arthroplasty [68].

Antithrombin is a thrombin and factor Xa inhibitor, and its activity is mediated by heparin [69, 70]. Inherited deficiencies are uncommon but can be qualitative or quantitative [70]. When greater than 5 g/day of protein is lost through urine in nephrotic syndrome, acquired antithrombin III (ATIII) deficiency can be observed, along with increased consumption during DIC [71]. These are things to keep in mind for orthopaedic surgeons considering operative solutions. Antithrombin III can be administered to patients undergoing orthopaedic surgery with a hereditary deficiency. It was found that ATIII may have a shorter half-life during and after surgery, suggesting a higher rate of utilization of the ATIII during these times [72].

All hereditary thrombotic conditions should be considered in the assessment by orthopaedic surgeons. Patients with thrombophilia undergoing orthopaedic surgery are at an elevated risk for postoperative VTE. The use of a combination of pharmacological interventions and mechanical measures holds paramount significance, especially for individuals with hereditary thrombophilia. The choice and duration of chemical prophylaxis following orthopaedic surgery should not be influenced by underlying thrombophilia [68, 70]. Management of patients with inherited thrombophilia who are on anticoagulation for VTE during the perioperative period can be challenging and depends on bleeding and thromboembolic risks and the specific anticoagulant used. In such cases, seeking expertise from other specialties such as hematology or cardiology is advisable. Minimizing the interruption of anticoagulation is crucial, particularly for those with high-risk thrombophilia (e.g., protein C and S deficiencies) who are at a significantly elevated perioperative risk of venous thromboembolism [68, 70, 71].

Antiphospholipid Antibody Syndrome

Antiphospholipid syndrome (APLS) is characterized by the presence of antibodies against phospholipid-binding proteins including lupus anticoagulant, anticardiolipin, and anti-beta2glycoprotein I antibodies, which lead to an increased risk for thrombosis in effected patients [73, 74]. Thrombosis can occur in any organ system and within both venous and arterial vasculature, with venous thromboses being more common than arterial thromboses. The most prevalent sites of thrombosis are the lower limbs, followed by cerebral arterial circulation [73]. In addition to thrombotic complications, obstetric complications such as recurrent pregnancy losses are frequently observed in patients with antiphospholipid syndrome [74]. The pathogenesis of thrombotic and obstetric complications is complex and complement activation has been associated with both [75]. Thrombotic complications have been linked to the activation of endothelial and immune cells and interaction between coagulation and fibrinolytic systems [76, 77].

Orthopaedic manifestations of APLS are under-recognized [78]. Cases reported in the literature suggest an association between osteonecrosis and primary APLS [79].. There is also evidence of osteonecrosis in secondary APLS associated with systemic lupus erythematosus, but this relationship requires further studies [80]. Bone marrow necrosis in patients with APLS has been reported in several case reports [81, 82].

The diagnostic criteria required for APLS were updated in 2006 [75]. The diagnosis requires at least one clinical and one laboratory criterion. Clinical criteria include vascular thrombosis that can be present in any tissue, an exception being a superficial venous thrombose, and it must be confirmed with objective validation criteria but without evidence of inflammation within the vessel walls [2, 75]. Another qualifying criterion is unexplained death of a morphologically normal fetus at or beyond 10 weeks, one or more premature births of a morphologically normal neonate before 34 weeks (due to either severe pre-eclampsia, eclampsia, or recognized features of placental insufficiency), and/or three or more unexplained consecutive spontaneous abortions before 10 weeks with some exclusions [75]. Exclusions include hormonal or anatomic abnormalities of the mother and chromosomal causes from either parent. The new laboratory criteria required that the antibodies must be present within the plasma at least 12 weeks apart to assure persistent antibodies [2, 75]. Thus confirmation of lupus anticoagulant in the plasma, anticardiolipin antibody IgG and/or IgM in serum or plasma must be present at medium or high titer, or Anti-beta2-glycoprotein I antibody IgG and/or IgM in serum or plasma at high titer must be at least 12 weeks apart [2].

For patients with antiphospholipid syndrome and thrombosis, warfarin is preferred over DOACs due to previous studies indicating a higher risk of thrombosis with DOACs compared to warfarin, especially in those with triple-positive serology and/or arterial thrombosis [83]. Given the elevated risk of recurrent thrombosis, bridging anticoagulation during the perioperative period it is recommended in patients with antiphospholipid syndrome to minimize interruptions in anticoagulation.

Cytochrome Interactions

A final consideration for selection of anticoagulation and prescription medications is the cytochrome system. Cytochromes are composed of a large class of enzymes which are primarily responsible for the breakdown of medications within the body. Orthopaedic patients are often on many medications to treat underlying health issues which may inhibit or enhance the cytochrome system [84]. These interactions

Table 10.1 Common CYP3A4 Substrates, Inducers and Inhibitors

Common CYP3A4 substrates, Inducers and Inhibitors		
CYP3A4 Substrates	CYP3A4 Inducers	CYP3A4 Inhibitors
Carbamazepine	Carbamazepine	Allopurinol
Ethosuximide	Corticosteroids	Amiodarone
Felbamate	Efavirenz	Amprenavir
Phenobarbital	Modafinil	Aprepitant
Phenytoin	Zonisamide	Atazanavir
Tiagabine	Nevirapine	Chloramphenicol
	Omeprazole	Cimetidine
	Oxcarbazepine	Clarithromycin
	Phenytoin	Cyclosporin
	Primidone	Darunavir
	Rifabutin	Dasatinib
	Rifampin	Delavirdine
	St. John's Wort	Diltiazem
		Erythromycin
		Fluconazole
		Fluoxetine
		Grapefruit juice
		Imatinib
		Indinavir
		Isoniazid
		Itraconazole
		Ketoconazole
		Nefazodone
		Nelfinavir
		Nifedipine
		Quinolones
		Ritonavir
		Saquinavir
		Tamoxifen
		Valproic acid
		Verapamil

Chart adapted from: Alreja G, Inayatullah S, Goel S, Braden G. [86]

can heavily influence the levels of anticoagulation medications in the body and thus lead to over or under coagulated states. Dabigatran, rivaroxaban, edoxaban, and apixaban are all anticoagulation medications that are affected by the permeability-glycoprotein (p-gp) which regulates both gastrointestinal uptake and excretion through the liver and kidneys [85]. Rivaroxaban, apixaban, dabigatran, and edoxaban all undergo metabolism by the CYP (cytochrome) proteins, most notably CYP 3A4 with minor contributions from other CYP isomers [85]. These interactions thus become critical when prescribing anticoagulation medications or medications to patients on anticoagulation. Tables 10.1 and 10.2 lists some of the common CYP and P-Gp inhibitors and inducers. Ideally, a warning system should exist that alerts the clinician of the cytochrome interactions and suggest need for alternative chemical anticoagulation medications. Thus, for example, a patient who is on Phenytoin (Dilantin) should avoid anticoagulation use of apixaban.

Table 10.2 Common Medications that affect P-glycoprotein (PGP)

Common Medications that affect P-glycoprotein (PGP)		
PGP substrates	PGP Inhibitors	PGP Inducers
Cyclosporine	Amiloride	Aspirin
Dipyridamole	Amiodarone	Cyclosporine
Digoxin	Atorvastatin	Paclitaxel
Diltiazem	Carvedilol	Reserpine
Ivermectin	Cyclosporine	
Losartan	Digoxin	
Quinidine	Diltiazem	
Tacrolimus	Dipyridamole	
	Doxazosin	
	Felodipine	
	Lidocaine	
	Lovastatin	
	Nifedipine	
	Propafenone	
	Propranolol	
	Quinidine	
	Simvastatin	
	Spironolactone	
	Verapamil	

Chart adapted from: Alreja G, Inayatullah S, Goel S, Braden G. [86]

Summary

The nature of orthopaedic surgery leads to an inmate relationship with the coagulation cascade and hematology. Nearly all orthopaedic patients fulfill at least part of Virchow's triad, and thus an orthopaedic physician must be aware of the coagulation pathway and difficulties that can present themselves in the clinical setting. Orthopaedic physicians can make valuable interventions in the coagulation pathway to prevent DVTs, Pes, and other complications, but this can also cause serious and life-changing harm if done incorrectly. This chapter reviewed the basic science of coagulation as well as common ways coagulation can go wrong. Unfortunately, there is no substitution for attention to many details.

Questions

1. What is the cause of death for this patient?

   This patient is suffering from Heparin-induced Thrombocytopenia. The key things to recognize are venous thrombosis and a drop in platelet count by over 50% from baseline after 1–3 days of heparin therapy.
2. What laboratory studies could have confirmed the diagnosis?

   As mentioned, a platelet drop of over 50% is critical to recognize. In an unclear diagnosis, a 4 T score can be calculated which considers thrombocytopenia, timing, complications, and alterative causes. Lastly, a serotonin release assay or PF4 immunoassay can be ordered to confirm only if needed.

3. What medication should the patient be switched to after identifying laboratory changes on postoperative day 6?

   The most important thing is to immediately stop the heparin product. The patient can then be switched to non-heparin products such as rivaroxaban, apixaban, dabigatran, or fondaparinux.

References

1. Scolaro JA, Taylor RM, Wigner NA. Venous thromboembolism in Orthopaedic trauma. J Am Acad Orthop Surg. 2015;23(1):1–6. https://doi.org/10.5435/JAAOS-23-01-1.
2. Vandevelde A, Devreese KMJ. Laboratory diagnosis of antiphospholipid syndrome: insights and hindrances. J Clin Med. 2022;11(8):2164. https://doi.org/10.3390/jcm11082164.
3. Stannard JP, Lopez-Ben RR, Volgas DA, Anderson ER, Busbee M, Karr DK, McGwin GR Jr, Alonso JE. Prophylaxis against deep-vein thrombosis following trauma: a prospective, randomized comparison of mechanical and pharmacologic prophylaxis. J Bone Joint Surg Am. 2006;88(2):261–6. https://doi.org/10.2106/JBJS.D.02932.
4. Sems SA, Levy BA, Dajani K, Herrera DA, Templeman DC. Incidence of deep venous thrombosis after temporary joint spanning external fixation for complex lower extremity injuries. J Trauma. 2009;66(4):1164–6.
5. Smith EB, Parvizi J, Purtill JJ. Delayed surgery for patients with femur and hip fractures-risk of deep venous thrombosis. J Trauma. 2011;70(6):E113–6.
6. SooHoo NF, Eagan M, Krenek L, Zingmond DS. Incidence and factors predicting pulmonary embolism and deep venous thrombosis following surgical treatment of ankle fractures. Foot Ankle Surg. 2011;17(4):259–62.
7. Nicholson M, Chan N, Bhagirath V, Ginsberg J. Prevention of venous thromboembolism in 2020 and beyond. J Clin Med. 2020;9(8):2467. https://doi.org/10.3390/jcm9082467.
8. Butenas S, Mann KG. Blood coagulation. Biochemistry (Mosc). 2002;67(1):3–12. http://protein.bio.msu.ru/biokhimiya/contents/v67/full/67010005.html.
9. Biga, L. M., Bronson, S., Dawson, S., Harwell, A., Hopkins, R., Kaufmann, J., LeMaster, M., Matern, P., Morrison-Graham, K., Oja, K., Quick, D., Runyeon, J., Oeru, O., & OpenStax. (2019). 18.5 hemostasis. Anatomy physiology. https://open.oregonstate.education/aandp/chapter/18-5-hemostasis/.
10. Garmo C, Bajwa T, Burns B. Physiology, clotting mechanism. In: StatPearls. Treasure Island (FL): StatPearls Publishing; 2023. https://www.ncbi.nlm.nih.gov/books/NBK507795/.
11. Coller BS, Beer JH, Scudder LE, Steinberg MH. Collagen-platelet interactions: evidence for a direct interaction of collagen with platelet GPIa/IIa and an indirect interaction with platelet GPIIb/IIIa mediated by adhesive proteins. Blood. 1989;74(1):182–92.
12. Sarratt KL, Chen H, Kahn ML, Hammer DA. Platelet receptor glycoprotein VI-mediated adhesion to type I collagen under hydrodynamic flow. Ann Biomed Eng. 2004;32(7):970–6. https://doi.org/10.1023/b:abme.0000032459.29696.65.
13. Gale AJ. Continuing education course #2: current understanding of hemostasis. Toxicol Pathol. 2011;39(1):273–80. https://doi.org/10.1177/0192623310389474.
14. McRae S. Physiological Haemostasis. In: Fitridge R, Thompson M, editors. Mechanisms of vascular disease: A reference book for vascular specialists. Adelaide (AU): University of Adelaide Press; 2011. p. 9. https://www.ncbi.nlm.nih.gov/books/NBK534253/.
15. Nacca CR, Shah KN, Truntzer JN, Rubin LE. Total knee arthroplasty in a patient with hypofibrinogenemia. Arthroplast Today. 2015;2(4):177–82. https://doi.org/10.1016/j.artd.2015.10.004
16. Chaudhry R, Usama SM, Babiker HM. Physiology, coagulation pathways. In: StatPearls. Treasure Island (FL): StatPearls Publishing; 2023. https://www.ncbi.nlm.nih.gov/books/NBK482253/.

17. Bailey JP, Kruger MP, Solano FX, Zajko AB, Rubash HE. Prospective randomized trial of sequential compression devices vs low-dose warfarin for deep venous thrombosis prophylaxis in total hip arthroplasty. J Arthroplast. 1991;6(Suppl):S29–35. https://doi.org/10.1016/s0883-5403(08)80053-8.
18. Chen AH, Frangos SG, Kilaru S, Sumpio BE. Intermittent pneumatic compression devices — physiological mechanisms of action. Eur J Vasc Endovasc Surg. 2001;21(5):383–92. https://doi.org/10.1053/ejvs.2001.1348.
19. Comerota AJ, Chouhan V, Harada RN, Sun L, Hosking J, Veermansunemi R, Comerota AJ Jr, Schlappy D, Rao AK. The fibrinolytic effects of intermittent pneumatic compression: mechanism of enhanced fibrinolysis. Ann Surg. 1997;226(3):306–13.; ; discussion 313–4. https://doi.org/10.1097/00000658-199709000-00010.
20. Christiansen M, Grove EL, Hvas AM. Contemporary clinical use of aspirin: mechanisms of action, current concepts, unresolved questions, and future perspectives. Semin Thromb Hemost. 2021;47(7):800–14. https://doi.org/10.1055/s-0041-1726096.
21. Falck-Ytter Y, Francis CW, Johanson NA, Curley C, Dahl OE, Schulman S, Ortel TL, Pauker SG, Colwell CW Jr. Prevention of VTE in orthopedic surgery patients: antithrombotic therapy and prevention of thrombosis, 9th ed: American College of Chest Physicians Evidence-Based Clinical Practice Guidelines. Chest. 2012;141(2 Suppl):e278S–325S. https://doi.org/10.1378/chest.11-2404.
22. Kamran SI, Downey D, Ruff RL. Pneumatic sequential compression reduces the risk of deep vein thrombosis in stroke patients. Neurology. 1998;50(6):1683–8. https://doi.org/10.1212/wnl.50.6.1683.
23. Oduah EI, Linhardt RJ, Sharfstein ST. Heparin: past, present, and future. Pharmaceuticals (Basel). 2016;9(3):38. https://doi.org/10.3390/ph9030038.
24. Mulloy B, Hogwood J, Gray E, Lever R, Page CP. Pharmacology of heparin and related drugs. Pharmacol Rev. 2016;68(1):76–141. https://doi.org/10.1124/pr.115.011247.
25. Warnock LB, Huang D. Heparin. In: StatPearls. Treasure Island (FL): StatPearls Publishing; 2023. https://www.ncbi.nlm.nih.gov/books/NBK538247/.
26. Estes JW. Clinical pharmacokinetics of heparin. Clin Pharmacokinet. 1980;5(3):204–20. https://doi.org/10.2165/00003088-198005030-00002.
27. Warner GT, Perry CM. Enoxaparin. Am J Cordiovosc Drugs. 2001;1:477–81. https://doi.org/10.2165/00129784-200101060-00010.
28. Farkas J. Unfractionated heparin (UFH), LMWH, Fondaparinux, Argatroban, and Bivalirudin. EMCrit Project, Resus Leadership Academy; 2023. emcrit.org/ibcc/heparin/.
29. Bethea A, Samanta D, Deshaies D, Richmond BK. Determination of optimal weight-based enoxaparin dosing and associated clinical factors for achieving therapeutic anti-Xa assays for deep venous thrombosis prophylaxis. J Am Coll Surg. 2019;229(3):295–304. https://doi.org/10.1016/j.jamcollsurg.2019.03.0.
30. Parikh S, Jakeman B, Walsh E, Townsend K, Burnett A. Adjusted-dose enoxaparin for VTE prevention in the morbidly obese. J Pharm Technol. 2015;31(6):282–8. https://doi.org/10.1177/8755122515593381.
31. Robinson DM, Wellington K. Fondaparinux Sodium. Am J Cardiovasc Drugs. 2005;5:335–46. https://doi.org/10.2165/00129784-200505050-00007.
32. Tun HN, Kyaw MT, Rafflenbeul E, Suástegui XL. Role of direct Oral anticoagulants for post-operative venous thromboembolism prophylaxis. Eur Cardiol. 2022;17:e11. https://doi.org/10.15420/ecr.2021.55.
33. Nopp S, Kraemmer D, Ay C. Factor XI inhibitors for prevention and treatment of venous thromboembolism: A review on the rationale and update on current evidence. Front Cardiovasc Med. 2022;9:903029. https://doi.org/10.3389/fcvm.2022.903029.
34. Neumann I, Rada G, Claro JC, Carrasco-Labra A, Thorlund K, Akl EA, Bates SM, Guyatt GH. Oral direct factor Xa inhibitors versus low-molecular-weight heparin to prevent venous thromboembolism in patients undergoing total hip or knee replacement: a systematic review

and meta-analysis. Ann Intern Med. 2012;156(10):710–9. https://doi.org/10.7326/0003-4819-156-10-201205150-00421.
35. Flevas DA, Megaloikonomos PD, Dimopoulos L, Mitsiokapa E, Koulouvaris P, Mavrogenis AF. Thromboembolism prophylaxis in orthopaedics: an update. EFORT Open Rev. 2018;3(4):136–48. https://doi.org/10.1302/2058-5241.3.170018.
36. Anderson DR, Dunbar M, Murnaghan J, Kahn SR, Gross P, Forsythe M, Pelet S, Fisher W, Belzile E, Dolan S, Crowther M, Bohm E, MacDonald SJ, Gofton W, Kim P, Zukor D, Pleasance S, Andreou P, Doucette S, Theriault C, Abianui A, Carrier M, Kovacs MJ, Rodger MA, Coyle D, Wells PS, Vendittoli PA. Aspirin or rivaroxaban for VTE prophylaxis after hip or knee arthroplasty. N Engl J Med. 2018;378(8):699–707. https://doi.org/10.1056/NEJMoa1712746.
37. Diep R, Garcia D. Does aspirin prevent venous thromboembolism? Hematology Am Soc Hematol Educ Program. 2020;2020(1):634–41. https://doi.org/10.1182/hematology.2020000150.
38. Stone J, Hangge P, Albadawi H, Wallace A, Shamoun F, Knuttien MG, Naidu S, Oklu R. Deep vein thrombosis: pathogenesis, diagnosis, and medical management. Cardiovasc Diagn Ther. 2017;7(Suppl 3):S276–84. https://doi.org/10.21037/cdt.2017.09.01.
39. Lee SY, Ro du H, Chung CY, et al. Incidence of deep vein thrombosis after major lower limb orthopedic surgery: analysis of a nationwide claim registry. Yonsei Med J. 2015;56(1):139–45. https://doi.org/10.3349/ymj.2015.56.1.139.
40. Motohashi M, Adachi A, Takigami K, Yasuda K, Inoue M, Sasaki S, Matsui Y. Deep vein thrombosis in orthopedic surgery of the lower extremities. Ann Vasc Dis. 2012;5(3):328–33. https://doi.org/10.3400/avd.oa.12.00049.
41. Kim HJ, Walcott-Sapp S, Leggett K, Bass A, Adler RS, Pavlov H, Westrich GH. Detection of pulmonary embolism in the postoperative orthopedic patient using spiral CT scans. HSS J. 2010;6(1):95–8. https://doi.org/10.1007/s11420-009-9128-5.
42. Righini M, Robert-Ebadi H, Le Gal G. Diagnosis of acute pulmonary embolism. J Thromb Haemost. 2017;15(7):1251–61. https://doi.org/10.1111/jth.13694.
43. Costello RA, Nehring SM. Disseminated intravascular coagulation. In: StatPearls. Treasure Island (FL): StatPearls Publishing; 2023. https://www.ncbi.nlm.nih.gov/books/NBK441834/.
44. Papageorgiou C, Jourdi G, Adjambri E, Walborn A, Patel P, Fareed J, Elalamy I, Hoppensteadt D, Gerotziafas GT. Disseminated intravascular coagulation: an update on pathogenesis, diagnosis, and therapeutics strategies. Clin Appl Thromb Hemost. 2018;24(9_suppl):8S–28S. https://doi.org/10.1177/1076029618806424.
45. Lim JWS, Zhang W, Park DH, AXR P. Disseminated intravascular coagulation following femoral nailing in a metastatic prostate carcinoma patient - A case report. Trauma Case Rep. 2021;36:100534. https://doi.org/10.1016/j.tcr.2021.100534.
46. Raphael BG, Lackner H, Engler GL. Disseminated intravascular coagulation during surgery for scoliosis. Clin Orthop Relat Res. 1982;162:41–6.
47. Hassmann GC, Keim HA. Disseminated intravascular coagulation (DIC) in orthopedic surgery. Case report and review of literature. Clin Orthop Relat Res. 1974;103:118–32. https://doi.org/10.1097/00003086-197409000-00070.
48. Ahmed I, Majeed A, Powell R. Heparin induced thrombocytopenia: diagnosis and management update. Postgrad Med J. 2007;83(983):575–82. https://doi.org/10.1136/pgmj.2007.059188.
49. Lovecchio. Heparin-induced thrombocytopenia. Clin Toxicol. 2014;52(6):579–83. https://doi.org/10.3109/15563650.2014.917181.
50. Arepally GM, Padmanabhan A. Heparin-induced thrombocytopenia: A focus on thrombosis. Arterioscler Thromb Vasc Biol. 2021;41(1):141–52. https://doi.org/10.1161/ATVBAHA.120.315445.
51. Perdomo J, Leung HHL, Ahmadi Z, Yan F, Chong JJH, Passam FH, Chong BH. Neutrophil activation and NETosis are the major drivers of thrombosis in heparin-induced thrombocytopenia. Nat Commun. 2019;10(1):1322. https://doi.org/10.1038/s41467-019-09160-7.
52. Cuker A, Arepally GM, Chong BH, Cines DB, Greinacher A, Gruel Y, Linkins LA, Rodner SB, Selleng S, Warkentin TE, Wex A, Mustafa RA, Morgan RL, Santesso N. American

Society of Hematology 2018 guidelines for management of venous thromboembolism: heparin-induced thrombocytopenia. Blood Adv. 2018;2(22):3360–92. https://doi.org/10.1182/bloodadvances.2018024489.
53. Olevsky OM, Rosove MH. "spontaneous" heparin-induced thrombocytopenia and thrombosis after Total knee arthroplasty: A report of 2 cases. Arthroplast Today. 2021;9:50–2. https://doi.org/10.1016/j.artd.2021.03.005.
54. Nichols WL, Hultin MB, James AH, Manco-Johnson MJ, Montgomery RR, Ortel TL, Rick ME, Sadler JE, Weinstein M, Yawn BP. von Willebrand disease (VWD): evidence-based diagnosis and management guidelines, the National Heart, Lung, and Blood Institute (NHLBI) expert panel report (USA). Haemophilia. 2008;14(2):171–232. https://pubmed.ncbi.nlm.nih.gov/18315614/
55. Sabih A, Babiker HM. Von Willebrand disease. In: StatPearls. Treasure Island (FL): StatPearls Publishing; 2023. https://www.ncbi.nlm.nih.gov/books/NBK459222/.
56. Kroonen LT, Gillingham BL, Provencher MT. Orthopedic manifestations, and management of patients with von Willebrand disease. Orthopedics. 2008;31(3):263–9. https://doi.org/10.3928/01477447-20080301-22.
57. Siboni SM, Biguzzi E, Solimeno LP, Pasta G, Mistretta C, Mannucci PM, Peyvandi F. Orthopaedic surgery in patients with von Willebrand disease. Haemophilia. 2014;20(1):133–40. https://pubmed.ncbi.nlm.nih.gov/23992395/.
58. Salen P, Babiker HM. Hemophilia A. In: StatPearls. Treasure Island (FL): StatPearls Publishing; 2023. https://www.ncbi.nlm.nih.gov/books/NBK470265/.
59. Konkle BA, Nakaya Fletcher S. Hemophilia B. 2000 Oct 2 [updated 2023 Feb 9]. In: Adam MP, Mirzaa GM, Pagon RA, et al., editors. GeneReviews®. Seattle (WA): University of Washington, Seattle; 2022. https://www.ncbi.nlm.nih.gov/books/NBK1495/.
60. Castaman G, Matino D. Hemophilia A and B: molecular and clinical similarities and differences. Haematologica. 2019;104(9):1702–9. https://doi.org/10.3324/haematol.2019.221093.
61. Steven MM, Yogarajah S, Madhok R, Forbes CD, Sturrock RD. Haemophilic arthritis. Q J Med. 1986;58(226):181–97.
62. Rodríguez-Merchán EC. The role of orthopaedic surgery in haemophilia: current rationale, indications, and results. EFORT Open Rev. 2019;4(5):165–73. https://doi.org/10.1302/2058-5241.4.180090.
63. Albagoush SA, Koya S, Chakraborty RK, et al. Factor V Leiden mutation. In: StatPearls. Treasure Island (FL): StatPearls Publishing; 2023. https://www.ncbi.nlm.nih.gov/books/NBK534802/.
64. Simone B, De Stefano V, Leoncini E, Zacho J, Martinelli I, Emmerich J, Rossi E, Folsom AR, Almawi WY, Scarabin PY, den Heijer M, Cushman M, Penco S, Vaya A, Angchaisuksiri P, Okumus G, Gemmati D, Cima S, Akar N, Oguzulgen KI, et al. Risk of venous thromboembolism associated with single and combined effects of factor V Leiden, prothrombin 20210A and Methylenetethraydrofolate reductase C677T: a meta-analysis involving over 11,000 cases and 21,000 controls. Eur J Epidemiol. 2013;28(8):621–47. https://doi.org/10.1007/s10654-013-9825-8.
65. Zambelli R, Nemeth B, Touw CE, Rosendaal FR, Rezende SM, Cannegieter SC. High risk of venous thromboembolism after orthopedic surgery in patients with thrombophilia. J Thromb Haemost. 2021;19(2):444–51. https://doi.org/10.1111/jth.15163.
66. Padda IS, Patel P, Citla Sridhar D. Protein C and S. In: StatPearls. Treasure Island (FL): StatPearls Publishing; 2023. https://www.ncbi.nlm.nih.gov/books/NBK557814/.
67. Boer CG, Szilagyi I, Nguyen NL, et al. Vitamin K antagonist anticoagulant usage is associated with increased incidence and progression of osteoarthritis. Ann Rheum Dis. 2021;80:598–604.
68. Thakkar SC, Streiff MB, Bruley DF, Mears SC. Case report: perioperative use of protein c concentrate for protein C deficiency in THA. Clin Orthop Relat Res. 2010;468(7):1986–90. https://doi.org/10.1007/s11999-009-1189-8.

69. Mourey L, Samama JP, Delarue M, Choay J, Lormeau JC, Petitou M, Moras D. Antithrombin III: structural and functional aspects. Biochimie. 1990;72(8):599–608. https://doi.org/10.1016/0300-9084(90)90123-x.
70. Patnaik MM, Moll S. Inherited antithrombin deficiency: a review. Haemophilia. 2008;14(6):1229–39. https://doi.org/10.1111/j.1365-2516.2008.01830.x.
71. Erworbene MG. Antithrombin III-Mangelzustände [acquired antithrombin III deficiency]. Z Gesamte Inn Med. 1992;47(2):74–7.
72. Mannucci PM, Boyer C, Wolf M, Tripodi A, Larrieu MJ. Treatment of congenital antithrombin III deficiency with concentrates. Br J Haematol. 1982;50:531–5. https://doi.org/10.1111/j.1365-2141.1982.00479.x-i1.
73. Bustamante JG, Goyal A, Singhal M. Antiphospholipid syndrome. In: StatPearls. Treasure Island (FL): StatPearls Publishing; 2023. https://www.ncbi.nlm.nih.gov/books/NBK430980/.
74. Sammaritano LR. Antiphospholipid syndrome. Best Pract Res Clin Rheumatol. 2020;34(1):101463. https://doi.org/10.1016/j.berh.2019.101463.
75. Di Prima FA, Valenti O, Hyseni E, Giorgio E, Faraci M, Renda E, De Domenico R, Monte S. Antiphospholipid syndrome during pregnancy: the state of the art. J Prenat Med. 2011;5(2):41–53.
76. Velásquez M, Rojas M, Abrahams VM, Escudero C, Cadavid ÁP. Mechanisms of endothelial dysfunction in antiphospholipid syndrome: association with clinical manifestations. Front Physiol. 2018;9:1840. https://doi.org/10.3389/fphys.2018.01840.
77. Krone KA, Allen KL, McCrae KR. Impaired fibrinolysis in the antiphospholipid syndrome. Curr Rheumatol Rep. 2010;12(1):53–7. https://doi.org/10.1007/s11926-009-0075-4.
78. Gorshtein A, Levy Y. Orthopedic involvement in antiphospholipid syndrome. Clin Rev Allergy Immunol. 2007;32:167–71. https://doi.org/10.1007/s12016-007-0006-y.
79. Tektonidou MG, Malagari K, Vlachoyiannopoulos PG, Kelekis DA, Moutsopoulos HM. Asymptomatic avascular necrosis in patients with primary antiphospholipid syndrome in the absence of corticosteroid use: A prospective study by magnetic resonance imaging. Arthritis Rheum. 2003;48:732–6. https://doi.org/10.1002/art.10835.
80. Haque W, Kadikoy H, Pacha O, Maliakkal J, Hoang V, Abdellatif A. Osteonecrosis secondary to antiphospholipid syndrome: a case report, review of the literature, and treatment strategy. Rheumatol Int. 2010;30(6):719–23. https://doi.org/10.1007/s00296-009-1269-9.
81. Paydas S, Koçak R, Zorludemir S, Baslamisli F. Bone marrow necrosis in antiphospholipid syndrome. J Clin Pathol. 1997;50(3):261–2. https://doi.org/10.1136/jcp.50.3.261.
82. Moore J, Ma DDF, Concannon A. Non-malignant bone marrow necrosis: A report of two cases. Pathology. 1998;30(3):318–20., https://www.sciencedirect.com/science/article/pii/S0031302516348966. https://doi.org/10.1080/00313029800169536.
83. Dufrost V, Risse J, Zuily S, Wahl D. Direct Oral anticoagulants use in antiphospholipid syndrome: are these drugs an effective and safe alternative to warfarin? A systematic review of the literature. Curr Rheumatol Rep. 2016;18(12):74. https://doi.org/10.1007/s11926-016-0623-7.
84. Hakkola J, Hukkanen J, Turpeinen M, Pelkonen O. Inhibition, and induction of CYP enzymes in humans: an update. Arch Toxicol. 2020;94(11):3671–722. https://doi.org/10.1007/s00204-020-02936-7.
85. Li A, Li MK, Crowther M, Vazquez SR. Drug-drug interactions with direct oral anticoagulants associated with adverse events in the real world: A systematic review. Thromb Res. 2020;194:240–5. https://doi.org/10.1016/j.thromres.2020.08.016.
86. Alreja G, Inayatullah S, Goel S, Braden G. Rhabdomyolysis caused by an unusual interaction between azithromycin and simvastatin. J Cardiovasc Dis Res. 2012;3:319–22.

Chapter 11
Lead Toxicity Due to Retained Bullet Fragments

Catherine Dong, Emily Kershner, Wilhelm A. Zuelzer, Matthew S. Smith, and Khalid Hasan

Case 1

A 20-year-old male sustained multiple gunshots during French class at a university—one bullet pierced his right shoulder, and three others became fragments in pelvis, and near but not within hips and left knee joints—more than 50 total bullet fragments. He stated he was told he would be fine for the long term. Ten years later, he noted fatigue and his mother had read a CDC report on retained bullet fragments (RBFs) and lead toxicity and suggested he get his blood tested for lead. His blood lead level (BLL) was 37 mcg/dL. He underwent surgery to remove a limited number of accessible bullet fragments, but this only slightly decreased his BLL. Additional surgery was felt not feasible to remove remaining 50 or more RBF. Thus, he has been placed on chelation therapy but whenever he stops chelation therapy, his BLLs rise [1].

C. Dong
Department of Emergency Medicine, Virginia Commonwealth University, Richmond, VA, USA
e-mail: Catherine.Dong@vcuhealth.org

E. Kershner
Division of Toxicology, Department of Emergency Medicine, Virginia Commonwealth University, Richmond, VA, USA
e-mail: Emily.Kershner@vcuhealth.org

M. S. Smith · K. Hasan (✉)
Department of Orthopaedic Surgery, Virginia Commonwealth University, Richmond, VA, USA
e-mail: Matthew.S.Smith@vcuhealth.org; khalid.hasan@vcuhealth.org

W. A. Zuelzer
Orthopaedic Surgery, Virginia Commonwealth University Medical School, Richmond, VA, USA
e-mail: wilhelm.zuelzer@vcuhealth.org

W. A. Zuelzer, S. Metikala (eds.), *Unusual Conditions That Every Orthopaedic Surgeon Should Know*, https://doi.org/10.1007/978-3-031-58946-1_11

Case 2

A 54-year-old black female had been followed in the arthritis clinic. She was seen in the emergency room with complaints of constipation and abdominal pain. She was treated symptomatically for constipation. She returned 3 weeks later with a complaint of black stools. Her guaiac test was 1+ positive. Sigmoidoscopy, barium enema, upper GI series, and oral cholecystogram were performed on an outpatient basis and all were negative. A routine blood count revealed a hemoglobin of 7.6 g% and a hematocrit of 23.9 vol%. She was admitted for work-up of her anemia. Her past medical history was significant for a gunshot wound to the right knee 5 months prior to admission. Physical examination revealed a blood pressure of 140/90 mmHg, pulse of 96/min, and respiratory rate of 16/min. She was afebrile with pale conjunctiva, clear chest, and a grade 2/6 systolic ejection murmur at the left sternal border. Stool guaiac was negative. Her laboratory revealed hemoglobin of 6.9 g%, hematocrit of 21.3 vol%, MCV (mean corpuscular volume) of 84 (considered low normal), and MCHC (mean corpuscular hemoglobin concentration) of 32.3 (considered low). The reticulocyte count was 5% (1% corrected) (inadequate response for RBC production in the face of anemia—reticulocytes are young immature non-nucleated red blood cells typically larger than normal red blood cells (RBC) and still contain RNA with reticulofilamentous appearance) and the peripheral smears were remarkable for basophilic stippling (basophilic granules—thought to be aggregates ribosomes dispersed in cytoplasm of red blood cells (RBC), mild anisocytosis (RBC varying sizes on blood smear) and poikilocytosis (RBC of varying shapes on blood smear), polychromasia (more immature RBC than normal), hypochromia (red blood cells have less color than normal), and target cells (thickened cell membrane-relative cell volume). Her white blood count was 5,500 with a normal differential. The platelet count was 388,000 (considered normal). She continued to complain of pain in her knees and abdominal pain. On the eighth hospital day, she was found unresponsive with her eyes tonically deviated to the right. Her vital signs were normal and neurological exam documented postictal confusion. No focal neurological signs were detected. The following morning, she had a grand mal seizure. Her serum electrolytes, serum calcium, and serum magnesium levels were within normal limits. A general toxicology screen was negative (did not include blood lead level). Lumber puncture revealed clear fluid with a protein of 130 ug/L, and glucose of 73 mg/dL. Cytology revealed no malignant cells. Bacterial cultures and VDRL were negative. On the 13th hospital day, the patient had four grand mal seizures, following which she was comatose with Cheyne-Stokes respirations. CT of the brain was compatible with diffuse cerebritis with possible compression of the left lateral ventricle. The following morning, she was found unresponsive without vital signs. Cardiopulmonary resuscitation was unsuccessful.

During the autopsy, it was suggested that the death may represent a case of lead poisoning based on clinically observed basophilic stippling. Analysis of blood obtained postmortem revealed lead levels of 5.3 mg/L (conversion roughly to 530 ug/dL). The antemortem blood obtained 5 days prior to death had lead levels of 5.1 mg/L (conversion roughly to 510 mg/dL). Blood level above 0.6 mg/L is considered toxic in adults in our laboratory. Microscopic examination of tissue and autopsy revealed characteristic eosinophilic intranuclear inclusion in hepatocytes and cells of the proximal tubules of the kidneys. Many perivascular spaces in the brain continued aggregates of periodic acid-Schiff (PAS) positive pink staining homogenous material (postmortem). X-rays taken at the time the deceased had been shot in the leg were obtained and reviewed. These showed flattened, deformed lead 0.32 caliber revolver bullets lodged in the soft tissue anterolateral to the distal femur immediately proximal to the condyle. Smaller fragments of lead were present adjacent to the main missile mass. The location of the bullet was consistent with it being in, or in communication with, the suprapatellar bursa (No other causes of plumbism were identified.). [2]

Questions
1. Why is it important to identify lead contamination early from projectiles?
2. What locations of projectiles predict higher lead contamination? What needs to be done to confirm diagnosis?
3. What is the management and goal of treatment? Why is it complicated?

Note: The term "RBF" will be used to describe one or multiple retained bullet fragments.

Introduction

Epidemiology of Retained Bullet Fragments

From 2009 to 2017, there are an estimated annual 85,000 survivors of firearm injuries, in addition to nearly 35,000 deaths from firearms in the United States [3]. Based on a cohort study comparing 6,498 survivors of firearm injuries matched to 32,490 control participants, the survivors of firearm injuries had a 40% increase in pain diagnoses, a 51% increase in psychiatric disorders, and an 85% increase in substance use disorders [4]. Bullet fragment removal is typically performed for specific reasons: (1) Palpable retained bullet fragments (RBF), (2) Visible RBF at surgery, (3) RBF found in (or near) joints, cerebrospinal fluid (CSF) or eye, (4) RBF-related nerve impingement, (5) RBF in lumen of vessel, or (6) medico-legal issues [5]. Thus, it is estimated that only between 2& and 10% of patients will have RBF removed [5, 6]. Another justification for RBF removal is the presence of abscess or infection involving the fragment, but this is surprisingly uncommon—in one study of 352 adults with low-energy extremity-only gunshot wounds, followed for at least 30-days post-injury, only 0.8% had deep infection requiring debridement [7]. One study of 298 patients, with the mean age of 29.5 years (range 6.1–62.1), who sustained nonfatal gunshot wounds, 75% (225 patients) had RBF at the time of presentation, and only 13% (27 patients) of this group had complete removal of RBF [6]. Additionally, there is always a possibility that the projectile will go through and through a body part. In a review of 244 children who were treated for gunshot injuries, 44% had retained RBF, 41% had through-and-thorough gunshot wounds, 9% had removal at time of injury, and 6% died of their injuries [8]. At follow-up, of the 107 patients with RBF, 10% had an abscess or cellulitis and only 13% underwent RBF removal. In conclusion, a conservative estimate can be made that between 50,000 and 60,000 patients injured by projectiles annually will have RBF after medical intervention in the United States.

RBF and Lead

Lead is used in the majority of bullets because it is cheap, has a relatively low melting point (621 °F), can easily be shaped into bullets and is malleable enough to fragment, but is dense (will thus "fly better") [9, 10]. Lead is found in easily accessible ore deposits throughout the world. Of the nine billion bullets manufactured in the United States each year, roughly 90% are made, at least in part, of lead [11]. Thus, a significant number of bullets, after entering a human, will contaminate that human with a potential "lead snowstorm." For animal hunting involving a high-power rifle, after a lead-core bullet enters an animal, the lead projectile expands, explodes, and a bullet fragment may be distributed up to 45 cm from the wound channel (bullet path) [12–14]. In addition, thousands of nanometer-sized lead particles may be distributed throughout the tissue, which are not detectable with our standard radiological instruments, and thus nearly impossible to remove [15].

Lead Pharmacology

Lead ($Pb^{2+}$and Pb^{4+} valence forms found in compounds) is a heavy metal that has no physiologic role and can negatively affect every organ system. The World Health Organization (WHO) 2021 update estimates that close to one million lives were lost due to lead poisoning in 2019 [16]. Lead is absorbed and distributed by binding to RBCs—in red blood cell wall and cytoplasm [17]. Lead in RBCs has a half-life estimated at 5 days, assuming no recycling back from surrounding tissue/bone back into blood [18]. Blood serves as the initial receptacle of absorbed lead before it distributes lead throughout the body [18–21] (see Fig. 11.1). Lead is stored primarily in bone and to a lesser extent in soft tissue (liver, bone marrow, kidneys, brain, teeth, and hair). It is predominately excreted renally into urine, but also through biliary clearance into the feces [21, 22]. Of the lead that is not excreted, the majority of it is stored in bone with a mean half-life of 10–30 years. (See Fig. 11.2) [22–24]. Thus, blood lead levels (BLL) typically reflect only a fraction of lead present in the body and not the cumulative body lead burden [25].

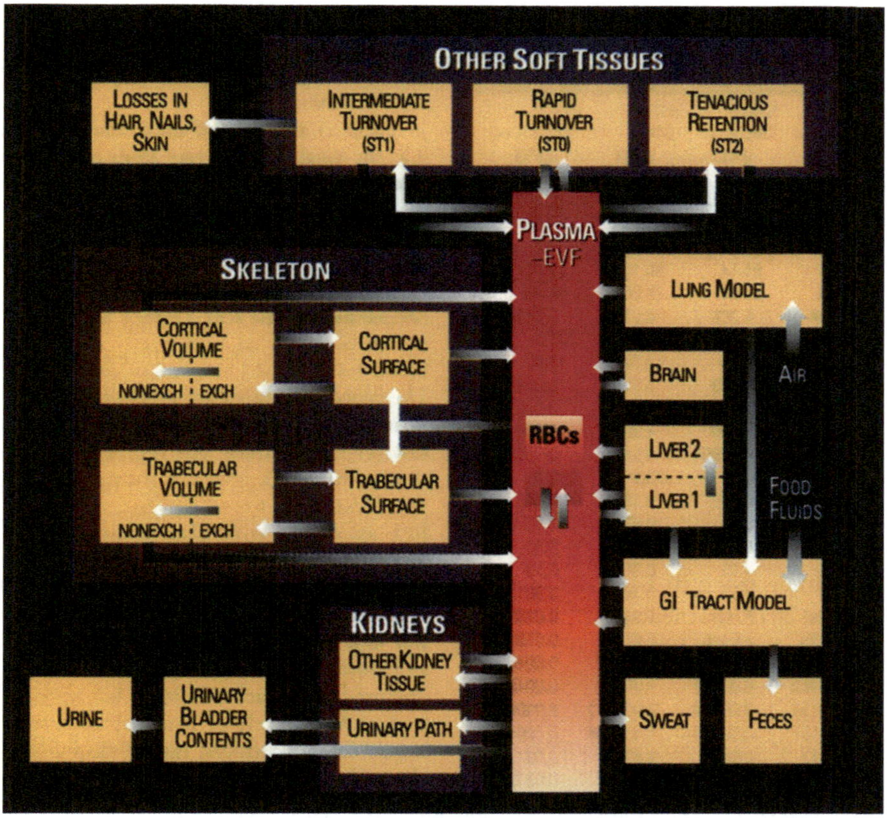

Fig. 11.1 Compartments and paths of movement in the biokinetic model for lead. Transfer rates for exchanges between compartments are age specific. Reproduced with permission from the author. Leggett R. An Age-specific Kinetic Model of Lead Metabolism in Humans. Environ Health Perspect (1993) 101:598-616 [18]

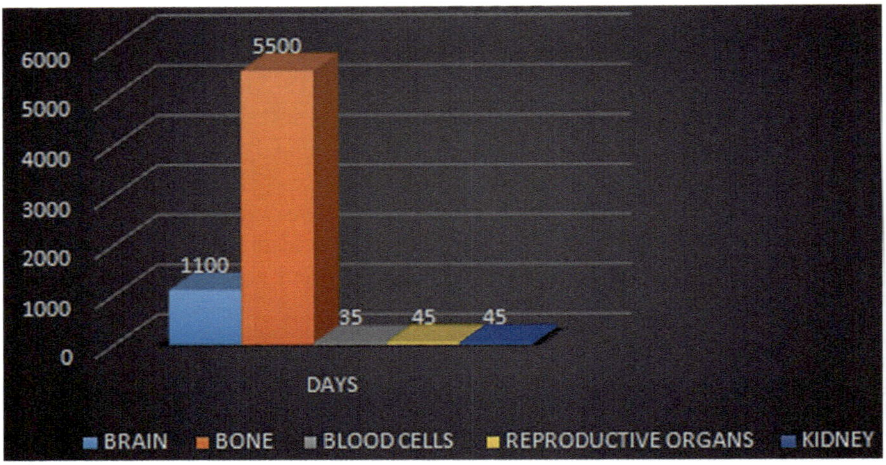

Fig. 11.2 Half-life of lead (*Reproduced with permission) from Collin M, Venkatraman S, Vijayakumar N, Kanimozhi V, Arbaaz S, Stacey R,* et al. *Bioaccumulation of lead (Pb) and its effects on human: A review. J Hazard Mater Adv. 2022 Aug 1; 7:100094* [23])

Review of BLL—Baseline Data

The Centers for Disease Control and Prevention (CDC) has stated that there is no safe BLL in children and recommends follow-up for all children with venous blood lead levels greater than 3.5 ug/dL [26–28]. There is demonstrable cognitive impact on children, even with lead levels below 10 ug/dL [28, 29]. Mothers with BLLs even lower than 5 ug/dL have an increased risk of reduced fetal growth [30]. The cognitive and neurobehavioral effects of lead observed in children have also been observed in adults [31, 32]. For adults, some state agencies also use the same threshold as children to indicate the need for follow-up (BLL greater than 3.5 ug/dL [33]), but others may differ, using BLL greater than or equal to 5 ug/dL [34, 35]. In a survey from 2015 to 2018, the median BLL for children ages 1 to 5 living in families with income below the poverty level was 0.8 ug/dL and for children living in families at or above the poverty level was 0.6 ug/dL [36]. In a survey from 2017 to 2018, adults 20 years and older had mean BLLs of 0.855 ug/dL [37]. The guideline for consideration for surgical and medical management, such as chelation, is critically dependent on BLL and clinical symptoms and signs. In general, chelation therapy is indicated for children with BLL greater than 45 ug/dL and adults with BLL greater than 70 ug/dL [38].

Mechanism of Lead Toxicity (Brief Overview)

Lead generates free radicals which damage DNA, cell membranes, and critical enzymes (see Fig. 11.3) [23, 39, 40]. Calcium is the main promoter of neurotransmission, which is the basis for cognition [41]. Lead mimics calcium and

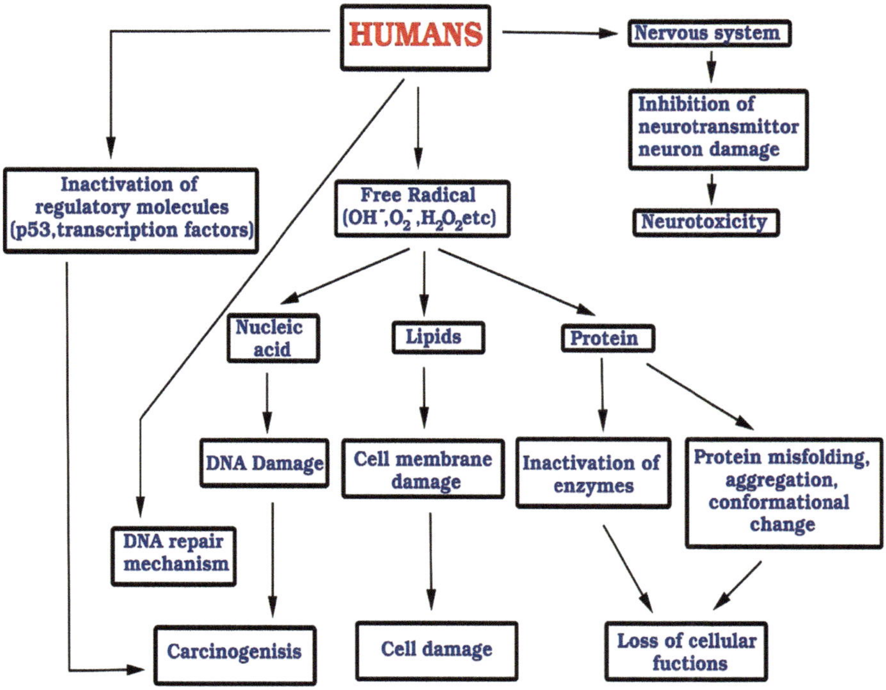

Fig. 11.3 Effects of heavy metal accumulation in human body (*Reproduced with permission from Collin MS, Venkatraman SK, Vijayakumar N, Kanimozhi V, Arbaaz SM, Stacey RGS,* et al. *Bioaccumulation of lead (Pb) and its effects on human: A review. J Hazard Mater Adv. 2022 Aug 1; 7:10094*) [23]

thus interferes with calcium-dependent cellular processes, disrupting cell membrane transport systems, and ultimately impairing neurotransmission [20, 40, 41].

Brain Function

The brain is the organ most vulnerable to lead poisoning. Lead has a significant impact on synapse formation in the cerebral cortex of a developing child's brain [42, 43]. It disrupts the formation of neurochemicals, including neurotransmitters, as well as the organization of ion channels. Lead poisoning also causes neuron myelin sheath loss, a decrease in the number of neurons, interferes with neurotransmission, and reduces neuronal growth. Because lead can substitute for calcium ions and be taken up by calcium-ATPase pumps, it can pass through the blood–brain barrier, interfering with synapse development [42, 43]. Elevated BLL is correlated with headaches, delayed reaction time, irritability, concentration difficulty, and typically motor nerve more than sensory function [43, 44].

Anemia/Red Blood Cells

Lead inhibits many enzymes essential to heme synthesis and ultimately, RBC production. It impairs the activity of the enzyme ferrochelatase, which catalyzes the integration of iron into the protoporphyrin ring. Iron is inserted into the middle of protoporphyrin as the last step in the formation of heme, a necessary component of hemoglobin, which is responsible for carrying oxygen [45]. If in lead intoxication, ferrochelatase is blocked or if there is insufficient iron available, zinc is substituted for iron and zinc protoporphyrin concentrations rise, which can be measured in blood. Lead also is a potent inhibitor of another important enzyme, delta-aminolaevulinic acid dehydratase, by displacing and accordingly changing the structure of the enzyme [46]. This enzyme is involved in the second step of biosynthesis of heme, catalyzing the condensation of delta-aminolaevulinic acid to promote the synthesis of the porphobilinogen ring, involved in RBC formation. Impairment of this enzyme will result in elevation of serum and urine delta-aminolaevulinic acid since it will not be condensed [47]. Lead also reduces the lifespan of RBCs by increasing the fragility of cell membrane, resulting in hemolysis [48, 49]. Thus, lead decreases the amount of hemoglobin in the blood by impairing synthesis and causing hemolysis eventually resulting in chronic anemia [45]. The anemia is typically mild, with peripheral smears demonstrating either normochromic or hypochromic and microcytic RBCs. Basophilic stippling is occasionally present—typically in patients who have been exposed to lead for a prolonged period [48, 49]. The stippling is due to aggregation of RNA and ribosomal and represents iron/heme disorder (See Fig. 11.4). Basophilic stippling is not pathognomonic of lead poisoning—differential diagnoses may include normal patients, and patients with blood disorders, such as hemoglobinopathies (thalassemia, sickle cell disease), megaloblastic anemia due to vitamin B12 or folate deficiency, benzene poisoning, chronic alcohol use, liver disease, infection, or myelodysplastic syndromes [48, 50, 51].

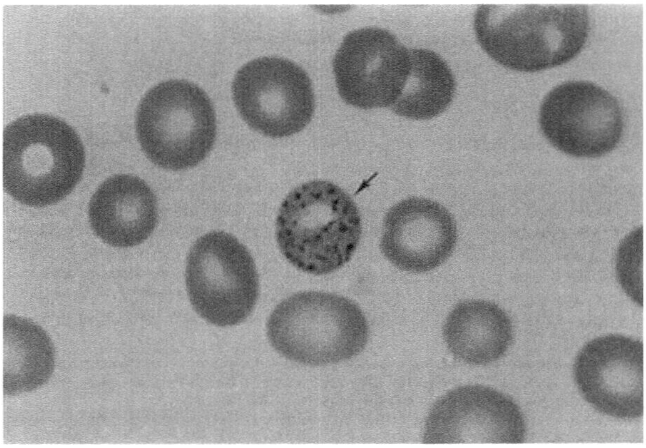

Fig. 11.4 Basophilic stippling (*Reproduced with permission from Cheson B, Rom W, Webber R. Basophilic Stippling of Red Blood Cells: A Nonspecific Finding of Multiple Etiology. American J of Industrial Medicine (1984)5(4): 327-334*) [50]

Renal Function

The proximal tubular lining cells are inhibited by lead toxicity. Lead toxicity can cause abnormalities such as aminoaciduria, phosphaturia, and glycosuria (Fanconi-like syndrome). Chronic lead nephropathy can develop after years of lead exposure, as evidenced by mild localized atrophy, loss of proximal tubules, and tubulointerstitial fibrosis in kidney biopsy [52]. "Saturnine" gout can be a consequence of lead toxicity by a combination of increased uric acid production or decreased uric acid excretion and is often associated with renal impairment [53].

Blood Pressure

Lead substitutes for calcium in blood vessels lead to stiffening of vessels and increasing blood pressure [54]. Lead also increases the level of reactive oxygen species that subsequently enhance the inactivation of nitric oxide, leading to hypertension [55].

Bone

Lead indirectly affects bone cell activity by reducing 1,25-dihydroxyvitamin D-3 concentrations and by inhibiting osteocalcin, which may impede new bone formation as well as the functional coupling of osteoblasts and osteoclasts [56]. It can inhibit the cells' capacity to manufacture or secrete other bone matrix components like collagen. In growing children, increased calcium deposition on the hydroxyapatite crystal preferentially in the zone of provisional calcification produces radiodense metaphyseal bands [56–58]. Lead inhibits osteoclastic remodeling but has a limited effect on osteoblasts. Thus, the thickness and number of trabeculae at the metaphysis result in increased dense metaphyseal bands (see Fig. 11.5). Dense metaphyseal bands are not pathognomonic for lead toxicity—differential diagnoses include adverse effects of chemotherapy (methotrexate), chronic anemia, leukemia, healing renal osteodystrophy and rickets [58]. It is estimated that about 50% of trabecular bone is lost over a lifetime, and thus there is a potential for higher BLL during periods of rapid bone turnover (i.e., osteoporosis, pregnancy, lactation) [59].

Clinical Signs/Symptoms of Lead Toxicity

Signs and symptoms of lead poisoning may be subtle, leading to a delay in diagnosis and treatment. The continuum of signs and symptoms is dependent on BLL, duration and frequency of lead exposure, mobilization of lead from bone, and individual susceptibility [60]. The main organ systems affected by lead intoxication are

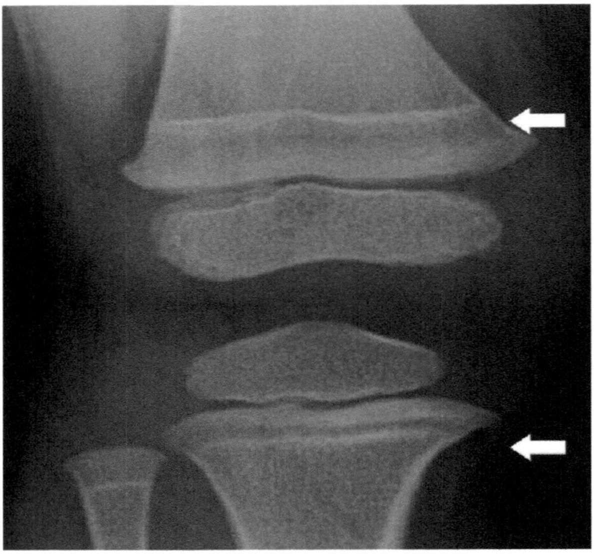

Fig. 11.5 X-ray of the patient showing "lead lines" (bands of increased metaphyseal density on radiographs of long bones in young children). (*Reproduced with permission from Lau K, Chow T, Chan C,* et al. *Hong Kong Poison Information Centre: Annual report 2017. Hong Kong Journal of Emergency Medicine. 2018;25(6):313-323. doi:10.1177/1024907918798997*) *Multiple lines are associated with repeated exposure to lead* [61]

the neurologic, gastrointestinal, renal, cardiovascular, hematologic, and musculoskeletal systems. However, it can be challenging to correlate these symptoms with the index RBF injury, which may have occurred remotely [61, 62]. It is crucial that orthopaedic surgeons are aware of the possibility of lead toxicity in RBF patients. Many of these patients can present with vague symptoms for years before being diagnosed with lead poisoning.

Suspicion of lead toxicity in a patient with RBF should arise when there is history of weight loss, weakness, fatigue, joint pain, myalgias, gastrointestinal discomfort including loss of appetite and constipation, memory loss, irritability, weakness, trembling, tingling limbs, change in mood, daylight drowsiness or anemia [63–66]. Table 11.1 and Fig. 11.6 summarize the clinical signs and symptoms that can be observed in patients with lead toxicity [67, 71, 72]. The key requirement is for the clinician to consider the diagnosis in anyone with history of RBF through careful history-taking. For example, one can inquire about subtle behavioral changes, such as chronic fatigue or irritability. There is a higher risk of fragility hip fractures in patients with elevated BLLs [73]. Microcytic anemia, as noted in the case presentation, is related to the impact of lead on RBC production, but anemia is typically mild. Classically, lead toxicity is associated with peripheral motor neuropathy, with children presenting with foot drop and adults with wrist drop [74]. However, sensory impairment is also well reported [67].

Table 11.1 Clinical signs and symptoms of lead toxicity CDC Agency for Toxic Substances and disease Registry/CDC Review May 24 2023 [67]. Also modified from Samarghandian S, Shirazi F, Saeedi F, et al. A systematic review of clinical and laboratory findings of lead poisoning: lessons from case reports. Toxicology and Applied Pharmacology (2021)429:115681 [68]

Neurological: Children	Decreased cognitive function characterized by learning deficits, impaired memory, verbal cognition, ADHD or hyperactivity, impaired speech and hearing, lower IQ, irritability, lethargy, fatigue, myalgia or paresthesia, encephalopathy, seizures, coma, paresis or paralysis, tremor, headaches, microcephaly, bulged anterior fontanelle, developmental retardation, dilated lateral ventricle, dysplastic aortic valve
Neurological: Adult	Decreased cognitive function including impaired memory and learning, altered mood and behavior, fatigue, headaches, and decreased peripheral nerve conduction velocity, encephalopathy, seizures, coma, paresis or paralysis, tremor, progressive hearing loss, peripheral neuropathy, rapid motor neuropathy
Renal	Decreased GFR, proteinuria, renal colic, gout, SIADH
Cardiovascular	Increased blood pressure, tachycardia, atherosclerosis, altered cardiac conduction, increased risk of heart disease, and increased mortality from cardiovascular disease
Hematologic effects	Facial pallor, decreased hemoglobin with hypochromic, microcytic, or normocytic anemia, basophilic stippling, low vitamin D levels
Hepatic effects	Increased liver enzymes and cholesterol, hepatomegaly and increased gallbladder wall thickness, jaundice
Gastrointestinal	Anorexia, abdominal pain/colic, nausea, vomiting, constipation, diarrhea, associated weight loss, loss of sphincter control
Musculoskeletal	Arthralgia, osteoporosis, motor neuropathy (upper motor neuron typically), wrist or foot drop, generalized weakness, numbness, paresthesia, myalgia, gout, wrist widening, absent reflexes LE and normal UE, progressive weakness of extremities, dense metaphyseal bands
Dental	"Lead lines" (see Fig. 11.7), metallic taste
Psychiatric	Anxiety, bizarre behavior, aggression, delirium, agitation, labile mood, and restlessness

Risk Assessment of RBF for Lead Toxicity

Once a history of gunshot wound with RBF has been established, additional factors can aid the clinician in assessing the risk of lead toxicity including number of fragments, location of the RBF, presence of adjacent fracture, hypermetabolic states, and characteristics of the bullet. It is logical that increasing number of RBF in a patient increases the risk of systemic lead toxicity. There is no established correlation between duration of RBF presence and higher BLL [62, 64, 75]. This may be due to deposition of lead in bone and additional leaching of lead from the RBF and/or bone is variable. However, the risk of lead toxicity is significantly higher if the RBF is in an area with a rich vascular supply and in the presence of a suitable solvent such as adipose or body fluids. The acidic nature of synovial fluid intensifies lead solubility substantially—thus RBF near or in a joint place the patient at higher risk for lead toxicity and should be managed by expeditiously removing all

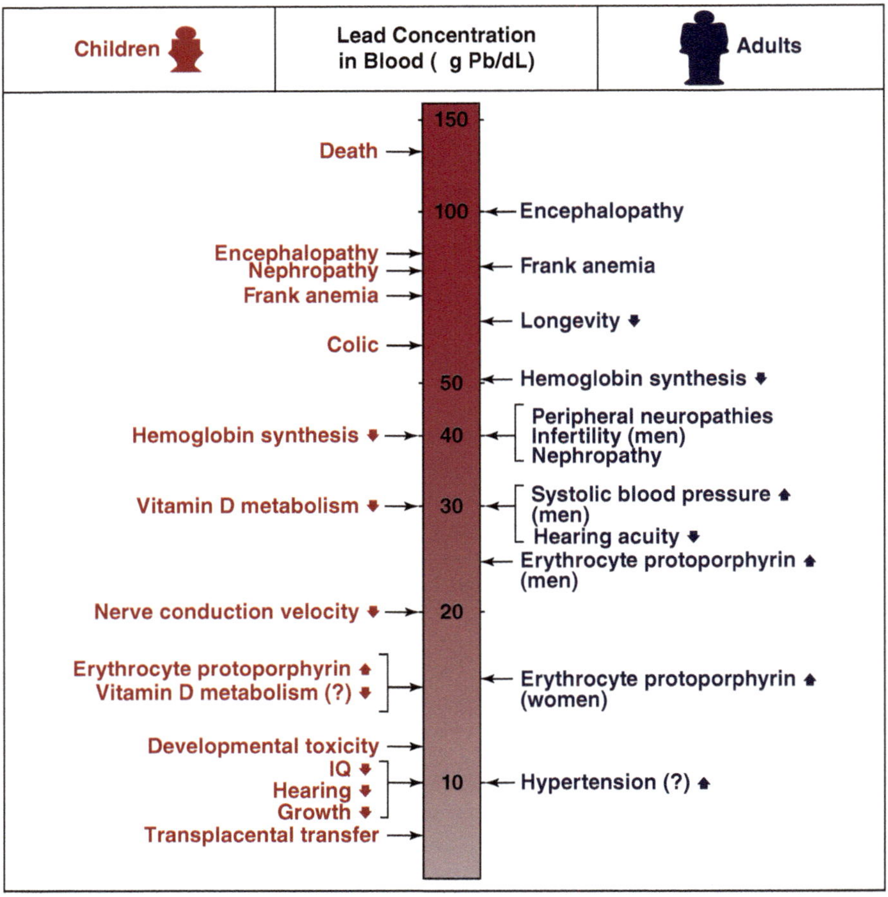

Fig. 11.6 Effects of inorganic lead on children and adults *(Public domain)* [68]. (Reproduced with permission: Effects of inorganic lead on children and adults (lowest observable adverse-effect levels) [70)])

fragments, if feasible, from this location [59, 60, 76]. In addition, the frictional forces in the joint space can increase RBF fragmentation and lead dispersion [77]. It has also been reported that RBF near/in bones have statistically higher chances of elevating lead concentrations (see Fig. 11.8) [62, 64, 78–80]. The likelihood of lead toxicity with RBF in only soft tissue is significantly lower as they may become encapsulated in fibrous tissue, effectively limiting them from exposure to body fluids and blood supply [78, 81, 82].

The presence of an associated fracture is correlated with higher BLL (see Fig. 11.9) [62, 64]. This has been attributed to a tissue inflammatory response activated by fractures and leads to increased lead absorption [78, 80]. Higher BLLs are noted in recent fractures in patients who have a history of prior RBF [83, 84]. It has

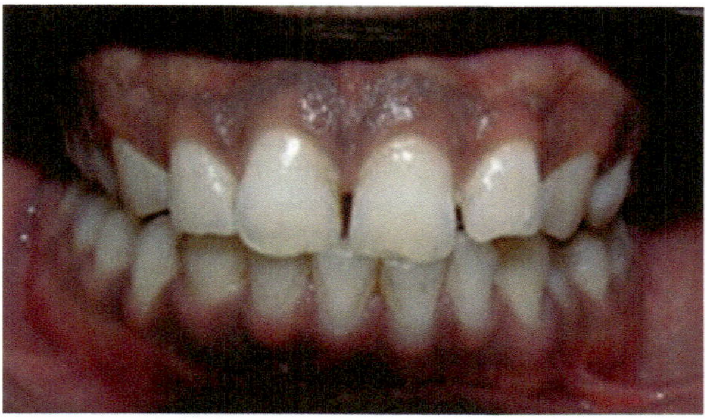

Fig. 11.7 Lead Lines on gingiva *(Public domain)* [67]. *The blue-purplish lines on gum are knowns as Burton's lines, created by a reaction between circulating lead and sulfur ions released during oral bacterial activity* [69]

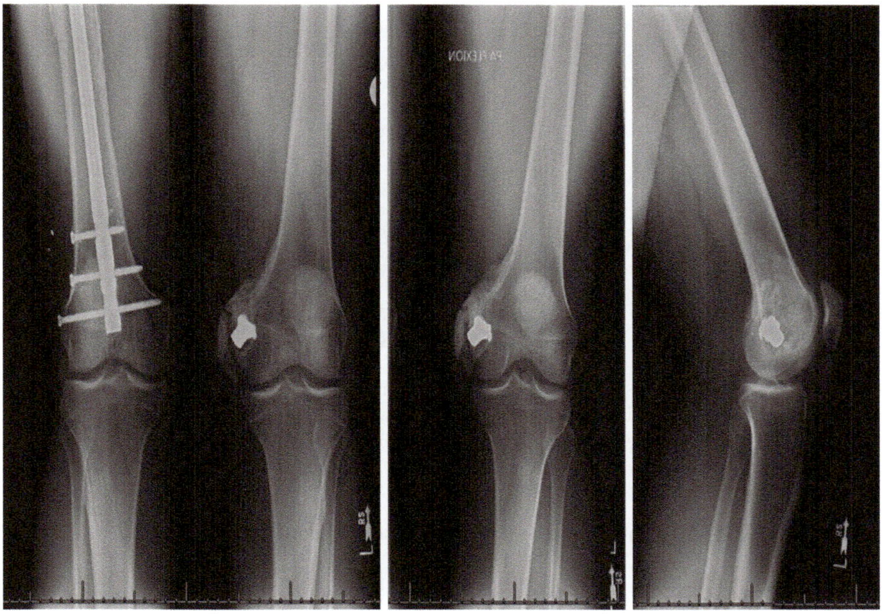

Fig. 11.8 Plain radiograph of a 39-year-old gentleman with a retained bullet in the distal femur

also been reported that RBF size of more than 20% of cortical width negatively impact bony union significantly (see Fig. 11.10) [85]. RBF with smaller fragment size is associated with higher BLL. Similarly, increased surface area of lead due to numerous pellets or more RBFs increases the risk that the lead will be absorbed [86]. Bullets that are unjacketed or partially coated also have increased risk of being absorbed and therefore result in higher BLL [87]. Increased metabolic rate of a patient, from conditions such as systemic inflammation, increased bone turnover, acidosis, pregnancy, hyperthyroidism, and infection, is associated with increased BLL [26] (Table 11.2).

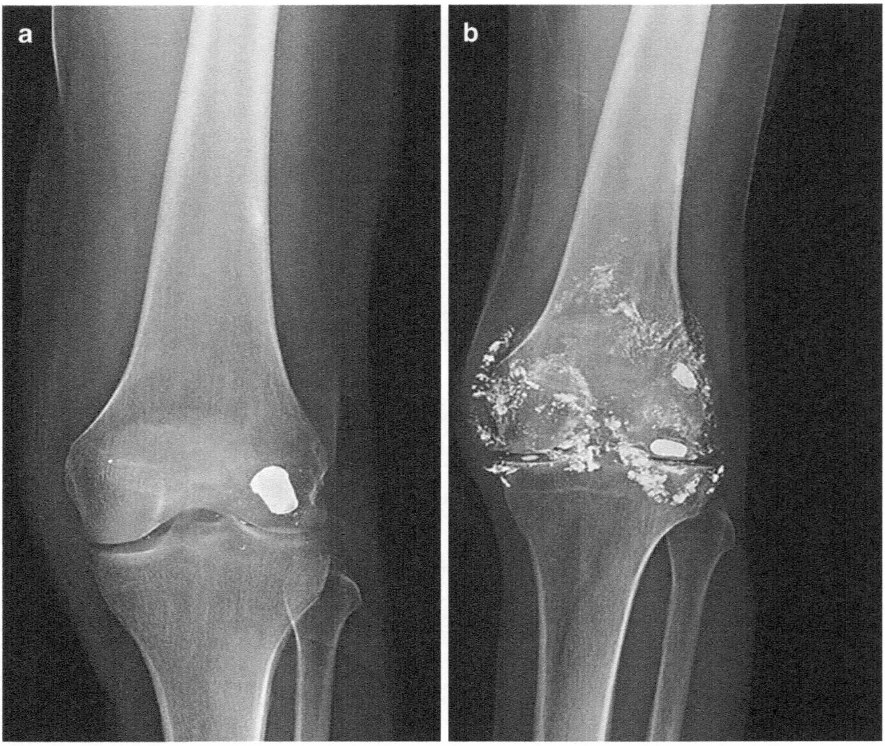

Fig. 11.9 Plain radiographs of the left knee were taken about 14 years apart. Image A was taken at age 32 at the time of initial gunshot wound injury, whereas image B was taken at age 46 with complaints of chronic knee pain. (*Reproduced with permission from Marquez JI, Schindlbeck MA. Lead Toxicity from a Retained Bullet. N Engl J Med. 2018 Dec 20;379(25):2451–2451*) [77]

Special Patient Populations at Increased Risk of Lead Toxicity

If a woman of child-bearing age has significant total body lead burden, the bone resorption during pregnancy potentially will, via RBCs, expose her fetus to significant amount of lead. Reiss et al. [25] noted that early in pregnancy, only trabecular bone with typically lower lead content is resorbed, whereas in late pregnancy, resorption of cortical bone with typically higher lead content will lead to increased maternal BLLs. Starting at 12 weeks of gestation, lead can cross the placenta and affect the developing fetus. This may increase the risk for miscarriage, and premature delivery, and result in neurologic and renal abnormalities in the fetus/neonate [25]. Thus, the key is to identify lead exposure early to minimize, if possible, the total amount of lead from RBFs incorporated in the soft tissues and bone. Not only does the lead do damage per se in each tissue, but lead, stored in the patient's bone, may be distributed to and cause additional damage to the liver, kidney, bone marrow and brain of the patient, and the neonate [88, 89, 90]. This will be additive to any continued absorption of lead directly from RBFs. During pregnancy, calcium and iron supplementation may decrease the release of lead from bone stores [91, 92].

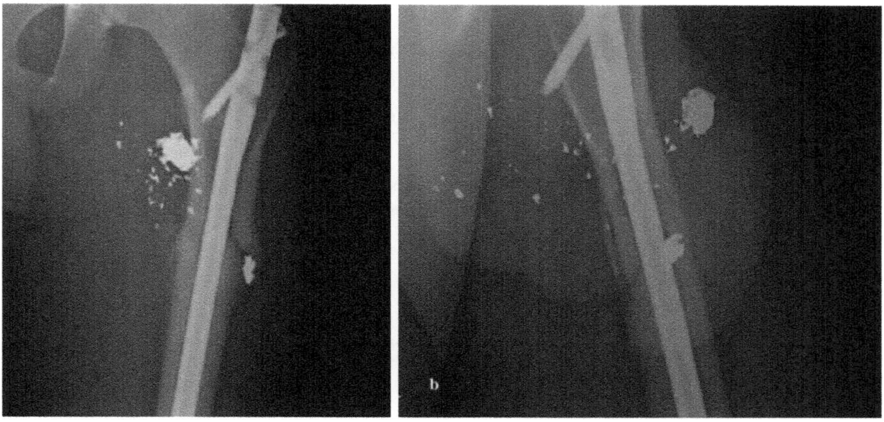

Fig. 11.10 Postoperative imaging from a hollow point bullet gunshot injury. The expanding bullet nose is observed as well as multiple secondary projectiles. (*Reproduced with permission from Riehl JT, Connolly K, Haidukewych G, Koval K. Fractures Due to Gunshot Wounds: Do Retained Bullet Fragments Affect Union? Iowa Orthop J. 2015;35:55-61. PMID: 26361445; PMCID: PMC4492146)*[85]

Table 11.2 RBF characteristics associated with increased BLL

Location of bullet	– Joint space – Intravertebral disc – Blood vessel – Body fluid compartment (pleural/peritoneal)
Size/volume of bullet fragments	– Multiple pellets – Fragmented
Characteristic of bullet	– Unjacketed
Associated conditions	– Fracture – Pregnancy – Infection – Hyperthyroidism – Acidosis

RBFs in pregnant patients and women with desired future fertility should be managed in an interdisciplinary approach with orthopaedics, obstetrics, and toxicology [91, 93].

Management and Surveillance of Patients with RBF

General Overview

Management of patients with RBFs can be complex. There is limited evidence to provide guidelines regarding appropriate surveillance or treatment of patients with lead toxicity secondary to RBFs. Most of the evidence available on surveillance and medical management of lead toxicity is based on environmental or occupational lead exposures. Tables 11.3 and 11.4 provide a general overview of management of elevated BLLs and are not specific to patients with RBFs. For all cases of lead toxicity, the first goal is always to eliminate or reduce exposure to lead sources. In the case of RBFs, this means early surgical removal of the

Table 11.3 Health-based recommendation for lead-exposed adults [94]

Blood lead level (μg/dL)	Short-term risks (lead exposure < 1 year)	Long-term risks (lead exposure ≥ 1 year)	Management
< 5	None documented	None documented	None indicated
5–9	Possible spontaneous abortion Possible postnatal developmental delay	Possible spontaneous abortion Possible postnatal developmental delay Possible hypertension and kidney dysfunction	Discuss health risks Reduce lead exposure for women who are or may become pregnant
10–19	Possible spontaneous abortion Possible postnatal developmental delay Reduced birth weight	Possible spontaneous abortion Reduced birth weight Possible postnatal developmental delay Hypertension and kidney dysfunction Possible subclinical neurocognitive deficits	As above for BLL 5–9 μg/dL, plus: Decrease lead exposure Increase biological monitoring Consider removal from lead exposure to avoid long-term risks if exposure control over an extended period does not decrease BLL < 10 μg/dL, or if medical condition present that increases risk with continued exposure[a]
20–29	Possible spontaneous abortion Possible postnatal developmental delay Reduced birth weight	Possible spontaneous abortion Possible postnatal developmental delay Reduced birth weight Hypertension and kidney dysfunction Possible subclinical neurocognitive deficits	Remove from lead exposure if repeat BLL measured in 4 weeks remains ≥ 20 μg/dL
30–39	Spontaneous abortion Possible postnatal developmental delay Reduced birth weight	Spontaneous abortion Reduced birth weight Possible postnatal developmental delay Hypertension and kidney dysfunction Possible neurocognitive deficits Possible nonspecific symptoms[b]	Remove from lead exposure
40–79	Spontaneous abortion Reduced birth weight Possible postnatal developmental delay Nonspecific symptoms[b] Neurocognitive deficits Sperm abnormalities	Spontaneous abortion Reduced birth weight Possible postnatal developmental delay Nonspecific symptoms[b] Hypertension Kidney dysfunction/nephropathy Subclinical peripheral neuropathy Neurocognitive deficits Sperm abnormalities Anemia Colic Possible gout	Remove from lead exposure Refer for prompt medical evaluation Consider chelation therapy for BLL > 50 μg/dL with significant symptoms or signs of lead toxicity
≥ 80	Spontaneous abortion Reduced birth weight Possible postnatal developmental delay Nonspecific symptoms[b] Neurocognitive deficits Encephalopathy Sperm abnormalities Anemia Colic	Spontaneous abortion Reduced birth weight Possible postnatal developmental delay Nonspecific symptoms[b] Hypertension Nephropathy Peripheral neuropathy Neurocognitive deficits Sperm abnormalities Anemia Colic Gout	Remove from lead exposure Refer for immediate/urgent medical evaluation Probable chelation therapy

BLL, blood lead level.

[a]Medical conditions that may increase the risk of continued exposure include chronic renal dysfunction (serum creatinine > 1.5 mg/dL for men and > 1.3 mg/dL for women, or proteinuria), hypertension, neurologic disorders, and cognitive dysfunction. [b]Nonspecific symptoms may include headache, fatigue, sleep disturbance, anorexia, constipation, arthralgia, myalgia, and decreased libido.

Public Health Services, US Dept of Health and Human

Table 11.4 WHO guideline for clinical management of exposure to lead: executive summary [95]. Geneva: World Health Organization; 2021. License: CC BY-NC-SA 3.0 IGO. There is no suggestion that WHO endorses these proposals. (Modified) Surveillance *of Patients with RBFs*

No.	Recommendation	Strength of recommendation
1	In all cases of suspected or confirmed lead exposure the patient or caregiver should educated about potential sources of lead exposure, methods for reducing continuing exposure and the importance of good nutrition, in particular, adequate dietary intake of iron and calcium	Recommended
2	For an individual with a blood lead concentration ≥ 5 μg/dL, the source(s) of lead exposure should be identified, and appropriate action taken to reduce and terminate exposure	Strong
3	For a non-pregnant adolescent girl or woman of child-bearing age who has a blood lead concentration of 45–70 μg/dL but who does not show clinical features of lead poisoning, oral chelation therapy should be considered	Very low-certainty evidence
4	For a male patient aged ≥11 years or a woman who is no longer of child-bearing age who has a blood lead concentration of 45–70 μg/dL but who does not show clinical features of lead poisoning, chelation therapy is not indicated. The patient should, however, be re-evaluated within 2–4 weeks to ensure that the blood lead concentration is decreasing, and the patient remains well	Very low-certainty evidence
5	For a non-pregnant adolescent or adult with a blood lead concentration of 45–70 μg/dL and who has mild–moderate clinical features of lead poisoning (such as abdominal pain, constipation, arthralgia, headache, lethargy), chelation therapy is suggested.	Very low-certainty evidence
6	An adolescent or an adult with a blood lead concentration > 70–100 μg/dL should be closely monitored for signs of clinical deterioration, regardless of whether chelation therapy is given	Recommended
7	For a non-pregnant adolescent or an adult with a blood lead concentration > 70–100 μg/dL but who does not show significant neurological features of toxicity, chelation therapy is suggested.	Very low-certainty evidence
8	For a non-pregnant adolescent or adult with a blood lead concentration > 70–100 μg/dL and with significant neurological features of lead toxicity (e.g., irritability, drowsiness, ataxia, convulsions, coma) or lead encephalopathy), urgent parenteral chelation therapy is recommended.	Strong
9	For a pregnant woman with lead encephalopathy, regardless of trimester, urgent chelation therapy is recommended. The preferred chelation agent depends on the stage of the pregnancy and available data on safety of use in pregnancy	Strong
10	For a pregnant woman with a blood lead concentration ≥ 45 μg/dL, with or without clinical features of lead poisoning, but without lead encephalopathy: 1. In the first trimester: The guideline development group could not make a recommendation because of an uncertain balance of risks and benefits 2. In the second or third trimester: Chelation therapy is recommended	No recommendation Strong

RBF. For patients with RBF, the onset of clinical lead toxicity following the initial injury remains unpredictable across multiple studies [96]. Symptoms of lead toxicity are often nonspecific, subtle, and can appear years after sustaining a gunshot wound, which can delay diagnosis. The considerable variation in clinical presentations of lead toxicity is, in part, attributable to differences in historical onset and duration of exposure. Additionally, individual intrinsic variations in response to the insult can also contribute to the diverse manifestations of lead toxicity [46, 47]. The median latency to clinical lead poisoning with known symptoms was 7 years, with the longest delay being 52 years from the time of the index injury, according to a recent systematic review [62, 64]. In some cases, an autopsy was required to determine the presence of lead intoxication from an RBF [2]. Moreover, patients who have RBF for an extended length of time may continue to redistribute lead from bone, resulting in elevated BLLs even after delayed surgical removal of RBFs because over 90% of systemically absorbed lead gets incorporated into bone over the course of several months [96–98]. Given this variability in presentation of lead toxicity and its potential catastrophic effects, orthopaedic surgeons should clearly educate the patient on signs and symptoms of lead toxicity, increased risk of toxicity with bedrest, and counsel female patients about the risk of infertility, toxicity to the fetus, and potential need for early intervention [94, 99]. Early surgical removal of the RBF appears critical to prevent continued degradation of the bullet and further systemic absorption of lead. Of course, clinicians can revisit RBF removal after monitoring for elevated BLL and symptoms of lead toxicity, but it is reasonable to anticipate that patients with delayed management may exhibit elevated total body lead levels due to storage in bone and need continued surveillance. In a recent systematic review, of 79 patients who received delayed surgical removal of RBF, 61% had improvement in symptoms with no deaths. Of the 34 patients who did not receive surgery, 12% died, and only 23% had an improvement in symptoms [98]. The efficacy of aggressive early removal of RBF requires additional validation.

In the following section, we will cover the limited evidence available for surveillance, surgical, and medical management in patients with RBF. Overall, it is important for orthopaedic surgeons to recognize patients at increased risk of lead toxicity due to RBF, the need for surveillance, and the importance of interdisciplinary management in those with elevated BLLs. Another consideration is that even low BLL may have clinical consequences. Clinicians caring for patients with RBF and elevated BLLs should discuss management with a toxicologist on a case-by-case basis. If there is no toxicology service available, the Poison Control Center (1-800-222-1222) is a national service that always has a toxicologist on call to assist. In the case of lead toxicity from RBFs, it is imperative to consider removal of the source of lead. This is especially true in cases that are higher risk for systemic lead absorption as previously discussed (in contact with synovium or body fluids). The patient or guardian must also be educated on the possible consequences and treatment options.

Laboratory Studies

Baseline BLL, complete blood count (CBC), creatinine, and blood pressure should be obtained at the time of the initial injury [98]. An initial zinc protoporphyrin (ZPP) level is considered a low cost, rapid test that can aid in establishing the patient's baseline chronic lead exposure. Zinc protoporphyrin is a complex that is formed when heme production is inhibited by lead or lack of iron, and lags behind BLL by 2–3 months [100]. Therefore, it is expected to be elevated in patients chronically exposed to lead. In the assessment of a patient suspected of chronic lead exposure from RBF, an elevated BLL coupled with a low ZPP may suggest the presence of a newer, alternative source of lead [98]. However, ZPP levels are associated with significant individual variability [100]. ZPP may be elevated in iron-deficiency anemia, and anemia of chronic disease, and its role in patients with prolonged history of RBFs is debatable [98, 100]. Lead toxicity should be included in the differential diagnosis of any patient who develops anemia. Chronic lead toxicity can alter blood pressure and renal function, so monitoring is reasonable. Obtaining baseline liver function tests is recommended if chelation is planned for treatment.

BLL Monitoring

McQuirter et al. recruited 502 subjects with acute RBF, over 7 years of age (20% aged 7–18), without prior history of RBF, who received medical care in Los Angeles, California, from 2000 to 2002 [64]. The peak BLL occurred at 3 months post injury. Of the 365 patients who had BLL checked at 3 months, the prevalence of BLL above 10 mcg/dL was 38.1%, and BLL above 20 mcg/dL was 11.8%. Of the 309 patients with available BLL measurements at 1 year, 20.1% had BLL above 10 mcg/dL and 2.6% BLL above 20 mcg/dL. The Council of State and Territorial Epidemiologists (CSTE) recommends monitoring BLL in adult equal to or above 3.5 mcg/dL [101]. Most guidelines were established for occupational exposure. Annual BLL measurement has been recommended in a multidisciplinary workshop at Veterans Affairs Walter-Reed Hospital for patients with RBFs [102]. Other authors have also suggested regular BLL monitoring for only those who have led in contact with body fluids [62, 102–104]. Routine monitoring in asymptomatic patients more than 1 year after firearm injury has not been validated as the half-life of lead in blood is so short [18, 64]. However, clearly there are case report of patients presenting with onset of clinical lead toxicity years after sustaining RBF [105]. We do not know whether screening within 1 year of RBF injury would have identified these at-risk patients. Another critical issue is lead bone storage is significant and resorption of bone with bed rest, pregnancy, or trauma (such as new fracture) may be the trigger that raises the BLL significantly.

The first goal is always to eliminate or reduce exposure to lead. Symptoms of lead toxicity are often nonspecific, subtle, and can appear years after sustaining a gunshot wound. The variation in clinical presentations of lead toxicity is significant, in part, at least, due to differences in acute and chronic dosing, historical and continued duration of exposure, and individual intrinsic variations in response to the insult [41]. The correlation, noted in Fig. 11.2, between BLL and symptoms is low [42]. In general, the higher the BLL, the more likely symptoms will develop. Again, BLL does not directly measure an individual total body lead content. In most cases, BLL measures current exposure to lead and endogenous contribution from prior exposures. The body can accumulate lead clearly over the lifetime from the presence of a projectile in a patient [43].

We recommend all asymptomatic adults with RBFs be considered for routine BLLs at admission, 2 weeks, 6 weeks, 3 months, 6 months, and annually post injury thereafter [62, 64, 71]. Asymptomatic children with RBFs should have similar initial BLL follow-ups and then be tested per CDC guidelines (See Table 11.5) [106].

Radiology

Obtaining appropriate radiographs is essential in patients with a history of bullet injury. By examining the location and quantity of bullet fragments as well as potential migration, radiographs can be helpful in estimating total body lead burden and serial imaging over time can determine fragment changes, including dissolution and foreign body reactions which may portend higher BLL [102]. Digital radiography in two planes can identify fragments as small as 0.1 mm in size [102]. In cases of chronic retained bullets in a joint space, a phenomenon known as "lead arthrogram" can be seen where the metal is seen coating the joint cavity due to partial dissolution of lead in the synovium (See Fig. 11.11) [59, 107]. Lead lines, which are lines of increased density on the metaphysis of the bone, show radiological growth retardation, a phenomenon seen in children (see Fig. 11.5). For evaluation of chronic exposure, techniques for bone lead measurements using fluorescence emissions exist though are not readily available. An X-ray fluorescence machine utilizes low-level gamma radiation to provoke emission of fluorescent photons from bone. This focused energy to a lead atom causes ejection of electrons from the inner K or L shells of the atom, which in turn makes the atom unstable. Accordingly, the atom restores stability by transferring electrons from the other shells to the inner shells, and this emits a photon which can be detected and analyzed [108, 109]. This method is widely used to measure elemental composition. It must be carefully performed

Table 11.5 CDC recommendation for follow-up lead blood testing in children (Public domain)

Venous blood lead levels (μg/dL)	Early follow up testing (2–4 tests after initial test above specific venous BLLs)	Later follow up testing after BLL declining
≥ 3.5–9	3 months	6–9 months
10–19	1–3 months	3–6 months
20–44	2 weeks–1 month	1–3 months
≥ 45	As soon as possible	As soon as possible

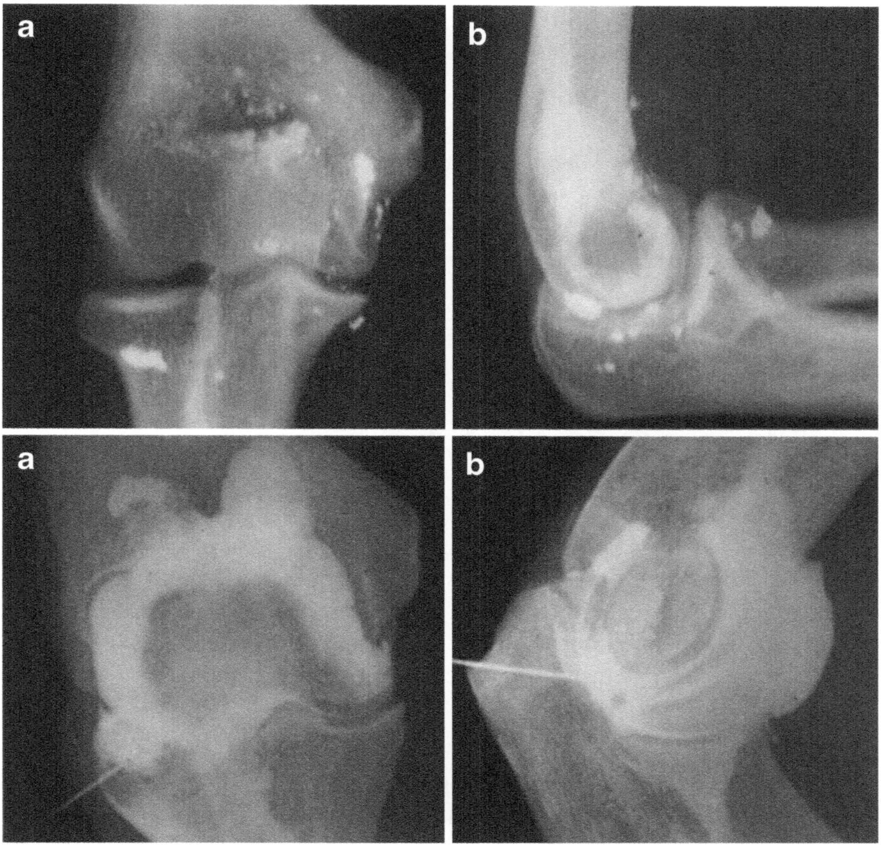

Fig. 11.11 (Top): Lead arthrogram. Numerous small fragments of lead have entered the synovial cavity of the elbow joint. The joint capsule is distended by an effusion, but no fracture is detected. (Bottom): Normal arthrogram of elbow joint. (*Reproduced with permission from Weston WJ. The lead arthrogram—Plumbography. Skeletal Radiol. 1978 Feb 1;2(3):169–70*) [107]

and requires a dedicated facility. Computed tomographic scan (CT) requires modification to minimize metal artifacts and give ideal three-dimensional localization of projectile/s [102]. Ultrasound scans (US) have been reported to be used for identification and intraoperative retrieval of RBFs [110, 111].

Recently, dual-energy CT has been used to differentiate bullets made with and without lead components [112]. This technology may be more valuable if lead bullets become the exception and not the rule. It should be noted that RBF may subsequently travel in the patient along facial planes or within or adjacent to veins or arteries, or even to the heart and lungs. Therefore, accounting for initial location of each projectile acutely is ideal and repeat radiographs to evaluate for migration of projectiles is reasonable [110, 111, 113]. One case report identified movement of a projectile from the distal third of the thigh to the left knee joint, documented over 4 years after initial projectile injury [114].

Management of Elevated BLLs and Lead Toxicity

Surgical removal of lead, nutrition, and chelation are the mainstays of management of lead poisoning secondary to RBF. Any patient who develops signs or symptoms of lead toxicity (Fig. 11.6) or an elevated BLL (Table 11.4) should be managed in collaboration with a toxicologist. Each case will likely vary with regard to the feasibility of surgery versus the risks and benefits of chelation therapy. As previously discussed, special patient populations (pregnant women, pediatric patients) should have an early referral to toxicology. Additionally, it is important to identify, even if RBF exist in a patient, alternative sources for lead toxicity (Table 11.6).

Nutrition

It is recommended that all patients with RBF consume adequate amounts of zinc, calcium, iron, Vitamins B1, B6, and C [129]. There is also a recommendation that individuals at risk should consume fruits and vegetables on a regular basis, such as berries, grapes, tomatoes, garlic, and onions, because of their theoretical antioxidant properties [46, 130]. Additional studies to validate the true benefits are needed—these are based largely on animal research and theoretical benefits.

Table 11.6 Additional sources of lead exposure

Lead-based paint	Homes built before 1978 (when lead-based paints were banned) may contain lead-based paint. When the paint peels and cracks, it creates lead dust. Children can be exposed to lead when they ingest or inhale lead dust/paint [115].
Soil	Soil and road dust may contain naturally occurring lead as well as lead from industrial sources, deteriorated paint, and the combustion of leaded gasoline and aviation fuel [116, 117]
Water	Older water pipes may contain lead or lead-based solder, as well as cooking utensils and water coolers [118]
Air	Lead in outdoor air comes mainly from industrial sources (e.g., smelters, waste incinerators, utilities, and lead-acid battery manufacturers)
Foods, cosmetics, and supplements	Lead can contaminate candies, chili powder, and tamarind. It can also contaminate Ayurvedic (traditional medicine native to India), herbal, and homeopathic remedies [119–121]. Traditional eye makeup (*kohl, kajal, tiro,* or *surma*) worn in Asia, Africa, and the Middle East may contain lead [122]
Toys and jewelry	Lead can be found in some inexpensive children's toys and jewelry, particularly older toys made of tin, brass, or pewter alloys [123]
Occupations and hobbies	Certain occupations and hobbies involve working with lead-based products, such as stained-glass work, painting, lead smelting or mining, automotive repair, plumbing, welding, and construction may cause parents to bring lead into the home [124, 125, 126]. Exposure may also occur from inhalation of lead in shooting ranges environs [116]
Illicit substance use	Ingestion of lead-contaminated drugs such as opium or homemade alcohol (moonshine) can result in lead poisoning [127, 128]

Surgery

Surgical removal of RBF can be classified into early versus delayed and can also be combined with pre- and/or postoperative chelation therapy. There are no set guidelines on when and which RBF should be surgically removed. Less than 15% of surgeons have reported institutional policies on bullet removal [131]. Nevertheless, there are specific instances when removal of RBF has been advocated by most authors. Clearly, early removal is justified if fragments are intraarticular, located within a vessel lumen, or causing nerve impingement [5, 85, 132]. There is significant risk of lead toxicity and joint destruction with intraarticular RBFs [133–135]. Lead may be more soluble in joint spaces than serum due to the synovial fluid's acidic composition. Additionally, frictional forces experienced by RB in the joints and bone itself might cause bullet fragmentation and lead dispersion [80, 107, 134, 136, 137]. Successful arthroscopic removal of bullet fragments from joint spaces have been reported in literature [138, 139].

The literature supports that high-velocity or severely contaminated injuries be surgically washed out and debrided as much as possible, while low-velocity gunshot wounds associated with fracture can be managed nonoperatively [140]. However low-velocity RBF can result in clinically significant lead toxicity. Surgical removal of RBF is currently supported if there is concern for continued systemic absorption of lead. Improvement of clinical symptoms and subsidence of BLL have been observed in most studies after delayed surgical intervention [63, 78, 133, 137, 141]. However, it is also advised that delayed surgical removal of RBF may not eliminate lead from the body as it stores in bone over time. Postoperative chelation may be needed as the bone will continue to disperse lead into the blood and should be discussed with a toxicologist [62, 141–143]. Repeat BLLs after surgical treatment are recommended by the World Health Organization (WHO) to ensure BLL is appropriately monitored and addressed [71].

Although rare, migration of an RBF from one part of the body to another has also been reported in the literature and treating physicians and surgeons need to be mindful of this [111, 114, 141]. There have been a few cases reported where the bullet embolized into the heart or even into the intracranial space through the vasculature [144, 145].

It may be necessary to obtain additional imaging in suspected cases of migration for surgical planning. It is important to correlate the number of bullet punctures (entrance versus entrance and exit where appropriate) with the number of RBFs visible on radiographs. RBF may rarely be transported significant distances from the initial resting location. Removal of RBFs from the spine have not been recommended as the surgical risks often overweigh the benefits in this region. Exceptions are the presence of neurologic signs, bullet in spinal canal/disc space, and continued high BLL on regular screening [146–148]. RBFs in the soft tissue are less often associated with high BLL and therefore not routinely recommended for surgical removal. However, even low levels of lead may be clinically consequential. It is hoped that the soft tissue forms a fibrous coating around the bullet, therefore limiting further the release of lead into the circulation [149–151]. As noted previously, other indications of surgical removal of RBF may include if it is relatively superficial and causing patient discomfort, if it impinges on nerve or nerve root and causes pain to the patient, or if it is lodged in the blood vessel and causing any ischemia [5]. Abscess formation related to RBF, entrance and even exit wound contamination is a definite indication for surgical debridement and excision regardless of where the trapped bullet is located. Often, dirt, clothing, smoke particulates, and bacterial organisms are pushed inside along the bullet track by the impact of the projectile, from contamination of the bullet itself, and recoil from the exit portion of a through and through wound. It is surprising how low the percentage of abscess formation is—it is assumed that the inoculum must be small [5, 152].

Chelation

Chelators are designed to form chemically inert and non-toxic complexes with lead that can then be excreted from the body though use is limited by availability, cost, and adverse reactions [153, 154]. The indications for chelation therapy are based on patient age, BLL, and clinical symptoms. In the United States, the three major chelators used in lead poisoning are dimercaprol (BAL), edetate calcium disodium ($CaNa_2EDTA$), and succimer. BAL and $CaNa_2EDTA$ are used parenterally in the event of severe lead poisoning (such as lead encephalopathy), whereas succimer is orally available for milder cases. Chelation therapy should not be initiated without consultation with a toxicologist (Table 11.7). Chelation is a relatively inefficient process, reducing total body burden of lead by only 1–2% [155, 156]. It is yet unproven if there is significant improvement to subclinical end-organ dysfunction after chelation therapy. A VAMC workshop patients with RBF regarding the risk-benefit balance of chelation recommended consideration of chelation for patients with significant symptoms and BLL above 50 mcg/dL, and for those without symptoms who have BLLs of 80 mcg/dL or higher [102]. Routine chelation therapy is generally not indicated in cases of asymptomatic and minimally symptomatic intoxication. This includes adults with BLL less than 70 mcg/dL, and children with BLL less than 45 mg/dL, and it is not recommended to be used as a preventative measure or in the event of ongoing exposure.

Many studies noted that repeated chelation regimens failed to reduce BLL, whereas subsequent surgical removal successfully reduced BLL [77–79]. Even if chelation greatly lowers the BLL, the effect is likely temporary as lead from the any remaining RBF and bone may continue to be released into the blood [157–159]. Thus, future BLL monitoring is required. Chelation only treatment has been suggested as a life-saving measure in cases where surgical treatment is otherwise contraindicated or to reduce the risk of postoperative elevation of BLL due to surgical manipulation of lead particles.

Some authors have recommended preoperative chelation in the past in patients with high BLL with a plan for surgical RBF removal. This is based on the

Table 11.7 Summary of Chelation Agents [147]. (*Reprinted with Permission: Towner JE, Pieters TA, Maurer PK. Lead Toxicity From Intradiscal Retained Bullet Fragment: Management Considerations and Recommendations. World Neurosurg. 2020 Sep;141:377-382. doi: 10.1016/j.wneu.2020.05.112. Epub 2020 May 19. PMID: 32442733*)

Summary of Chelation Agents

Common Name	Compound	Common Administration Route	FDA approval for Lead Chelation	Solubility	Excretion	Elements Chelated
Dimercaptosuccinic acid (DMSA)	2,3-bis(sulfanyl)butanedioic acid	Oral	Yes	Hydrophilic	Urine	Lead, Arsenic, Mercury, Camium, Silver, Tin, Copper
Ethylenediaminetetraacetic acid (EDTA)	2-[2-[bis(carboxymethy) amino]ethyl-(carboxymethyl) amino]acetic acid	IV	Yes	Hydrophilic	Urine and Bileent + F12	Lead, Cadmium, Zinc
Dimercaprol; British anti-Lewisite (BAL)	2,3-bis(sulfanyl)propan-1-ol	IM	Yes	Lipophilic	Urine	Arsenic, Gold, Mercury, Lead
Sodium dimercaptopropanesulfonate (DMPS)	Sodium 2,3-bis(sulfanyl) prpane-1-sulfanate	Oral, IV, IM	No	Hydrophilic	Urine and Bile	Mercury, Arsenic, Lead, Cadmium, Tin, Silver, Copper, Selenium, Zinc, Magnesium
Pencillamine	(2S)-2-amino-3-methyl-3-sulfanylbutanoic acid	Oral	No	Hydrophilic	Urine	Copper, Arsenic, Zinc, Mercury, Lead

FDA US Food and Drug Administration, *IM* intramuscular, *IV* intravenous theoretical hypothesis that mobilization of lead during surgical procedure can lead to even more increased BLL [63, 160]. The literature is inconclusive of its clinical and practical implication. However, there are postoperative deaths reported with high BLL [161]. Thus, a team approach with toxicologist/internist is very reasonable with preoperative planning and patient preparation. As discussed by Kershner et al., it is reasonable to preoperatively chelate for patients with symptoms of lead toxicity or BLL greater than 70 mcg/dL and pediatric patients with BLL greater than 45 mcg/dL [98]. There is no specific goal BLL as an endpoint for therapy. A typical course of succimer is 19 days and is generally well tolerated.

Recommendations

In reviewing the literature, there is a consensus that RBF patients should undergo BLL monitoring and even radiologic follow-up [62]. There is a need for additional studies and guidance. Currently, there are three options available for management of patients with RBF.

1. Educate the patient on clinical symptoms and risks of lead toxicity, with clinician (e.g., primary care) follow-up as needed.
2. Educate the patient on clinical symptoms and risks of lead toxicity and measure serial BLL on higher risk RBF patients (see Table 11.2).
3. Educate and monitor serial BLL on all RBF patients.

Our experience is that despite a vigorous education, including risk and discussion with the patient, follow-up is unpredictable. Therefore, we recommend the third option, with serial monitoring of all patients with RBF. The goal is to limit the total amount of lead absorption early, if feasible by early removal of RBFs, and thus reduce the amount of lead in the heart, liver, kidney, brain, bone marrow and especially reduce bone storage. We recommend early removal of RBF as much as is reasonable—including palpable RBF, all visible RBFs at surgery, RBF found in (or near) joints, RBF in or near cerebrospinal fluid (CSF) or eye, RBF-related nerve impingement, RBF adjacent or in lumen of vessel, RBF involved with infection, and for medico-legal issues. We are also advocating for early RBF removal in patients with elevated BLL. Clinicians should educate patients and document clinical features of lead toxicity and its association with retained bullets or bullet. There should be awareness of increased risk of hypermetabolic states and pregnancy. When pregnancy is possible, the patient should be advised about effects of lead poisoning on fetal, neonatal, and child development (see Annex 1). This is in accordance with CDC recommendation for persons with RBFs [162]. The patient should be given appropriate written information (see Annex 11.1).

The risk-benefit relationship of RBF removal and chelation, and deficiency in our knowledge base should be discussed with the patient. There is very little literature about the advantage of early aggressive RBF removal. There are clearly situations where excision is unrealistic (such as widely distributed shot gun pellets, and multiple fragments distributed deep in soft tissues). Initial investigations that should be obtained in all patients with RBF should include:

- Complete blood count.
- Venous blood lead levels (BLLs).
- Renal function test.
- Plain radiographs of RBF and confirm location of the anticipated number of bullets.

In asymptomatic patients with RBF, even with venous blood levels within normal limits, regular surveillance and BLL at hospital admission or discharge, 2 weeks, 6 weeks, 3 months, 6 months, 1 year is a reasonable protocol. If BLLs remains low and stable, revisit critical sign and symptoms of lead poisoning with patients before discharge at the 1-year follow-up. Repeat CBC and BLL should occur at every visit. Surgical management including removal of RBFs should be considered and discussed with patients in following situations:

- Elevated or rising BLL.
- RBFs near or in joints, near or in bone.
- Prior to pregnancy.
- Hypermetabolic states.

Most states request or require reporting of elevated BLL. Thus, consultation with a local health department, poison control center (800-222-1222), or experienced clinician, particularly a toxicologist, is recommended.

Conclusion

Lead toxicity due to RBFs is an uncommon but known complication. Unfortunately, delayed or missed diagnosis can lead to consequences, rarely including death. Nonfatal firearm injuries are common and thus vigilance, as demonstrated in Case 2, will be required to identify a patient with remote injury with RBFs. It is recommended that the surgeon discuss the consequence of lead exposure with the patient, discuss possible clinical symptoms, and recommend BLL measurements near the time of initial injury, 2 weeks, 6 weeks, 3 months, 6 months, and 1 year after initial injury. It is reasonable to prospectively monitor the patient, as even low BLL may be associated with clinical dysfunction. Consultation with an experienced physician (such as a toxicologist) in dealing with elevated BLL is highly recommended.

The CDC has stated that even low levels of BLL are associated with measurable adverse outcomes—state agencies have lowered over past many years the threshold for recommended follow-up to either BLL > 3.5 ug/dL or > 5 ug/dL, for both children and adults. There is clearly a substantial number of the population that has undergone lead inoculation by projectiles, and it is reasonable to presume that elevated BLL above these thresholds are underdiagnosed and underreported [163]. Publications suffer from multiple deficiencies including 1. bias toward publishing lead toxicity case, 2. control series with low numbers, 3. prospective series with significant loss of follow-up, 4. BLL measurements does not reflect acuteness or chronicity of lead contamination or total lead load of a patient, 5. focus on ruling out of other sources for BLL and toxicity, and 6. limited validated assessments of clinical lead toxicity associated symptoms [98] (see Table 11.8). The follow-up of RBF patients is clearly challenging. In one study, 60% of children with RBF failed to follow-up and another study in adults, 42% of patients failed to follow-up [64, 168]. Regardless, the fundamental change over the years is the realization that low levels

Table 11.8 Review of available literature of RBF with follow-up including, if available, BLL

Author	Locale	RBF w/o Removal	% F/U	BLL	Mo post injury/ symptom BLL
Mazotas et al. 2012 [8]	Retrospective children hospital	107 pts No consistent BLL	65% at least one post injury visit	3% (3 pts) criterion GSW abdomen 9–47 ug/dL	3–17 months f/u Hard to assess symptoms/ inconsistent follow-up
Moazeni et al. 2014 [65]	Case control Iran Av:35.6 age GSW more than 3 months ago	25 RBF/25 control Volunteer		RBF mean 29 (14.4–71.5) ug/ dL Control mean 25.3 (14.5–39.7)	Av 38.6 (3–70) f/u Neither group has symptoms lead toxicity
Magos 1994 [164]	Case studies age 4–66 years old England pts with signs and symptoms lead poisoning	10 pts BLL <80 ug/dL versus 15 pts BLL > 80 ug/ dL		BLL range 18–920 ug/dL	1/8 –40 years f/u 24/25 with potential projectile/lead symptoms
Edetanlen B, Saheeb B 2016 [86]	Case control age 19–65 prospective GSW to craniomaxillofacial region, Nigeria	26 pts RBF/26 year Control BLL 3 days and 3 months post injury		RBF 3 months 6.2 ug/dL (2.49–12.2 ug/ dL) versus Control 0–1.24 ug/dL	3 days and 3 mo post injury versus control
Nguyen et al. 2005 [82]	Case control >18 years age prospectively Chicago asked pt whether had RBF on ED visit versus control	120 pt with extra-articular retained missiles versus 120 control pt		5/120 pts with RBF had BLL greater 20 ug/ dL RBF BLL: 6.7 ug/dL (5.68–7.74) versus control 3.16 (2.79–3.53)ug/ dL	Missiles retention 4.6 years (1 day to 51 years) No significant difference comparing symptoms

Table 11.8 (continued)

Author	Locale	RBF w/o Removal	% F/U	BLL	Mo post injury/ symptom BLL
deAraujo et al. 2015 [165]	Case control >18 years age/ males, Brazil	45 RBF more than 6 months post injury versus 45 matched controls		RBF BLL 9.01 ug/dL (6.07–11.96) versus control 2.17 ug/dL (1.71–2.63) highest 61.8 ug/ dL intraarticular	11 statistically significant symptoms in RBF group compared control
McQuirter et al. 2000 [64]	Prospective: >18 year old 28 pts out of recruited 48 pts with RBF follow-up 8 months post injury Los Angeles BLL and in vivo bone lead measurement Questionnaire to exclude other sources lead	28 pts first BLL near or within 6 months injury and then second BLL 5 to 234 days after first BLL (mean 63.1 days later)	At least two post injury visits	Geometric mean first BLL 5.1 with range 8–42.5 ug/dL Second BLL 7.7 ug/dL with range 2.3 to 50 ug/dL	BLL went up over time only with fracture-associated RBF
McQuirter et al. 2004 [166]	Prospective 502 subjects RBF, with BLL, bone lead measurements, radiographs, risk questionaries, mean age 24 (range 9–70), Los Angeles	451 RBF pts with BLL 426 seen 0 days/414 at 18 days, 365 at 3 months, 309 at 12 months	Mean follow-up time post injury 0.3, 3.1, 18.7, 94.5, 188.3, and 349.4 days	First lab 1.9 ug/ dL Highest percentage BLL > 10 ug/ dL and 20 ug/ dL at 3 month Rapid increase BLL over first 25 days post injury	Head, face, neck fractures, increasing age and weapon type associated significant odds of inc BLL >20 ug/dL BLL higher with increased number of RBF Higher BLL if RBF near or in bone/joint bone lead calcaneus at 18 days higher BLL and fragmentation RBF associated with higher BLL, higher RBF in humerus

(continued)

Table 11.8 (continued)

Author	Locale	RBF w/o Removal	% F/U	BLL	Mo post injury/ symptom BLL
Farrell et al. 1998 [105]	Control case series 15 pts with RBF and 15 control ED patients time since RBF 1–45 years			RBF BLL mean 17 ug/dL (7–50 ug/dL) Control BLL mean 7 ug/dL (0–16 ug/dL)	
Andrade et al. (2022) [167]	Trauma 1 center in 2017 674 pts presented GSW	394 with RBF versus 280 without RBF 65 mortalities	ED visit 31.7% within 1 year	5.1% with RBF has subsequent GSW, bullet moving 4.8%, pain 73.6%	

of lead may have clinical consequences. Thus, it is reasonable to consider a change in management of a patient with RBFs.

There is a great need for additional studies to validate using BLL above a "to be determined lower threshold" as a justification, per se, for early aggressive RBF removal. McQuirter et al. study of 451 RBF patients followed for a least 3 months, found the rapid increase of BLL is over first 18 days post projectile injury [166]. It is reasonable to monitor patients with BLL early (starting within 1 weeks of initial RBF inoculation), and where appropriate, consider aggressive RBF surgical removal, with the goal of predictably and meaningfully averting lead-associated symptoms, and averting elevated bone level. Clearly operative open removal of RBFs itself has risks and traumatizes tissue. In addition to traditional open surgery, ultrasound or even CT guidance can facilitate percutaneously removing RBFs. There is a need to identify lead detection units and enhanced metal capture devices. Identifying high lead content fragments which may help adjust the risk benefit ratio prior to a surgical procedure [169].

There have been many models which predict distribution of lead between blood and soft tissues and bone [21–23]. We need to continue to understand the relationship between duration of lead exposure to bone, brain and other tissue lead levels, and relationship of duration of lead exposure to clinical consequence. It is the red blood cells and blood serum that carry lead throughout the body. Chelation has small impact in reducing total body lead levels, and thus addressing RBF bullets months later after projectile injury, one would expect the patients would have higher total body lead levels. Another issue is that a patient may be clinically fine until they exhibit lead toxicity 30 years after projectile event, associated with, for example, being immobilized, becoming pregnant, suffering a fracture, or develop thyroid issues. The threshold of BLL levels that should trigger early aggressive intervention with patient benefits is unknown. We need more studies. However regardless, early aggressive removal should be discussed with patient balancing risks and the unfortunately more theoretical benefits.

Questions

1. Why is it important to identify lead contamination early from projectiles? Earlier intervention may reduce the total amount of lead distributed and stored in the patient. Patient care can be tailored to the clinical symptoms and/or lead level. The patient has the right to be informed about this condition.
2. What locations of projectiles predict higher lead contamination? Projectiles in joint space, intervertebral disc, blood vessel, GI tract, pleural and peritoneal cavity, multiple bullets, fragmented bullets, unjacketed bullets, bullets associated with fracture and/or near bone, patient with pregnancy, infection and hyperthyroidism,
3. What needs to be done to confirm diagnosis of lead toxicity? Review of the patient's symptoms and measurement of whole blood lead levels is a good start.
4. What is the management and goal of treatment of lead toxicity? To eliminate symptoms and remove as much lead from the patient as possible in a safe fashion.
5. Why is it complicated? Bullet removal may not be feasible because surgery may cause per se significant damage trying to remove lead. Chelation removes only a small amount of whole-body lead content and thus will have limited impact if there is continued lead absorption or if lead stored in patient is significantly high.

Annex 1

Handout to Patient

Lead has no value in the human body, and it is ideal to have no or very low levels of lead in your body. You have been identified as having retained bullet fragment which may have exposed you to lead. Not everyone needs or should have removal of the bullet or its fragments. Surgery may have significant risks and itself may inadvertently cause injury. Often, the lead bullet may become walled off and not cause issues with lead absorption. However, lead may sometimes be absorbed from the bullet into the body. Lead elevation is associated with symptoms, and among others may include:

Tiredness/fatigue.
Joint and muscle pain.
Headache.
Abdominal discomfort or pain, nausea, vomiting, constipation, and weight loss.
High blood pressure.
Trouble concentrating/trouble sleeping.
Memory problems, dysfunction in learning and cognitive processing.
Lethargy, irritability, and other mood changes.
Tremo
Decreased libido.
Miscarriage, stillbirth, or premature birth.

We are recommending that you monitor yourself for these and any new symptoms. Regardless, please allow us to obtain blood lead levels roughly near the time of injury, 2 weeks after injury, 6 weeks after injury and then 3 and 6 months and finally 1 year after the injury, even if you have no symptoms. If any of these symptoms or other new symptoms arise, please discuss them with your assigned physician at the time you notice them (do not wait until follow-up). Although most patients do not develop problems, some do. It is necessary to monitor lead levels even if you do not have any clinical signs or symptoms, and especially if you might be or become pregnant. The blood lead level should be reviewed with your physician after being obtained. We have treatments available if lead levels require treatment.

Date__________________ Name (print) __________________

Signature ____________ Physician Signature _________________.

References

1. Chan M. They survived mass shootings. Years later, the bullets are still trying to kill them, Time Magazine, 2019.
2. DiiMaio V, DiMaio S, Garriott J, Simpson P. A fatal case of lead poisoning due to a retained bullet. Am J Forensic Med Pathol. 1983;4(2):165–9.
3. Kaufman E, Wiebe D, Xiong R, Morrison C, Seamon M, Delgado M. Epidemiologic trends in fatal and nonfatal firearm injuries in the US, 2009-2017. JAMA Intern Med. 2021;181(2):1–8.
4. Song Z, Zubizarreta J, Giuriato M, Paulos E, Koh K. Changes in health care spending, use, and clinical outcomes after nonfatal firearm injuries among survivors and family members: a cohort study. Ann Intern Med. 2022;175(6):795–803.
5. Dienstknecht T, Horst K, Sellei R, Berner A, Nerlich M, Hardcastle T. Indications for bullet removal: overview of the literature, and clinical practice guidelines for European trauma surgeons. Eur J Trauma Emerg Surg. 2012;38(2):89–93.
6. Nee N, Inaba K, Schellenberg M, et al. Retained bullet fragments after nonfatal gunshot wounds: epidemiology and outcomes. J Trauma Acute Care Surg. 2021;90:973–9.
7. Nguyen M, Savakus J. Simske N et al single dose IV antibiotic for low-energy extremity gunshot wounds: a prospective protocol. Ann Surg Open. 2022;3(1):e136.
8. Mazotas I, Hamilton N, McCubbins M, Keller M. The Long -term outcome of retained foreign bodies in pediatric gunshot wounds. J Trauma Nurs. 2012;19(4):240–5.
9. McTee M, Parish C, Jourdonnais C, Ramsey P. Weight retention and expansion of popular lead-based and lead-free hunting bullets. Sci Total Environ. 2023;904:166288.
10. McVean, A. (2019). Lead bullets can harm in more ways than one. www.mcgill.ca. https://www.mcgill.ca/oss/article/lead-bullets-can-harm-more-ways-one.
11. Minick J. Get the Lead out of bullets. The New York Times; 2018. https://www.nytimes.com/2018/11/01/opinion/get-the-lead-out-of-bullets.html
12. Stewart CM, Veverka NB. The extent of Lead fragmentation observed in deer culled by sharpshooting. J Wildl Manag. 2011;75(6):1462–6.
13. Grund MD, Cornicelli L, Carlson LT, Butler EA. Bullet fragmentation and lead deposition in white-tailed deer and domestic sheep. Hum-Wildl Interact. 2010;4(2):12. https://doi.org/10.26077/72ts-6n20.
14. Hunt W, Watson R, Oaks J, et al. Lead bullet fragments in venison from rifle-killed deer: potential for human dietary exposure. PLoS One. 2009;4(4):e5330.

15. Leontowich A, Panahifar A, Ostrowski R. Fragmentation of hunting bullets observed with synchrotron radiation: lighting up the source of a lesser-known lead exposure pathway. PLoS One. 2022;17(8):e0271987.
16. World Health Organization: WHO. (2023). Lead poisoning. ; https://www.who.int/news-room/fact-sheets/detail/lead-poisoning-and-health.
17. Desilva P. Determination of lead in plasma and studies on its relationship to lead in erythrocytes. British J Industrial Medicine. 1981;38:209–17.
18. Leggett R. An age-specific kinetic model of Lead metabolism in humans. Environ Health Perspect. 1993;101(7):598–616.
19. Bert J, van Dusen J, Grace J. A generalized model for the prediction of Lead body burdens. Environ Res. 1989;48:117–27.
20. Radulescu A. Lundgren S a pharmacokinetic model of lead absorption and calcium competitive dynamics. Sci Rep. 2019;9(1):14225.
21. Kehoe R, Thamann F, Cholak J. Normal Absorption and Excretion of Lead JAMA. 1935;104(2):90–2.
22. Barbosa F, Tanus-Santos J, Gerlach R, Parsons P. A critical review of biomarkers used for monitoring human exposure to lead: advantages, limitations, and future needs. Environ Health Perspect. 2005;113(12):1669–74.
23. Collin M, Venkatraman S, Vijayakumar N, Kanimozhi V, Arbaaz S, Stacey R, et al. Bioaccumulation of lead (Pb) and its effects on human: a review. J Hazard Mater Adv. 2022;7:100094.
24. Rabinowitz M. Toxicokinetics of bone Lead. Environ Health Perspect. 1991;91:33–7.
25. Riess M, Halm J. Lead poisoning in an adult: Lead mobilization by pregnancy. JGIM. 2007;22:1212–5.
26. Needleman H. Lead poisoning. Annu Rev Med. 2004;55:209–22.
27. Wani AL, Ara A, Usmani JA. Lead toxicity: a review. Interdiscip Toxicol. 2015;8(2):55–64.
28. CDC CDC updates blood lead reference value to 3.5 μg/dL. 2022. CDC.gov. https://www.cdc.gov/nceh/lead/news/cdc-updates-blood-lead-reference-value.html.
29. Hu H, Teliez-Rojo M, et al. Fetal Lead exposure at each stage of pregnancy as a predictor of infant mental development. Environ Health Perspect. 2006;114:1730–5.
30. Rodosthenous R, Burris H, Svensson K, et al. Prenatal Lead exposure and fetal growth: smaller infants have heightened susceptibility. Environ Int. 2017;99:228–33.
31. Fenga C, Gangemi S, et al. Relationship between lead exposure and mild cognitive impairment. J Prev Med Hyg. 2016;57(4):E205–10.
32. Rocha a, Trujillo K. Neurotoxicity of low-level lead exposure: history, mechanisms of action, and behavioral effects in humans and preclinical models. Neurotoxicology. 2019;73:58–80.
33. California Department of Public Health. (n.d.). Occupational lead poisoning prevention program. https://www.cdph.ca.gov/Programs/CCDPHP/DEODC/OHB/OLPPP/Pages/OLPPP.aspx.
34. CDC's Adult Blood Lead Epidemiology and Surveillance (ABLES) Adult Blood Lead Epidemiology and Surveillance. https://wwwn.cdc.gov/NIOSH-WHC/source/ables.
35. Elevated blood lead levels in adults - epidemiology. 2023. Epidemiology https://www.vdh.virginia.gov/epidemiology/epidemiology-fact-sheets/elevated-blood-lead-levels-in-adults/.
36. Biomonitoring - Lead | US EPA. 2023. US EPA. https://www.epa.gov/americaschildrenenvironment/biomonitoring-lead.
37. Blood lead levels. 2022. EPA ROE Lead indicator. https://cfpub.epa.gov/roe/indicator.cfm?i=63.
38. Lead (PB) toxicity: How should patients exposed to lead be treated and managed? | Environmental Medicine | ATSDR. 2023. https://www.atsdr.cdc.gov/csem/leadtoxicity/patient_treatment.html.
39. Kasten-Jolly J, Lawrence DA. Sex-specific effects of developmental lead exposure on the immune-neuroendocrine network. Toxicol Appl Pharmacol. 2017;334:142–57.

40. Simons T. Lead-calcium interactions in cellular lead toxicity. Neurotoxicology. 1993;14:77–85.
41. Cory-Slechta D. Relationships between lead-induced learning impairments and changes in dopaminergic, cholinergic, and glutamatergic neurotransmitter system functions. Annu Rev Pharmacol Toxicol. 1995;35:391–415.
42. Goldstein G. Lead poisoning and brain cell function. Environ Health Perspect. 1990;89:91–4.
43. Neal A, Guilarte T. Molecular neurobiology of Lead (Pb^{2+}):effects on synaptic function. Mol Neurobiol. 2010;42(3:151–60.
44. Shobha N, Taly A, Sinha S, Venkatesh T. Radial neuropathy due to occupational lead exposure phenotypic and electrophysiological characteristics of five patients. Ann Indian Acad Neurol. 2009;12(2):111–5.
45. Lubran M. Lead toxicity and Heme biosynthesis. Ann Clin Lab Sci. 1980;10(5):402–13.
46. Qader A, Rehman K, Akash M. Genetic susceptibility of delta-ALAD associated with lead (Pb) intoxication: sources of exposure, preventive measures, and treatment intervention. Environ Sci Pollut Res. 2021;28:44818–32.
47. Scinicariello F, Murray H, Moffett D, et al. Lead and Delta-Aminolevulinic acid dehydratase polymorphism: where does it Lead? A Meta-Analysis. Environ Health Perspect. 2007;115(1):35–41.
48. Sanchez J, Lunch D. Histology, basophilic stippling. In: Stat pearls. Treasure Island (FL): Stat Pearls Publishing; 2022.
49. George J, Duncan J. The hematology of Lead poisoning in man and animals. Vet Clin Pathol. 1979;8:23–30.
50. Cheson B, Rom W, Webber R. Basophilic stippling of red blood cells: a nonspecific finding of multiple etiology. Am J of Ind Med. 1984;5(4):327–34.
51. Lead (PB) toxicity: Clinical assessment - Diagnostic tests and imaging | Environmental Medicine | ATSDR. 2023. https://www.atsdr.cdc.gov/csem/leadtoxicity/diagnostic_testing.html.
52. Benjelloun M, Tarrass F, Hachim K, Medkouri G, Benghanem MG, Ramdani B. Chronic lead poisoning: a "forgotten" cause of renal disease. Saudi J Kidney Dis Transplant. 2007;18(1):83–6.
53. Farkas WR, Stanawitz T. Effects of plumbous ion on guanine metabolism. J Inorg Biochem. 1979;11(1):31–8.
54. Nawrot TS, Thijs L, Den Hond EM, Roels HA, Staessen JA. An epidemiological re-appraisal of the association between blood pressure and blood lead: a meta-analysis. J Hum Hypertens. 2002;16(2):123–31.
55. Ding Y, Vaziri ND, Gonick HC. Lead-induced hypertension. Environ Res. 1998;76(2):107–13. https://doi.org/10.1006/enrs.1997.3796.
56. Pounds J, Long G, Rosen J. Cellular and molecular toxicity of Lead in bone. Environ Health Perspect. 1991;91:17–32.
57. Blickman J, Wilkinson R, Graef J. The radiologic "lead band" revisited. Am J Roentgenol. 1986;146(2):245–7.
58. Kearns C. Dense metaphyseal bands (differential). Radiopaedia; https://radiopaedia.org/articles/dense-metaphyseal.
59. Silbergeld EK, Schwartz J, Mahaffey K. Lead and osteoporosis: mobilization of lead from bone in postmenopausal women. Environ Res. 1988;47:79–94.
60. U.S Department of Health and Human Services Agency for Toxic Substances and Disease Registry Division of Toxicology and Environmental Medicine Environmental Medicine Branch. Last reviewed May 24, 2023.
61. Lau K, Chow T, Chan C, et al. Hong Kong poison information Centre: annual report 2018. Hong Kong J Emerg Med. 2018;25(6):313–23.
62. Apte A, Bradford K, Dente C, Smith RN. Lead toxicity from retained bullet fragments: a systematic review and meta-analysis. J Trauma Acute Care Surg. 2019;87(3):707–16.

63. Linden MA, Manton WI, Stewart RM, Thal ER, Feit H. Lead poisoning from retained bullets. Pathogenesis, diagnosis, and management. Ann Surg. 1982;195(3):305–13.
64. McQuirter JL, Rothenberg SJ, Dinkins GA, Manalo M, Kondrashov V, Todd AC. The effects of retained lead bullets on body lead burden. J Trauma. 2001;50(5):892–9.
65. Moazeni M, Mohammad Alibeigi F, Sayadi M, Poorya Mofrad E, Kheiri S, Darvishi M. The serum Lead level in patients with retained Lead pellets. Arch Trauma Res. 2014;3(2):e18950.
66. Beazley WC, Rosenthal RE. Lead intoxication 18 months after a gunshot wound. Clin Orthop. 1984;190:199–203.
67. Lead (PB) toxicity: Signs and symptoms I Environmental Medicine I ATSDR. 2023. https://www.atsdr.cdc.gov/csem/leadtoxicity/signs_and_symptoms.html.
68. Samarghandian S, Shirazi F, Saeedi F, et al. A systematic review of clinical and laboratory findings of lead poisoning: lessons from case reports. Toxicol Appl Pharmacol. 2021;429:115681.
69. Pearce J. Burton's line in lead poisoning. Eur Neurol. 2007;57:118–9.
70. Williams R, Erickson T. Evaluating Lead, and iron intoxication in an emergency setting. Lab Med. 1998;29(4):224–30.
71. Guideline for clinical management of exposure to lead. 2023. https://www.who.int/publications-detail-redirect/9789240037045.
72. Garcés J, Artuz R. Lead poisoning due to bullets lodged in the human body. Colomb Médica (Cali). 2012;43(3):230–4.
73. Khalil N, Cauley JA, Wilson JW, Talbott EO, Morrow L, Hochberg MC, et al. Relationship of blood Lead levels to incident nonspine fractures and falls in older women: the study of osteoporotic fractures. J Bone Miner Res. 2008;23(9):1417–25.
74. Brown J. Smith, E peripheral neuritis due to lead. J Pediatr. 1937;10(5):656–65.
75. Rhee J, Martin R. The management of retained bullets in the limbs. Injury. 1997;28(Suppl.3):S-C23–8.
76. Morton L. The solution of lead by synovial fluid. Clin Orthopaedics and Related Research. 1969;64:255–61.
77. Marquez JI, Schindlbeck MA. Lead toxicity from a retained bullet. N Engl J Med. 2018;379(25):2451.
78. Mahan ST, Murray MM, Woolf AD, Kasser JR. Increased blood lead levels in an adolescent girl from a retained bullet. A case report. J Bone Joint Surg Am. 2006;88(12):2726–9.
79. Begly J, Lajam C. Systemic Lead toxicity secondary to retained intraosseous bullet a case report and review of literature. Bull Hosp Jt Dis. 2013;74(3):229–33.
80. Jensen SP, Richardson ML, Conrad EU, Lazerte GD. Case report 608: retention of a bullet fragment within a traumatic pseudarthrosis, resulting in lead arthropathy and lead intoxication. Skeletal Radiol. 1990;19(3):233–5.
81. Ganocy K, Lindsey RW. The management of civilian intraarticular gunshot wounds: treatment considerations and proposal of a classification system. Injury. 1998;29(Suppl 1):SA1–6.
82. Nguyen A, Schaider JJ, Manzanares M, Hanaki R, Rydman RJ, Bokhari F. Elevation of blood lead levels in emergency department patients with extra-articular retained missiles. J Trauma. 2005;58(2):289–99.
83. Switz D, Elmorshidy M, Deyerle W. Bullets, joints, and lead intoxication. A remarkable and instructive case. Arch Intern Med. 1976;136(8):939–41.
84. Smith K, Shafer M, Weiss D, Anderson H, Gorski P. High-precision (MC-ICPMS) isotope ratio analysis reveals contrasting sources of elevated blood Lead levels of an adult with retained bullet fragments, and of his child, in Milwaukee, Wisconsin. Biol Trace Elem Res. 2017;177(1):33–42.
85. Riehl J, Connolly K, Haidukewych G, Koval K. Fractures due to gunshot wounds: do retained bullet fragments affect union? Iowa Orthop J. 2015;35:55–61.
86. Edetanlen B, Saheeb B. Blood lead concentrations as a result of retained lead pellets in the craniomaxillofacial region in Benin City. Nigeria Br J Oral Maxillofac Surg. 2016;54(5):551–5.

87. Wunnapuk K, Durongkadech P, Minami T, Ruangyuttikarn W, Tohno S, Vichairat K, et al. Differences in the element contents between gunshot entry wounds with full-jacketed bullet and lead bullet. Biol Trace Elem Res. 2007;120(1–3):74–81.
88. Lead (Pb) toxicity: what is the biological fate of Lead in the body? Environmental Medicine|ATSDR. 2023. ; https://www.atsdr.cdc.gov/csem/leadtoxicity/biologic_fate.html.
89. Ettinger A, Lamadrid-Figueroa H, et al. Effect of calcium supplementation on blood Lead levels in pregnancy: a randomized placebo-controlled trial. Environ Health Perspect. 2009;117(1):26–31.
90. Overview of childhood Lead poisoning prevention. 2023. CDC. https://www.cdc.gov/nceh/lead/overview.html.
91. CDC division of environmental health science and practice. NCEH|CDC. 2022. https://www.cdc.gov/nceh/ehsp/default.html.
92. Mahaffey KR. Environmental lead toxicity: nutrition as a component of intervention. Environ Health Perspect. 1990;89:75–8.
93. Cleveland LM, Minter ML, Cobb KA, Scott AA, German VF. Lead hazards for pregnant women and children: part 1: immigrants and the poor shoulder most of the burden of lead exposure in this country. Part 1 of a two-part article details how exposure happens, whom it affects, and the harm it can do. Am J Nurs. 2008;108(10):40–9.
94. Kosnett M, Wedeen R, Rothenberg S, et al. Recommendations for medical management of adult Lead exposure. Environ Health Perspect. 2007;115(3):463–71.
95. WHO guideline for clinical management of exposure to lead: executive summary. Geneva: World Health Organization; 2021. License: CC BY-NC-SA 3.0 IGO. There is no suggestion that WHO endorses these proposals. (Modified) *Surveillance of Patients with RBFs.*
96. Milkovic-Kraus S, Restek-Samarzija N, Samarzija M, Kraus O. Individual variation to response to Lead exposure: a dilemma for the occupational health physician. Am J Ind Med. 1997;31:631–5.
97. Silbergeld EK, Sauk J, Somerman M, Todd A, McNeill F, Fowler B, et al. Lead in bone: storage site, exposure source, and target organ. Neurotoxicology. 1993;14(2–3):225–36.
98. Kershner EK, Tobarran N, Chambers A, Wills BK, Cumpston KL. Retained bullets and lead toxicity: a systematic review. Clin Toxicol (Phila). 2022;60(10):1176–86.
99. Nally E, Jelinek J, Bunning RD. Quadriparesis caused by Lead poisoning nine years after a gunshot wound with retained bullet fragments: a case report. PM R. 2017;9(4):411–4.
100. Martin C, Werntz C, Ducatman A. The interpretation of zinc protoporphyrin changes in lead intoxication: a case report and review of the literature. Occup Med. 2004;54:587–91.
101. Council of State and Territorial Epidemiologists Technical Supplement: 22-EH-0.
102. Gaitens J, Potter B, D'Alleyrand J, Overmann A, Gochfeld M, Smith D, et al. The management of embedded metal fragment patients and the role of chelation therapy: a workshop of the Department of Veterans Affairs-Walter Reed National Medical Center. Am J Ind Med. 2020;63(5):381–93.
103. Coon T, Miller M, Shirazi F, Sullivan J. Lead toxicity in a 14-year-old female with retained bullet fragments. Pediatrics. 2006;117(1):227–30.
104. Nickel WN, Steelman TJ, Sabath ZR, Potter BK. Extra-articular retained missiles; is surveillance of Lead levels needed? Mil Med. 2018;183(3–4):e107–13.
105. Farrell SE, Vandevander P, Schoffstall JM, Lee DC. Blood lead levels in emergency department patients with retained lead bullets and shrapnel. Acad Emerg Med Off J Soc Acad Emerg Med. 1999;6(3):208–12.
106. Recommended actions based on blood lead level. 2022 CDC. https://www.cdc.gov/nceh/lead/advisory/acclpp/actions-blls.htm.
107. Weston WJ. The lead arthrogram—Plumbography. Skeletal Radiol. 1978;2(3):169–70.
108. Hu H, Aro A, Rotnitzky A. Bone lead measured by x-ray fluorescence: epidemiologic methods. Environ Health Perspect. 1995;103(Suppl. 1):105–10.

109. Gherase M, Serna B, Kroeker S. A novel calibration for L-shell x-ray fluorescence measurements of bone lead concentration using the strontium KBeta/Kalpha ratio. Physiol Meas. 2021;42(4):04501.
110. Rizaldy R, Janitra G. Ultrasound with needle guiding exploration as a real-time modality for exploration of air rifle bullet close to cervical spine: a case report. Int J Surg Case Rep. 2021;81:105730.
111. Meena S, Singla A, Saini P, Mittal S, Chowdhary B. Spontaneous migration of bullet from arm to forearm and its ultrasound guided removal. J Ultrasound. 2013;16(4):223–5.
112. Gascho D, Zoelch N, Richter H, Buehlmann A, Wyss P, Schaerli S. Identification of bullets based on their metallic components and X-ray attenuation characteristics at different energy levels on CT. Am J Roentgenol. 2019;213(3):W105–13.
113. Genetics: Iron transporter gene, Mani M, Dsouza V, Dsouza H. Evaluation of divalent metal transporter 1(DMT1) (rs224589) polymorphism on blood lead levels of occupationally exposed individuals. Toxicol Lett. 2021;353:13–9.
114. Gutiérrez V, Radice F. Late bullet migration into the knee joint. Arthroscopy. 2003;19(3):E15.
115. O-Connor D, Hou D, Ye J, et al. Lead-based paint remains a major public health concern: a critical review of global production, trade, use, exposure, health risk, and implications. Environ Int. 2018;121:85–101.
116. Mills A, Peckham S. Lead exposure from general aviation emissions in the UK: a review and call for action. Public Health Chall. 2022;1:e27.
117. Zahran S, Mielke H, Filippelli MES, GM, Laidlaw M Taylor M. Determining the relative importance of soil sample locations to predict risk of child lead exposure. Environ Int. 2013;60:7–14.
118. Moore MR. Lead in drinking water in soft water areas—health hazards. Sci Total Environ. 1977;7(2):109–15.
119. Duan Y, Yan L, Gao Z, Gou Y. Lead poisoning in a 6-month-old infant: a case report. Front Public Health. 2022;11:1132199.
120. Parry C, Eaton J. Kohl: a lead-hazardous eye makeup from the third world to the first world. Environ Health Perspect. 1991;94:121–3.
121. Tamayo-Ortiz M, Sanders A, Rosa M. Lead concentrations in Mexican candy: a follow-up report Ann glob. Health. 2020;86(1):20.
122. FDA. Kohl, Kajal, Al-Kahal, Surma, Tiro, Tozali, or Kwalli: by any name, beware of lead poisoning. U.S. Food And Drug Administration; 2022; https://www.fda.gov/cosmetics/cosmetic-products/kohl-kajal-al-kahal-surma-tiro-tozali-or-kwalli-any-name-beware-lead-poisoning.
123. Muscat M. A tarnished toy story. JIFCC. 2020;31(2):174–6.
124. van der Kuijp TJ, Huang L, Cherry CR. Health hazards of China's lead-acid battery industry: a review of its market drivers, production processes, and health impacts. Environ Health. 2013;3(12):61.
125. Bartrem C, Tirima S, von Lindern I, von Braun M, Worrell MC, Mohammad Anka S, et al. Unknown risk: co-exposure to lead and other heavy metals among children living in small-scale mining communities in Zamfara state. Nigeria Int J Environ Health Res. 2014;24(4):304–19.
126. Laidaw M, Flippelli G, et al. Lead exposure at firing ranges— a review. Environ Health. 2017;16:34.
127. Mirzaei S, Akbari A, Mehrpour O, Zamani N. Lead toxicity due to ingestion of led contaminated opium in a patient presenting with motor neuropathy and upper limb paresis: a case report. Sultan Qaboos Univ Med J. 2018;18(4):e529–32.
128. Halle J, Ball G. Saturnine gout: a review of 42 patients. Semin Arthritis Rheum. 1982;11(3):307–14.
129. Simon J, Hudes E. Relationship of ascorbic acid to blood lead levels. JAMA. 1999;282(24):2289–93.
130. Mumtaz S, Ali S, Khan R, et al. Therapeutic role of garlic and vitamins C and E against toxicity induced by lead on various organs. Environ Sci Pollut Res. 2020;27:8953–64.

131. Smith RN, Tracy BM, Smith S, Johnson S, Martin ND, Seamon MJ. Retained bullets after firearm injury: a survey on surgeon practice patterns. J Interpers Violence. 2022;37(1–2):NP306–26.
132. Omid R, Stone MA, Zalavras CG, Marecek GS. Gunshot wounds to the upper extremity. J Am Acad Orthop Surg. 2019;27(7):e301–10.
133. Meade A, Hembd A, Cho MJ, Zhang AY. Surgical treatment of upper extremity gunshot injures: an updated review. Ann Plast Surg. 2021;86(3S Suppl 2):S312–8.
134. Sclafani SJ, Vuletin JC, Twersky J. Lead arthropathy: arthritis caused by retained intra-articular bullets. Radiology. 1985;156(2):299–302.
135. Ganocy K, Lindsey RW. The management of civilian intra-articular gunshot wounds: treatment considerations and proposal of a classification system. Injury. 1998;29 Suppl 1:SA1–6.
136. Bolanos AA, Demizio JP, Vigorita VJ, Bryk E. Lead poisoning from an intra-articular shotgun pellet in the knee treated with arthroscopic extraction and chelation therapy. A case report. J Bone Joint Surg Am. 1996 Mar;78(3):422–6.
137. Windler EC, SMith RB, Bryan WJ, Woods GW. Lead intoxication and traumatic arthritis of the hip secondary to retained bullet fragments. A case report. J Bone Joint Surg Am. 1978;60(2):254–5.
138. Berg EE, Ciullo JV. Arthroscopic debridement after intraarticular low-velocity gunshot wounds. Arthrosc J Arthrosc Relat Surg. 1993;9(5):576–9.
139. Lee GH, Virkus WW, Kapotas JS. Arthroscopically assisted minimally invasive intraarticular bullet extraction: technique, indications, and results. J Trauma. 2008;64(2):512–6.
140. Bartlett CS. Clinical update: gunshot wound ballistics. Clin Orthop. 2003;408:28–57.
141. Hanson TM, Nierenberg DW, LaRoche HB, Mead KC, Ames JB. Symptomatic Lead toxicity and joint pain because of migration of shotgun pellets into the hip 12 years after injury: a case report. JBJS Case Connect. 2021;11(2):e20.00751.
142. Rehani B, Wissman R. Lead poisoning from a gunshot wound. South Med J. 2011;104(1):57–8.
143. Bédry R, Brun P, Sudre E, Kandji M, Sarram-Nadjimi N, Mesli S, et al. Massive lead poisoning from a gunshot with high soft lead charge; 2018. p. 490. https://unilim.hal.science/hal-01990965.
144. Shannon JJ, Vo NM, Stanton PE, Dimler M. Peripheral arterial missile embolization: a case report and 22-year literature review. J Vasc Surg. 1987;5(5):773–8.
145. Dadsetan MR, Jinkins JR. Peripheral vascular gunshot bullet embolus migration to the cerebral circulation. Report and literature review. Neuroradiology. 1990;32(6):516–9.
146. Rentfrow B, Vaidya R, Elia C, Sethi A. Lead toxicity and management of gunshot wounds in the lumbar spine. Eur Spine J. 2013;22(11):2353–7.
147. Towner JE, Pieters TA, Maurer PK. Lead toxicity from Intradiscal retained bullet fragment: management considerations and recommendations. World Neurosurg. 2020;141:377–8.
148. Grogan DP, Bucholz RW. Acute lead intoxication from a bullet in an intervertebral disc space. A case report. J Bone Joint Surg Am. 1981 Sep;63(7):1180–2.
149. Stromberg BV. Symptomatic lead toxicity secondary to retained shotgun pellets: case report. J Trauma. 1990;30(3):356–7.
150. Windler EC, Smith RB, Bryan WJ, Woods GW. Lead intoxication and traumatic arthritis of the hip secondary to retained bullet fragments. A case report. J Bone Joint Surg Am. 1978;60(2):254–157.
151. Tosti R, Rehman S. Surgical management principles of gunshot-related fractures. Orthop Clin North Am. 2013 Oct;44(4):529–40.
152. Kobbe P, Frink M, Oberbeck R, Tarkin IS, Tzioupis C, Nast-Kolb D, et al. Treatment strategies for gunshot wounds of the extremities. Unfallchirurg. 2008 Apr;111(4):247–54.
153. Kim J, Kim Y. Kumar V heavy metal toxicity: an update of chelating therapeutic strategies. J Trace Elem Med Biol. 2019;54:226–31.
154. Centers for Disease Control and Prevention (CDC). Deaths associated with hypocalcemia from chelation therapy—Texas, Pennsylvania, and Oregon, 2003-2005. MMWR Morb Mortal Wkly Rep. 2006;55(8):204–7.

155. Chisolm J, Harrison H. The treatment of acute lead encephalopathy in children. Pediatric. 1957;19(1):2–20.
156. Mortensen M, Walson P. Chelation therapy for childhood lead poisoning: the changing scene in the 1990s. Clin Pediatr (Phila). 1993;32(5):284–91.
157. Dietrich KN, Ware JH, Salganik M, Radcliffe J, Rogan WJ, Rhoads GG, et al. Effect of chelation therapy on the neuropsychological and behavioral development of lead-exposed children after school entry. Pediatrics. 2004;114(1):19–26.
158. Mortensen ME, Walson PD. Chelation therapy for childhood lead poisoning. The changing scene in the 1990s. Clin Pediatr (Phila). 1993;32(5):284–91.
159. Rogan WJ, Dietrich KN, Ware JH, Dockery DW, Salganik M, Radcliffe J, et al. The effect of chelation therapy with succimer on neuropsychological development in children exposed to lead. N Engl J Med. 2001;344(19):1421–6.
160. Meggs WJ, Gerr F, Aly MH, Kierena T, Roberts DL, Shih R, et al. The treatment of lead poisoning from gunshot wounds with succimer (DMSA). J Toxicol Clin Toxicol. 1994;32(4):377–85.
161. CDC. Deaths associated with hypocalcemia from chelation therapy—Texas, Pennsylvania, and Oregon, 2003-2005. JAMA. 2006;295(18):2131.
162. Weiss D. Elevated blood Lead levels associated with retained bullet fragments — United States, 2003–2012. MMWR Morb Mortal Wkly Rep. 2017;66(5):130–3;https://www.cdc.gov/mmwr/volumes/66/wr/mm6605a2.htm.
163. Weiss D, Lee D, Feldman R, Smith KT. Severe lead toxicity attributed to bullet fragments retained in soft tissue. Case Reports. 2017;2017:bcr2016217351.
164. Magos L. Lead poisoning from retained lead projectiles. A critical review of case reports. Hum Exp Toxicol. 1994;13(11):735–42.
165. deAraujo G, Mourao N, Pinheiro I, et al. Lead toxicity risks in gunshot victims. PLoS One. 2015;10(10):e0140220.
166. McQuirter JL, Rothenberg SJ, Dinkins GA, Kondrashov V, Manalo M, Todd AC. Change in blood Lead concentration up to 1 year after a gunshot wound with a retained bullet. Am J Epidemiol. 2004;159(7):683–92.
167. Andrade E, Uberoi M, Hayes J, Thornton M, Kramer JB, Punch L. The impact of retained bullet fragments on outcomes in patients with gunshot wounds. Am J Surg. 2022;223(4):787–91.
168. Fleenor T, Haupt J. Richard K et al characteristics of pediatric patients with retained bullet fragments and need to follow-up blood Lead monitoring. South Med J. 2020;113(1):23–8.
169. Grasso I, Blattner M, Short T, Downs JW. Severe systemic lead toxicity resulting from extra-articular retained shrapnel presenting as jaundice and hepatitis: a case report and review of the literature. Mil Med. 2017;182(3):e1843–8.

Chapter 12
Methyl Methacrylate-Related Issues in Geriatric Hip Fractures (Bone Cement Implantation Syndrome)

Madana Mohana Vallem, Khalid Hasan, Jacob Farrar, Daniel Layon, and Gregory Golladay

Clinical Vignette: 1
A 94-year-old Caucasian woman sustained an oblique fracture of the shaft of femur that extended distal to a previously inserted Austin Moore prosthesis (Fig. 12.1a). The fracture of the shaft was treated with an open reduction and internal fixation, and the hemiarthroplasty was revised to a cemented long-stem bipolar prosthesis.

The femur was exposed through an extended posterolateral approach incorporating the previous incision. The Austin Moore prosthesis was successfully removed, the fracture was carefully reduced and secured with cerclage wires, and the femur was reamed with flexible reamers to accommodate a long-stem femoral component. The femur was prepared by placing a large cement-restrictor, followed by injecting three units of methyl methacrylate cement into the intramedullary canal using a cement-injection gun and the prosthesis was inserted into the femur. The patient experienced a sudden drop in blood pressure and went into cardiac arrest immediately after the prosthesis was placed in the acetabulum. While the patient was still in lateral decubitus position external cardiac massage was initiated, followed by a rapid closure of the wound. The patient was placed in a supine position and effectively resuscitated using intravenous fluids, epinephrine infusion through a central line, and external cardiac massage.

When the patient was transferred to the recovery room, an idioventricular rhythm was present, with runs of ventricular tachycardia, and she still required moderate support with vasopressors. Her condition showed gradual improvement after

M. M. Vallem (✉) · K. Hasan · J. Farrar · D. Layon · G. Golladay
Department of Orthopaedic Surgery, Virginia Commonwealth University, Richmond, VA, USA
e-mail: madana.vallem@vcuhealth.org; khalid.hasan@vcuhealth.org; jacob.farrar@vcuhealth.org; Daniel.layon@vcuhealth.org; gregory.golladay@vcuhealth.org

W. A. Zuelzer, S. Metikala (eds.), *Unusual Conditions That Every Orthopaedic Surgeon Should Know*, https://doi.org/10.1007/978-3-031-58946-1_12

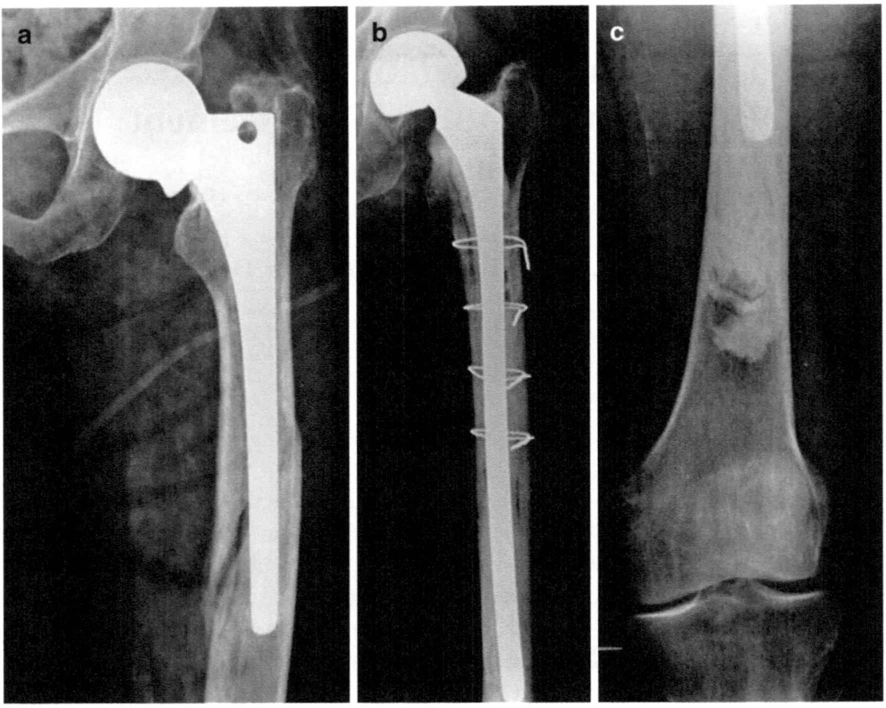

Fig. 12.1 (**a**–**c**): Case1. (**a**) preoperative radiograph showing a fracture distal to an Austin Moore prosthesis. (**b**) Radiograph made after a hemiarthroplasty with cementing of a long-stem component. The interdigitation of bone with cement is very good in the distal part of the canal, a radiograph sign of pressurization of the methyl methacrylate. (**c**) Postoperative radiograph revealed that pressurization of the cement caused distal migration of the cement-restrictor and filling of the distal diaphyseal region with methyl methacrylate. Case 1, 2 and radiographs reproduced with permission from Patterson BM, Healey JH, Cornell CN, Sharrock NE. Cardiac arrest during hip arthroplasty with a cemented long-stem component. A report of seven cases. J Bone Joint Surg Am. 1991 Feb;73 [1]:271–7 [2]

spending several days in the intensive-care unit. The postoperative radiographs (Fig. 12.1b and c) revealed evidence of high pressurization of the methyl methacrylate in the distal part of the canal. On the fifteenth day following surgery, the patient was discharged.

Clinical Vignette:2

A 109-year-old woman suffered a left femoral neck fracture after a fall at home. She underwent uncemented hemiarthroplasty and sustained an intraoperative periprosthetic fracture. Two days later, she was transferred to a higher level of care with a dislocated bipolar prosthesis and a periprosthetic fracture from the lesser trochanter to the distal third of the femur. She underwent revision surgery with epidural anesthesia and invasive monitoring, including a Swan-Ganz catheter and continuous blood pressure monitoring with an arterial line.

After removal of the prosthesis, the fracture was anatomically reduced and fixed with cerclage wires. The femur was then prepared to accept long-stem femoral component. On placement of cement-restrictor, the patient's blood pressure suddenly dropped to zero, and electromechanical dissociation of the heart developed. Chest compressions were initiated, and she was turned to the supine position and successfully resuscitated with the administration of epinephrine, bicarbonate, and chest compressions. Arterial blood gasses showed a pH of 7.35, a pCO_2 of 40 mm of mercury, and a PO_2 of 400 mm of mercury with the patient on 100% inspired oxygen. The presumed cause of the cardiac arrest was an air embolism although no air could be aspirated from the Swan-Ganz catheter after the initial event.

The patient was monitored in the operating theater for 30 min, during which time she remained stable despite discontinuation of vasopressors. The femoral canal was irrigated with a pulse irrigation system and packed with rolled gauze. 120 g of methyl methacrylate was injected into the canal, but pressurization was not attempted. As the prosthesis was advanced into the intramedullary space, the methyl methacrylate was allowed to escape proximally. No extrusion of cement was noted distally along the site of the fracture.

As the femoral component was seated, the patient had a second cardiac arrest, but she was again resuscitated with external compressions of the chest and the administration of 3 mg of epinephrine. The pulmonary artery pressure increased to 25 mm of mercury and remained elevated. The cardiovascular status remained unstable, and large doses of epinephrine and norepinephrine were required to maintain blood pressure. The prosthesis was relocated into the acetabulum, and the wound was closed. Evaluation of arterial blood gasses after the second arrest indicated mild metabolic acidosis and severe hypoxemia, despite the use of 100% inspired oxygen. The patient died in the recovery room, approximately 1 h postoperatively. No postmortem examination was performed.

Questions

1. How is bone cement implantation syndrome (BCIS) diagnosed intraoperatively?
2. What can be done to reduce the incidence or prevent BCIS?
3. How is BCIS treated?

Introduction

Fragility fractures of the hip are a global concern that affects the quality of life of elderly patients and has a significant impact on the socioeconomic burden on healthcare systems. Globally, the incidence of hip fractures is projected to rise from 1.7 million in 1990 to 6.3 million in 2050, primarily due to an aging population [1, 3]. Approximately 50% of hip fractures are intracapsular and require surgical intervention. Cemented hemiarthroplasty is widely regarded as a treatment choice for geriatric displaced intracapsular femur neck fractures though some patients may be treated with total hip arthroplasty.

Studies have proven that cemented hemiarthroplasty has a significantly better outcome, a lower incidence of periprosthetic fractures, a reduced incidence of reoperation, and a lower mortality rate compared to uncemented hemiarthroplasty [4–6]. Consequently, there is an increased interest in cemented hemiarthroplasty in elderly patients with intracapsular hip fractures.

Additionally, hybrid total hip arthroplasty for primary osteoarthritis is an appealing alternative to press-fit stems due to decreased rates of periprosthetic fracture and thigh pain [7].

Bone cement implantation syndrome (BCIS) is a specific complication associated with cemented hip arthroplasty. The incidence of BCIS varies widely in the literature between 28% and 37%; this large variance is mainly due to the fact that there has been no uniform definition of BCIS in the literature up to now [8, 9]. Severe BCIS has a huge impact on early and late mortality.

Bone Cement Implantation Syndrome (BCIS)

BCIS is a spectrum of conditions ranging from mild hypoxia and hypotension to severe pulmonary vascular resistance (PVR) resulting in cardiac arrest. Due to the lack of a specific diagnosis, it is often poorly reported. It is a primarily intraoperative and early postoperative complication during and after implanting a cemented prosthesis.

BCIS is characterized by hypoxia, hypotension, or both, and/or an unexpected loss of consciousness occurring around the time of cementation, prosthesis insertion, reduction of the joint, or, occasionally, limb tourniquet deflation in a patient undergoing cemented bone surgery [10].

A grading system for BCIS has been proposed in the literature, as outlined in Table 12.1.

Table 12.1 Grading system for BCIS

Grade 1:	Drop in oxygen saturation < 94%; drop in systolic blood pressure > 20%
Grade II:	Drop in oxygen saturation < 88%; drop in systolic blood pressure > 40%, unconsciousness of the awake patient
Grade III:	Cardiopulmonary resuscitation required

Etiology and Pathogenesis

Several mechanisms have been suggested to cause BCIS.

Methyl Methacrylate Monomer Mediated

Multiple hypotheses have been proposed for the etiology of BCIS. In vitro studies focused on the concentration of methyl methacrylate (MMA) cement monomers causing vasodilation, [11] but in vivo animal studies did not support this hypothesis because serum monomer concentrations are much lower than the concentrations required to cause significant cardiovascular and pulmonary effects [12, 13].

Pulmonary Emboli

It has been proposed that an increase in intramedullary pressure during pressurization of cement may lead to pulmonary emboli, which can cause decreased oxygen saturation and increased pulmonary vascular resistance, leading to secondary cardiovascular events [14].

Since then, researchers have increased their focus on pulmonary embolization in BCIS. Emboli were detected using an echocardiogram in the RA, RV, and pulmonary arteries during surgery [15–17]. Postmortem examinations of patients who died as a result of cemented arthroplasty have also revealed pulmonary emboli [2, 18, 19]. Pulmonary emboli could be due to fat, marrow [13, 20] cement particles, [18] air, [21] bone particles, [22] and aggregates of platelets and fibrin [23]. The physiological consequences of embolization are due to both mechanical and mediator-release [20].

Mechanism of Emboli Formation

Embolization occurs because of the high intramedullary pressures that develop during cementation and prosthesis insertion [14]. Pressures can reach 1000 mm of hg during cementation and implant insertion. The cement undergoes an exothermic reaction [24] and expands in the space between the prosthesis and bone, trapping air and medullary contents under pressure so that they are forced into the circulation [14, 25]. The temperature of the cement can increase as high as 96 °C 6 min after mixing the components [24].

Cementation is generally done with a cement gun. After introduction of cement, prosthesis insertion into the cemented femur is associated with considerably increased intramedullary pressure than introduction of cement alone. When cement is inserted into the femur using a cement gun, the pressures generated are almost double those seen when manual packing is used, though use of a cement gun is standard practice, as vacuum mixing and use of a cement gun is integral to optimum cementation technique [26, 27].

Transesophageal Echocardiography (TOE)

Several studies have demonstrated emboli in the heart using transesophageal echocardiography (TEE), and these vary greatly in size and number [28]. One study described the appearance of multiple small emboli as a "snow flurry." [16, 29] Emboli greater than 10 mm were demonstrable in approximately one-third of patients. In one patient, these were reported to be up to 5 cm in length [16]. In addition, TEE has demonstrated that the embolic load is greater in cemented compared with uncemented hip arthroplasty [17] (Fig. 12.2).

These findings were confirmed in a small study that observed emboli on TEE in all seven patients undergoing cemented and uncemented total hip arthroplasties. "Snow flurries" were visible on the TEE intermittently from the start of reaming until the end of the surgical procedure in both cemented and uncemented arthroplasty. In the cemented group, these were most marked during reaming of both the femur and acetabulum and during insertion of the femoral component and reduction of the hip joint. In the group undergoing uncemented arthroplasty, the incidence and duration of the flurries did not increase at any specific point during the procedure. Cardiorespiratory variables were minimally changed during these episodes [22].

Imperfections in the Embolic Model

The embolic model has become the predominant explanation for the cause of BCIS. Nevertheless, embolization does not account for all observed phenomena. Embolization is not always accompanied by hemodynamic changes, [17, 22] and the degree of embolism has a poor correlation with the severity of hypotension or hypoxemia [30, 31]. Studies utilizing TEE reveal that embolic events are common and well tolerated by most patients. One study found that the diameter of the emboli was less than that of the functional pulmonary gas exchange vessels (75 milli microns vs. 150 milli microns) The authors hypothesized that the small emboli would reside in the pulmonary vessels' terminal branches. The larger vessels that furnish the functional gas exchange units may be spared, maintaining a normal ventilation perfusion (V/Q) ratio. They were unable to exhibit V/Q mismatching 30 min after femoral prosthesis insertion [17].

Hypotension has been observed in patients who received polymethyl methacrylate (PMMA) cement in situations where a significant embolism is unlikely, such as

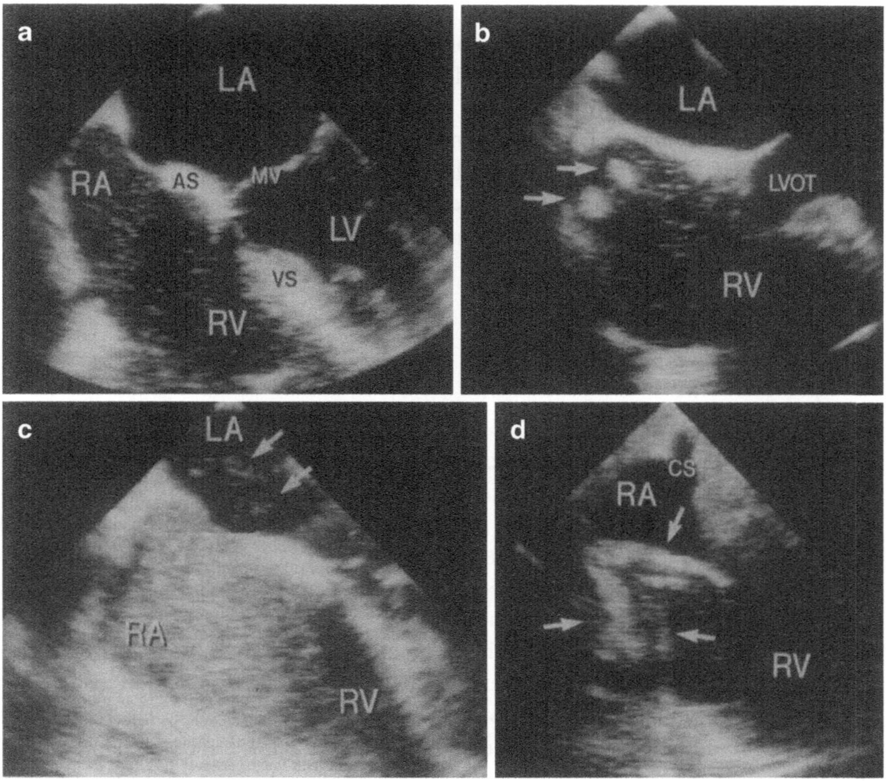

Fig. 12.2 Four-chamber transesophageal echocardiographic views showing embolism during total hip arthroplasty (**a**): Small emboli (less than 5 mm), filling less than half of the right atrium (score 1). (**b**): Medium-sized emboli (5–10 mm) (2 arrows) and small emboli filling more than half of the right atrium. (**c**): Small emboli (less than 5 mm) completely filling the right atrium multiple paradoxical emboli in the left atrium (arrows). (**d**): Large emboli (more than 10 mm) in the right atrium with delayed passage at the tricuspid valve *AS* atrial septum, *CS* coronary sinus, *LA* left atrium, *LV* left ventricle, *LVOT* left ventricular outflow tract, *MV* mitral valve, *RA* right atrium, *RV* right ventricle, *VS* ventricular septum. (Reproduced with permission from Ereth MH, Weber JG, Abel MD, Lennon RL, Lewallen DG, Ilstrup DM, Rehder K. Cemented versus noncemented total hip arthroplasty—embolism, hemodynamics, and intrapulmonary shunting. Mayo Clin Proc. 1992 Nov;67 (11):1066–74 [17])

percutaneous vertebroplasty [32]. Despite the possibility that micro-embolism contributes to BCIS, it is likely that other mechanisms must be involved.

Histamine Release and Hypersensitivity

Anaphylaxis (Type 1 hypersensitivity) has also been implicated as a potential cause for a fatal case of BCIS in 1972 [10]. Anaphylaxis and BCIS share various clinical similarities. A considerable increase in plasma histamine concentration has been demonstrated in hypotensive patients undergoing cementation [33]. It is unknown whether an IgE-mediated mechanism or a direct effect of the cement monomer is what causes the release of histamine. In one study, blocking histamine receptors with clemastin and cimetidine (H1 and H2 antagonists) appeared to confer protection, [33] but these results have not been replicated in subsequent studies [30, 31].

At least one case report of anaphylactic shock due to bone cement has been reported in a patient with a specific risk factor (underlying systemic mastocytosis) undergoing total hip arthroplasty during cementation of an acetabular component [34].

Complement Activation

The anaphylatoxins C3a and C5a are potent vasoconstriction and bronchoconstriction mediators. In contrast to uncemented hemiarthroplasty, cemented hemiarthroplasty is associated with an increase in C3a and C5a levels, indicating activation of the complement pathway [35]. In a small randomized, controlled, double-blind study, high-dose methylprednisolone (2 g) was demonstrated to reduce complement activation and hypoxia in patients undergoing cemented arthroplasty. It appeared that methylprednisolone prevented the production of anaphylatoxins and the onset of oxygen desaturation [36]. However, a few years later, Lewis and colleagues reported no substantial decline in C3 and C4 levels during the first 30 min after the cement was introduced in patients undergoing a standard cemented THR procedure [37].

A more recent study by Thordardottir and colleagues observed similar findings of complement activation through both classic and alternate pathways in 12 patients undergoing cemented total hip arthroplasty for osteoarthritis [38].

Multifactorial

It is likely that patients who develop BCIS do so as a result of a combination of the processes mentioned previously. Depending on an individual's physiological response, the degree to which each of these models contributes to clinical features may vary. The combined effects of BCIS on hemodynamic variables will depend on the relative magnitude of the alterations in peripheral vascular resistance (PVR), systemic vascular resistance (SVR), and myocardial contractility. It is reasonable to presume that the patient's comorbidities may alter the clinical presentation and severity of BCIS. For example, a patient with preexisting right ventricular dysfunction would be anticipated to be more susceptible to the effects of a sudden increase in PVR.

Table 12.2 Elevated risk factors for BCIS

Patient Factors:	• Advanced age • Cardiovascular disease (CHF, CAD) • Cardiovascular malformations (Patent foramen ovale or Atrial-Septal Defect) • Pulmonary hypertension • Presence of fracture of proximal femur
Other risk factors:	• Uninstrumented femoral canal • Presence of metastatic disease • Use of long-stem component

Risk Factors

Numerous patient-related risk factors have been implicated in the genesis of BCIS, including advanced age, osteoporosis, [2, 18] impaired cardiovascular function, [8, 18] preexisting pulmonary hypertension, metastatic bone disease, [39] and concomitant hip fractures, especially pathologic and intertrochanteric fractures. Patients with a patent foramen ovale or atrial-septal defect may be at increased risk of paradoxical emboli and neurological sequelae.

Patients with uninstrumented femoral canals and metastatic disease are at higher risk of developing BCIS [2, 8, 39]. Two possible mechanisms exist. First, an uninstrumented femur contains a greater volume of potentially embolic material. Second, once the canal has been instrumented and cemented, the interior surface of the femur becomes smooth and sclerotic, providing a surface that is less permeable. The use of a femoral component with a long stem increases the likelihood of developing BCIS [2, 39].

Risk factors are summarized in Table 12.2.

Treatment and Prevention

Intraoperative deaths during hip arthroplasty almost exclusively happen during cemented hip arthroplasty done for fracture [2, 18, 40, 41]. In a retrospective study done at the Mayo Clinic, [18] it was shown that patients undergoing cemented arthroplasty for a fracture diagnosis had a significantly higher mortality rate than patients without fractures. In addition, the incidence of mortality was significantly higher when the fracture type was intertrochanteric or was associated with an underlying malignancy. Although systemic hypotension and potentially other cardiorespiratory changes are frequently observed during cementation, the fatal nature of these changes in some patients but not in others may be influenced by several factors. The presence of severe cardiovascular disease in the preponderance of patients who died during cementing was one of the most striking findings of the study.

In high-risk cases, it is vital that the surgical and anesthesia teams communicate and plan effectively to mitigate risks wherever possible.

Anesthesia Risk Reduction

At the time of cementation, increasing the inspired oxygen concentration (FiO_2) should be considered for all patients, particularly in patients at high risk [2, 20, 41, 42]. Avoiding intravascular volume depletion may further reduce the severity of BCIS-related hemodynamic alterations [18, 39, 42, 43].

A decrease in systolic pressure may serve as an early warning sign of cardiovascular collapse. A sharp decline in end-tidal pCO_2 during general anesthesia may indicate right heart failure and/or a catastrophic reduction in cardiac output.

In addition to standard anesthetic monitoring, high-level hemodynamic monitoring—using transesophageal echocardiography [17, 20] or intraoperative pulmonary artery catheter [2, 18, 20] is suggested in high-risk patients undergoing cemented hip arthroplasty. Central venous pressure (CVP) monitoring further aids in volume supplementation and ionotropic administration if necessary.

At one institution, routine use of low-dose epinephrine became standard practice after observing a series of seven intraoperative cardiac arrests during hemiarthroplasty [2].

We recommend considering discussion with anesthesia that patients with one or more significant risk factors for developing BCIS receive intensive perioperative monitoring of their vital signs. This should involve invasive arterial pressure monitoring and the placement of a central venous catheter. Hypotension in BCIS may result from decreased systemic vascular resistance (SVR), decreased cardiac output (CO), or a combination of the two. CO monitoring with an assessment of cardiac filling, CO, and SVR should be considered in patients at high risk for BCIS. This would enable more appropriate management direction should BCIS develop [10].

Surgery Risk Reduction

The following surgical techniques have been used to reduce the risk of BCIS in cemented hip arthroplasty:

Thorough lavage helps to reduce the embolic load prior to cementation, thereby reducing the risk of BCIS.

Venting the femoral canal through a large diameter bore hole in the distal femur or through a plastic suction catheter in the medullary canal helps reduce intramedullary pressure. This phenomenon has been called medullary venting.

In animal models, venting through a 4.5-mm drill hole in the proximal femur decreased intramedullary pressure there by 70% and by 90% in the distal femur.

However, there are worries that cement may leak out of the vent hole, decreasing the cement mantle's thickness and integrity and possibly harming the nearby soft tissues [44]. In another study, it was noted that there is a higher incidence of a drop in oxygen tension and thrombocytes when a venting hole is not created compared to when a venting hole is made in the femur while cementing [45].

There is some evidence that femoral component cementation with low-viscosity cement lowers intramedullary pressure compared to higher viscosity cement without changing the pullout strength of the bone-cement-implant interface. This lowers the risk of BCIS [46].

Bone-Vacuum Cementing Technique

A suction of −800 millibars (−80,000 pascals) was applied to a proximal drainage cannula placed along the Linea aspera and a distal drainage cannula placed in the diaphysis to produce a vacuum in the medullary cavity of the femur during the application of cement and the insertion of the stem (see Fig. 12.3).

Questions

- How is BCIS diagnosed intraoperatively?

  Dyspnea or altered sensorium could be an early sign of BCIS in an awake patient under regional anesthesia undergoing cemented arthroplasty or A sharp decline in end-tidal pCO_2 during general anesthesia may be the first sign of clinically significant BCIS and indicate right heart failure and/or a catastrophic reduction in cardiac output. A fall in systolic pressure may serve as an early warning sign of cardiovascular collapse.
- What can be done to reduce the incidence or prevent BCIS?

  High-risk patients should be identified, and a high level of hemodynamic monitoring should be considered for all high-risk patients undergoing cemented arthroplasty. Communication between the anesthesiologist and surgeon throughout the procedure is critical, especially during cement implantation, prosthesis insertion, reduction of the prosthetic femoral head, or tourniquet release during total knee replacement. Thorough lavage prior to cementation helps reduce the embolic load. Using low-viscosity cement, avoiding excessive pressurization during cementation and insertion of prostheses, and venting the femoral canal through a large diameter bore hole in the distal femur should be considered. Alternative options, including uncemented arthroplasty, should be considered in high-risk patients.
- How is BCIS treated?

  If BCIS is suspected, the inspired oxygen concentration should be increased to 100%, and supplemental oxygen should be administered in the immediate postoperative period. Cardiovascular collapse in the context of BCIS has been suggested to be treated as RV failure with aggressive fluid resuscitation and inotropic agents.

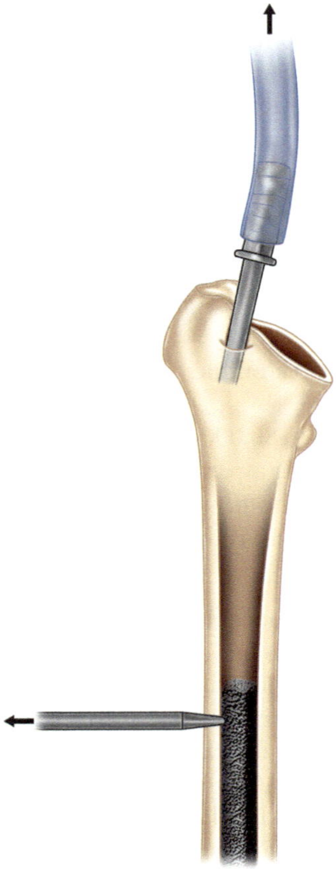

Fig. 12.3 Positions of the two cannulae used in the bone-vacuum cementing technique The proximal cannula is placed posteriorly between the greater and lesser trochanters along the projection of the linea aspera. A permeable synthetic plug is placed at the level of the distal unicortical venting hole and fixed to the threaded tip of the cannula. (Reproduced with permission from Pitto RP, Koessler M, Kuehle JW). Comparison of fixation of the femoral component without cement and fixation with use of a bone-vacuum cementing technique for the prevention of fat embolism during total hip arthroplasty. A prospective, randomized clinical trial. J Bone Joint Surg Am. 1999 Jun;81 [6]:831–43 [47]

Conclusion

BCIS is a source of morbidity and potential mortality during orthopaedic procedures which require cementation. Identification of high-risk patients, perioperative monitoring by the anesthesia team, and close communication between surgeon and anesthesiologist prior to and during cement implantation and prosthesis insertion may help reduce the risk of BCIS. During cementation, appropriate intravascular fluid resuscitation, and appropriate oxygenation are adjunct treatments which may reduce the risk of BCIS. Bone preparation should include thorough lavage of the medullary canal, consideration for limited pressurization in higher risk patients, when longer stems are used, and for previously uninstrumented femurs. Canal venting may also be considered. If BCIS occurs, FiO_2 should be increased to 100%, fluid bolus and inotropic agents should be administered as appropriate, and the team should be immediately prepared to initiate lifesaving resuscitation as needed.

References

1. Cooper C, Campion G, Melton LJ. Hip fractures in the elderly: a world-wide projection. Osteoporos Int. 1992;2(6):285–9.
2. Patterson BM, Healey JH, Cornell CN, Sharrock NE. Cardiac arrest during hip arthroplasty with a cemented long-stem component. A report of seven cases. J Bone Joint Surg Am. 1991;73(2):271–7.
3. Johnell O. The socioeconomic burden of fractures: today and in the 21st century. Am J Med. 1997;103(2):S20–6.
4. Fernandez MA, Achten J, Parsons N, Griffin XL, Png ME, Gould J, et al. Cemented or Uncemented Hemiarthroplasty for Intracapsular hip fracture. N Engl J Med. 2022;386(6):521–30.
5. Parker MJ, Cawley S. Cemented or uncemented hemiarthroplasty for displaced intracapsular fractures of the hip: a randomized trial of 400 patients. Bone Joint J. 2020;102-B(1):11–6.
6. Kristensen TB, Dybvik E, Kristoffersen M, Dale H, Engesæter LB, Furnes O, et al. Cemented or Uncemented Hemiarthroplasty for femoral neck fracture? Data from the Norwegian hip fracture register. Clin Orthop Relat Res. 2020;478(1):90–100.
7. González Della Valle A, Sharrock N, Barlow M, Caceres L, Go G, Salvati EA. The modern, hybrid total hip arthroplasty for primary osteoarthritis at the Hospital for Special Surgery. Bone Joint J. 2016;98-B(1 Suppl A):54–9.
8. Olsen F, Kotyra M, Houltz E, Ricksten SE. Bone cement implantation syndrome in cemented hemiarthroplasty for femoral neck fracture: incidence, risk factors, and effect on outcome. Br J Anaesth. 2014;113:800–6.
9. Weingärtner K, Störmann P, Schramm D, Wutzler S, Zacharowski K, Marzi I, et al. Bone cement implantation syndrome in cemented hip hemiarthroplasty—a persistent risk. Eur J Trauma Emerg Surg. 2022;48(2):721–9.
10. Donaldson AJ, Thomson HE, Harper NJ, Kenny NW. Bone cement implantation syndrome. Br J Anaesth. 2009;102(1):12–22.
11. Karlsson J, Wendling W, Chen D, Zelinsky J, Jeevanandam V, Hellman S, et al. Methylmethacrylate monomer produces direct relaxation of vascular smooth muscle in vitro. Acta Anaesthesiol Scand. 1995;39(5):685–9.
12. McLaughlin RE, DiFazio CA, Hakala M, Abbott B, MacPhail JA, Mack WP, et al. Blood clearance and acute pulmonary toxicity of methylmethacrylate in dogs after simulated arthroplasty and intravenous injection. J Bone Joint Surg Am. 1973;55(8):1621–8.
13. Modig J, Busch C, Waernbaum G. Effects of graded infusions of monomethylmethacrylate on coagulation, blood lipids, respiration and circulation. An experimental study in dogs. Clin Orthop Relat Res. 1975;113:187–97.
14. Orsini EC, Byrick RJ, Mullen JB, Kay JC, Waddell JP. Cardiopulmonary function and pulmonary microemboli during arthroplasty using cemented or non-cemented components. The role of intramedullary pressure. J Bone Joint Surg Am. 1987;69(6):822–32.

15. Chen HL, Wong CS, Ho ST, Chang FL, Hsu CH, Wu CT. A lethal pulmonary embolism during percutaneous vertebroplasty. Anesth Analg. 2002;95(4):1060–2. table of contents
16. Lafont ND, Kalonji MK, Barre J, Guillaume C, Boogaerts JG. Clinical features and echocardiography of embolism during cemented hip arthroplasty. Can J Anaesth. 1997;44(2):112–7.
17. Ereth MH, Weber JG, Abel MD, Lennon RL, Lewallen DG, Ilstrup DM, et al. Cemented versus noncemented total hip arthroplasty—embolism, hemodynamics, and intrapulmonary shunting. Mayo Clin Proc. 1992;67(11):1066–74.
18. Parvizi J, Holiday AD, Ereth MH, Lewallen DG. The frank Stinchfield award. Sudden death during primary hip arthroplasty. Clin Orthop Relat Res. 1999;369:39–48.
19. Kepes ER, Undersood PS, Becsey L. Intraoperative death associated with acrylic bone cement. Report of two cases. JAMA. 1972;222(5):576–7.
20. Byrick RJ, Forbes D, Waddell JP. A monitored cardiovascular collapse during cemented total knee replacement. Anesthesiology. 1986;65(2):213–6.
21. Hyland J, Robins RH. Cardiac arrest and bone cement. Br Med J. 1970;4(5728):176–7.
22. Hayakawa M, Fujioka Y, Morimoto Y, Okamura A, Kemmotsu O. Pathological evaluation of venous emboli during total hip arthroplasty. Anaesthesia. 2001;56(6):571–5.
23. Modig J, Busch C, Olerud S, Saldeen T, Waernbaum G. Arterial hypotension and hypoxaemia during total hip replacement: the importance of thromboplastic products, fat embolism and acrylic monomers. Acta Anaesthesiol Scand. 1975;19(1):28–43.
24. Frost PM. Cardiac arrest and bone cement. Br Med J. 1970;3(5721):524.
25. Michel R. Air embolism in hip surgery. Anaesthesia. 1980;35(9):858–62.
26. Tronzo RG, Kallos T, Wyche MQ. Elevation of intramedullary pressure when methylmethacrylate is inserted in total hip arthroplasty. J Bone Joint Surg Am. 1974;56(4):714–8.
27. McCaskie AW, Barnes MR, Lin E, Harper WM, Gregg PJ. Cement pressurisation during hip replacement. J Bone Joint Surg Br. 1997;79(3):379–84.
28. Lafont ND, Kostucki WM, Marchand PH, Michaux MN, Boogaerts JG. Embolism detected by transoesophageal echocardiography during hip arthroplasty. Can J Anaesth. 1994;41(9):850–3.
29. Bisignani G, Bisignani M, Pasquale GS, Greco F. Intraoperative embolism and hip arthroplasty: intraoperative transesophageal echocardiographic study. J Cardiovasc Med (Hagerstown). 2008;9(3):277–81.
30. Lamadé WR, Friedl W, Schmid B, Meeder PJ. Bone cement implantation syndrome. A prospective randomised trial for use of antihistamine blockade. Arch Orthop Trauma Surg. 1995;114(6):335–9.
31. Mitsuhata H, Saitoh J, Saitoh K, Fukuda H, Hirabayasi Y, Shimizu R, et al. Methylmethacrylate bone cement does not release histamine in patients undergoing prosthetic replacement of the femoral head. Br J Anaesth. 1994;73(6):779–81.
32. Vasconcelos C, Gailloud P, Martin JB, Murphy KJ. Transient arterial hypotension induced by polymethylmethacrylate injection during percutaneous vertebroplasty. J Vasc Interv Radiol. 2001;12(8):1001–2.
33. Tryba M, Linde I, Voshage G, Zenz M. Histamine release and cardiovascular reactions to implantation of bone cement during total hip replacement. Anaesthesist. 1991;40(1):25–32.
34. ten Hagen A, Doldersum P, van Raaij T. Anaphylactic shock during cement implantation of a total hip arthroplasty in a patient with underlying mastocytosis: case report of a rare intraoperative complication. Patient Saf Surg. 2016;10:25.
35. Bengtson A, Larsson M, Gammer W, Heideman M. Anaphylatoxin release in association with methylmethacrylate fixation of hip prostheses. J Bone Joint Surg Am. 1987;69(1):46–9.
36. Gammer W, Bengtson A, Heideman M. Inhibition of complement activation by high-dose corticosteroids in total hip arthroplasty. Clin Orthop Relat Res. 1988;236:205–9.
37. Lewis G. Viscoelastic properties of injectable bone cements for orthopaedic applications: state-of-the-art review. J Biomed Mater Res B Appl Biomater. 2011;98B(1):171–91.
38. Thordardottir S, Vikingsdottir T, Bjarnadottir H, Jonsson H Jr, Gudbjornsson B. Activation of complement following Total hip replacement. Scand J Immunol. 2016;83(3):219–24.

39. Herrenbruck T, Erickson EW, Damron TA, Heiner J. Adverse clinical events during cemented long-stem femoral arthroplasty. Clin Orthop Relat Res. 2002;395:154–63.
40. Burgess DM. Cardiac arrest and bone cement. Br Med J. 1970;3(5722):588.
41. Kallos T. Impaired arterial oxygenation associated with use of bone cement in the femoral shaft. Anesthesiology. 1975;42(2):210–5.
42. Pietak S, Holmes J, Matthews R, Petrasek A, Porter B. Cardiovascular collapse after femoral prosthesis surgery for acute hip fracture. Can J Anaesth. 1997;44(2):198–201.
43. Peebles DJ, Ellis RH, Stride SD, Simpson BR. Cardiovascular effects of methylmethacrylate cement. Br Med J. 1972;1(5796):349–51.
44. Issack PS, Lauerman MH, Helfet DL, Sculco TP, Lane JM. Fat embolism and respiratory distress associated with cemented femoral arthroplasty. Am J Orthop (Belle Mead NJ). 2009;38(2):72–6.
45. Engesæter LB, Strand T, Raugstad TS, Husebø S, Langeland N. Effects of a distal venting hole in the femur during total hip replacement. Arch Orth Traum Surg. 1984;103(5):328–31.
46. Rothberg DL, Kubiak EN, Peters CL, Randall RL, Aoki SK. Reducing the risk of bone cement implantation syndrome during femoral arthroplasty. Orthopedics. 2013;36(4):e463–7.
47. Pitto RP, Koessler M, Kuehle JW. Comparison of fixation of the femoral component without cement and fixation with use of a bone-vacuum cementing technique for the prevention of fat embolism during total hip arthroplasty. A prospective, randomized clinical trial. J Bone Joint Surg Am. 1999;81(6):831–43.

Chapter 13
Adrenal Insufficiency

Ritu Madan and Priyanka Majety

Case 1

A 55-year-old female with human immunodeficiency virus (HIV) gets knee replacement surgery. She had severe knee arthritis and was getting intra-articular triamcinolone (steroid injections) every 3 months for knee pain for last 12 months, last injection was 1 month ago. During the surgery, she gets hypotensive and blood pressure does not respond to intravenous hydration. There is no excessive loss of blood during surgery. She gets started on vasopressors and surgery needs to be abandoned prematurely, and she is moved to ICU intubated and on pressors. On examination, she is obese (BMI 35) with facial plethora. Her extremities are thin and she has bruises on her arms. Her husband reports that she has lower strength in her arms and legs than she used to. She has difficulty going upstairs. Besides HIV, she has sleep apnea. She has been taking HIV medications elvitegravir, cobicistat, emtricitabine, and tenofovir. For almost 2 years, she has been getting intra-articular steroid injections in the knee. Labs show TLC 12000, Hb 10, platelet count 400 k. Electrolytes Na 137, potassium 3.8, BUN 30, crt 1.5, Bicarb 26.

In the ICU, AI is suspected. She receives intravenous hydrocortisone. A random cortisol comes back at 2 mcg/dL. A random ACTH level comes back low at 5 pg/mL. With hydrocortisone on board, pressors are weaned off and she is able to go back to operating room to get the knee replacement.

Case 2

A 65-year-old male with primary adrenal insufficiency and diabetes type 1 is admitted to the hospital for right foot ulcer. He has had low grade fever of up to 100 °F for 7 days, has low appetite. Examination is unremarkable except for an ulcer around the first right metatarsophalangeal joint. Blood tests indicate WBC 15000,

R. Madan (✉) · P. Majety
Division of Endocrinology, Diabetes and Metabolism, Department of Medicine, Virginia Commonwealth University, Richmond, VA, USA
e-mail: Ritu.Madan@vcuhealth.org; Priyanka.Majety@vcuhealth.org

W. A. Zuelzer, S. Metikala (eds.), *Unusual Conditions That Every Orthopaedic Surgeon Should Know*, https://doi.org/10.1007/978-3-031-58946-1_13

neutrophils 70%, Hemoglobin 11, elevated ESR and CRP. MRI of the foot shows osteomyelitis. He is started on iv antibiotics and taken to OR on day 2 for debridement. After coming back from OR in the evening, he has fever of up to 102 °F, HR 95, BP 100/60. He is on iv cefazolin, oral hydrocortisone, fludrocortisone, insulin Levemir, insulin aspart. Patient starts to act confused at 10 pm. Fingerstick glucose check shows blood sugar as 54 mg/dL. He is treated for low sugars with 50% dextrose infusion and improves. Electrolytes at the time show Na 132, K+ 4.5, BUN 20, crt 1.2. At this time, his dose of hydrocortisone has changed to intravenous hydrocortisone 25 mg every 8 h. He does well the next day with no fever. By day 3, he is tapered down to home dose of hydrocortisone.

Case 3
A 54-year-old woman with history of psoriatic arthritis is admitted to the hospital after bilateral knee arthroplasty. Her operative course was complicated by popliteal artery occlusion for which she underwent urgent thrombectomy. She is started on heparin drip for thromboprophylaxis on postoperative day (POD) 1.

On POD 8, she developed nausea, abdominal pain, tachycardia, and orthostatic hypotension. Laboratory results show leukocytosis (23,000 cells/μL), thrombocytopenia (93,000 /μL), elevated D-dimer (20,000 ng/mL), and fibrinogen (643 mg/dL) levels. A CT scan done for evaluation of abdominal pain revealed bilateral hyperdense and enlarged adrenal glands. Adrenal hemorrhage was suspected, and she was treated for adrenal insufficiency. Later, a random cortisol drawn before treatment came back as 1.3 mcg/dL.

Questions
1. You are evaluating a patient for a knee replacement. He has been a kidney transplant recipient on prednisone 2.5 mg daily for 5 years. How should this be managed perioperatively?
2. You see a patient for carpal tunnel syndrome, he has history of long-standing adrenal insufficiency because of pituitary tumor resection. Patient is on hydrocortisone for adrenal hormone replacement. What instruction would you give to the patient for the day of surgery?
3. What HIV medication inhibits CYP 3A4 and thus decrease steroid metabolism?

Introduction

Adrenal crisis is a term used for acute decompensation of adrenal glands usually precipitated by stress from surgery, infection, or trauma due to inadequate adrenal hormones being available. The characteristic manifestation of adrenal crisis is circulatory shock, but patients often present with non-specific symptoms like nausea, vomiting, abdominal pain, fever or altered mental status. Cardiovascular symptoms include postural dizziness or syncope. Since the presenting symptoms of AI can be vague and since there is a significant overlap with many symptoms in the postoperative setting, the diagnosis of AI poses a clinical challenge to clinicians. A high index of suspicion is required to make a timely diagnosis.

Adrenal insufficiency (AI) is a term used for chronic lack of adrenal hormones, and this would usually present with malaise, fatigue, weight loss, arthralgia, and hyperpigmentation.

Background

Anatomy and Function of Adrenal Glands

A normal adrenal gland is 1 cm thick, 5 cm long, and 2 cm thick (Fig. 13.1). An adrenal gland is composed of two distinct parts: the outer part called the adrenal cortex and the inner adrenal medulla. Adrenal cortex produces glucocorticoids, mainly cortisol, mineralocorticoid mainly aldosterone and sex steroids that are mainly androgens. Adrenal medulla produces epinephrine norepinephrine and dopamine. Glucocorticoids are responsible for vascular reactivity to epinephrine, a vasoconstrictor. Glucocorticoids are responsible for gluconeogenesis, sodium and water retention, and maintenance of glomerular filtration rate. Mineralocorticoids are also responsible for sodium and water retention. Production of glucocorticoid hormones is regulated by pituitary adrenocorticotropic hormone and that in turn is regulated by hypothalamic corticotropic-releasing hormone (Fig. 13.2). Note the interplay between the brain adjusting the adrenal gland hormonal responses. The primary mineralocorticoid is aldosterone, and its production is regulated by the renin-angiotensin system (Fig. 13.3). Renin is a hormone that is released from juxtaglomerular cells in afferent arterioles in response to decreased renal perfusion and sympathetic activation. It cleaves peptide angiotensinogen in liver to produce angiotensin I. Angiotensin I is cleaved to form angiotensin II by angiotensin-converting enzyme (ACE), which is found predominantly within lung endothelium. Angiotensin II is a systemic vasoconstrictor and stimulates the release of aldosterone from adrenal glands.

Epinephrine and norepinephrine are produced in response to stress. They are responsible for fight and flight response, increase myocardial contractility, relax muscles of gastrointestinal tract, urinary bladder, bronchioles, and pupils and cause glycogenolysis and lipolysis.

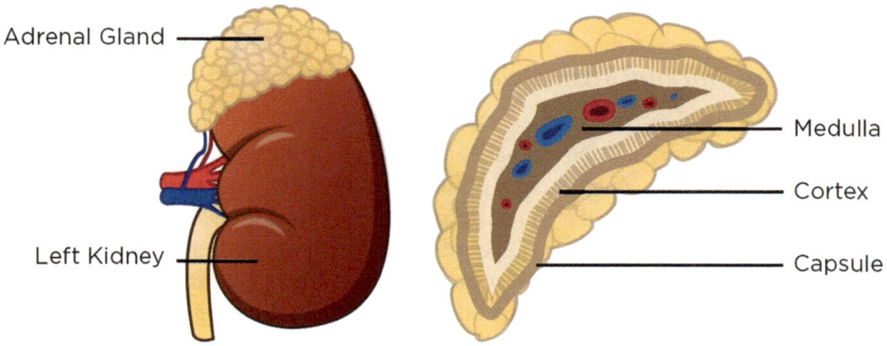

Fig. 13.1 Structure of adrenal gland

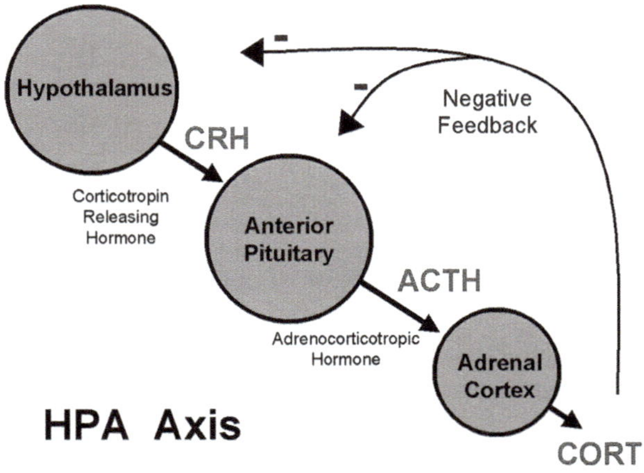

Fig. 13.2 Hypothalamic pituitary adrenal axis

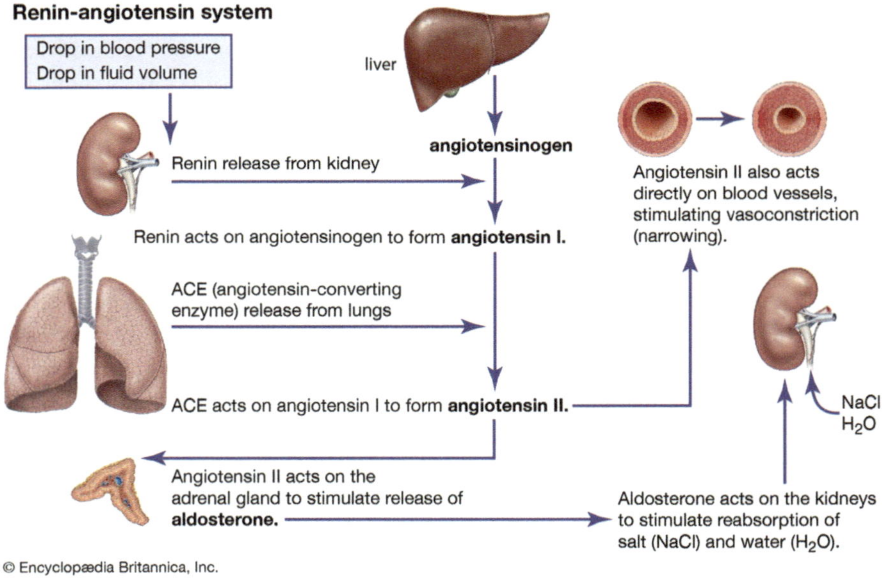

Fig. 13.3 Renin angiotensin aldosterone axis

Etiology of Adrenal Insufficiency

Adrenal insufficiency can be primarily caused by primary destruction of adrenal glands (Primary AI), secondary to a problem with pituitary gland called secondary adrenal insufficiency or tertiary to destruction of hypothalamus. Secondary and tertiary adrenal insufficiency can also be referred to as central adrenal insufficiency.

Most common cause of adrenal insufficiency is exogenous use of steroids leading to central or secondary or tertiary adrenal insufficiency. Exogenous steroids like prednisone, hydrocortisone, and dexamethasone suppress CRH and ACTH and thus decrease endogenous cortisol production. In the presence of stress, a suppressed HPA axis is unable to increase the cortisol production in response [1].

Most common cause of primary adrenal insufficiency in the developed world is autoimmune destruction of adrenal glands. 90% of both adrenal glands need to be destroyed to lead to AI. Autoimmune AI can be an isolated hormonal deficiency in an individual or occur in conjunction with other autoimmune endocrine disorders like hypothyroidism, and hypoparathyroidism. Vitiligo, mucocutaneous candidiasis, pernicious anemia, and primary hypogonadism can be seen in conjunction as well.

The second most common cause of primary adrenal insufficiency or maybe more common in the developing world is infectious infiltration by *Mycobacterium tuberculosis*, HIV and in immunocompromised individuals, infection with cytomegalovirus (CMV), fungi-like cryptococcus, histoplasma, and coccidioides. Adrenal infiltration with metastases from solid tumors, sarcoidosis, amyloidosis, hemochromatosis, and adrenal hemorrhage can completely destroy adrenal glands and lead to AI. Genetic disorders that lead to AI are adrenoleukodystrophy, congenital adrenal hyperplasia, congenital lipoid adrenal hyperplasia, adrenal hypoplasia congenita, and ACTH insensitivity syndrome. Usually, adrenal insufficiency from genetic disorders would be detected at birth or early childhood (Table 13.1).

The reasons for secondary and tertiary adrenal insufficiency other than steroid use are listed in Tables 13.2 and 13.3.

Clinical Presentation of Adrenal Insufficiency

It can present emergently with abdominal pain, nausea, vomiting, hypotension, or shock. The most common symptoms of adrenal insufficiency are fatigue and weight loss. In primary AI, there is lack of mineralocorticoid and sex steroid action in addition to glucocorticoid action. Individuals with chronic primary AI have more symptoms of dizziness, salt craving, and lack of axillary hair because of lacking all

Table 13.1 Primary AI

1	Autoimmune: Isolated or as part of Autoimmune Polyendocrine Syndromes APS I and II
2	Infectious: Tuberculosis, CMV, cryptococcus, histoplasma, and coccidioides
3	Adrenal metastases from cancer of lung, breast, colon, kidney, melanoma, lymphoma
4	Infiltrative disorders: Sarcoidosis, amyloidosis, hemochromatosis
5	Adrenal hemorrhage from sepsis (meningococcemia), antiphospholipid antibody syndrome, anticoagulants, trauma
6	Genetic disorders: Congenital adrenal hyperplasia, congenital adrenal hypoplasia
7	Genetic syndromes: Adrenoleukodystrophy
8	Iatrogenic: Surgical removal of adrenal glands
9	Inherited insensitivity to ACTH

Table 13.2 Causes of secondary AI

1	Tumors like pituitary adenoma, craniopharyngioma, meningioma, metastases, ependymoma
2	Surgery
3	Pituitary radiation
4	Pituitary apoplexy, e.g., Sheehan syndrome
5	Lymphocytic hypophysitis, e.g., postpartum or drug induced by CTLA4 inhibitor chemotherapy
6	Head trauma
7	Infiltrative disorders like sarcoidosis, histiocytosis X, Wegener granulomatosis
8	Genetic: Isolated congenital ACTH deficiency, pro-opiomelanocortin deficiency
9	Chronic opioid use [2]

Table 13.3 Causes of tertiary AI

1.	Radiation for brain tumors
2	Infiltrative disorders like sarcoidosis, histiocytosis X
3	Meningitis
4	Traumatic brain injury
5	Subarachnoid hemorrhage
6	Chronic opioid use

Table 13.4 Symptoms of chronic adrenal insufficiency

Symptom	Frequency
Weakness/fatigue	100%
Anorexia	100%
Nausea /vomiting	80–90%
Abdominal pain	
Arthralgia	
Dizziness	
Salt craving	22%, more in primary AI

hormones (Table 13.4). They also have hyperpigmented sun exposed areas, i.e., face, neck and back of hand, areas that are already pigmented get more pigment, i.e., nipple of areola, scrotum and labia, areas that undergo repeated trauma that is palmar folds, and mucosa of lip and palate. (Figs. 13.4 and 13.5).

Individuals with Central AI usually have a history of steroid use, pituitary tumors, irradiation, or insult.

Laboratory studies show hyponatremia and hyperkalemia. One may see acute kidney injury- elevated blood urea nitrogen and creatinine in adrenal crisis. Hypoglycemia is more commonly seen in children. Anemia and eosinophilia can also be seen in long-standing disease. Very rarely, one may see hypercalcemia (Table 13.5).

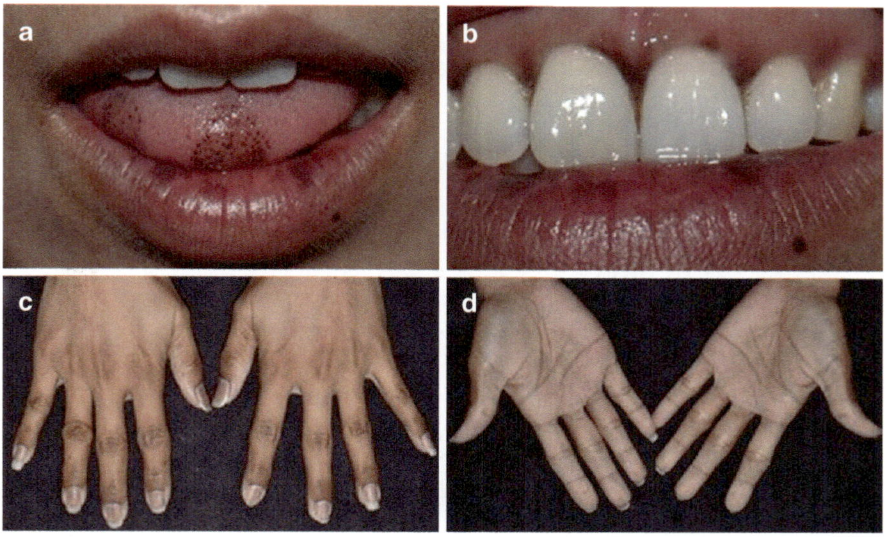

Fig. 13.4 (**a** and **b**) Multiple pigmented macules on oral mucosa, tongue, and lips. (**c** and **d**) Hyperpigmentation of bilateral hands, especially knuckles and periungual areas, nails, and palmar creases

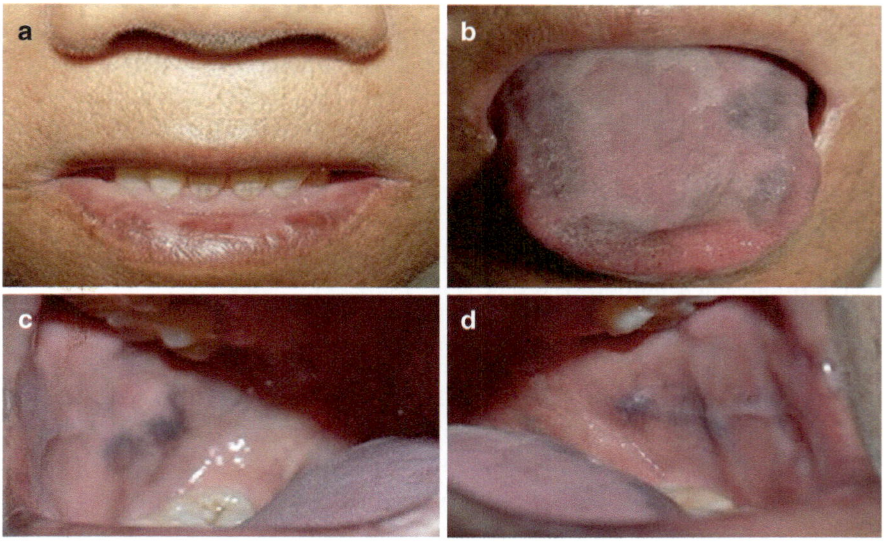

Fig. 13.5 Pigmented macules and patches over the (**a**) lips, (**b**) tongue, and (**c** and **d**) buccal mucosa. Chen H, Hsieh FN, Yang CC. Mucocutaneous hyperpigmentation as a clue to diagnose Addison disease—Two case reports. Dermatol Sin 2022;40:48-9 [3]

Table 13.5 Lab abnormalities in adrenal insufficiency

Abnormality	Frequency
Hyponatremia	85–90%
Hyperkalemia	More in primary AI 60–65%
Hypoglycemia	More common in children
Mild normochromic normocytic anemia	Primary AI
Eosinophilia	Primary AI
Lymphocytosis	Primary AI
Salt craving	

Diagnosis of Adrenal Insufficiency

Screening of AI can be done by an 8 am morning fasting cortisol levels. AM cortisol levels are preferred for diagnosis as ACTH and cortisol secretion follow circadian rhythm with highest levels in morning (Fig. 13.6). Levels less than 3 mcg/dL are diagnostic of adrenal insufficiency [5]. Levels between 3 and 8 mcg/dL using LCMS assays or monoclonal radioimmunoassay are in gray zone and will need additional testing called cosyntropin stimulation for diagnosis. Levels greater than 8 mcg/dL rule out the diagnosis [6]. If patient presents in a crisis, it is better to draw a random cortisol and proceed as one would for the treatment of AI. Definitive diagnosis can wait till patient is stable.

Cosyntropin stimulation test uses cosyntropin, which is a synthetic derivative of ACTH at a supraphysiological dose of 250 mcg intramuscularly or intravenously to stimulate the adrenal glands to produce cortisol. Cortisol levels are measured before the cosyntropin injection, 30 and 60 min later. A peak cortisol level of 16 mcg/dL rules out AI [7](Fig. 13.7). This test is not suitable for acute AI secondary to pituitary surgeries, pituitary apoplexy, or subarachnoid hemorrhage. Another caveat to this test is that since this test measures free plus bound cortisol, it is not reliable in patients who may have low cortisol-binding globulin as in patients with cirrhosis, malnutrition, and nephrotic syndrome (Fig. 13.8).

Case 1

A 55-year-old female with HIV gets knee replacement surgery. She had severe knee arthritis and has been getting intra-articular triamcinolone (steroid injections) every 3 months for knee pain for last 12 months. Her last injection was 1 month ago. During the surgery, she gets hypotensive and her blood pressure does not respond to intravenous hydration. There is no excessive loss of blood during surgery. She gets started on vasopressors and surgery needs to be abandoned prematurely, and she is moved to ICU intubated and on pressors. On examination, she is obese (BMI 35) with facial plethora. Her extremities are thin and she has bruises on her arms. Her husband reports that she has lower strength in her arms and legs than she used to. She has difficulty going upstairs. Besides HIV, she has sleep apnea. She has been taking HIV medications elvitegravir, cobicistat, emtricitabine, and tenofovir. For almost 2 years, she has been getting intra-articular steroid injections in the knee.

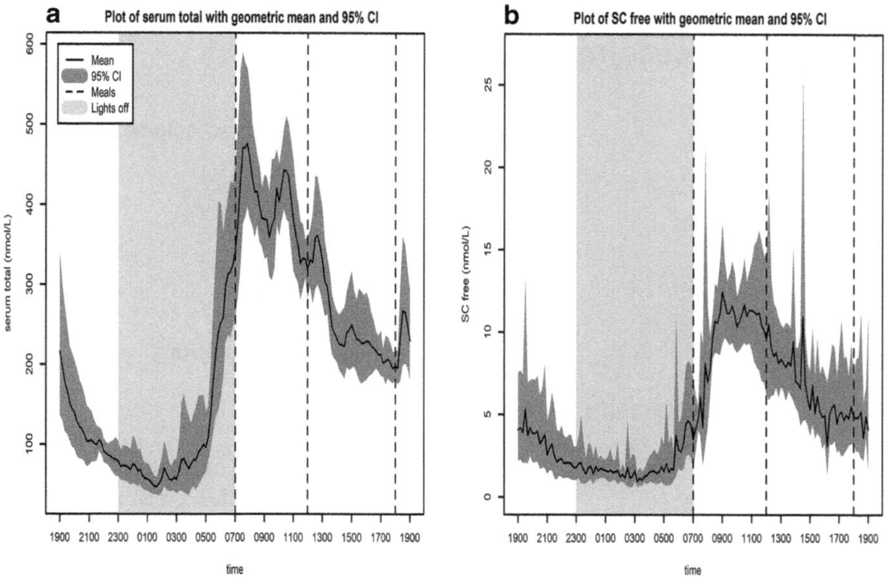

Fig. 13.6 Plot showing circadian rhythm of total cortisol (panel a) and free cortisol (panel b) [4]. (Review: Scenarios of adrenal insufficiency that can catch an orthopaedist by surprise)

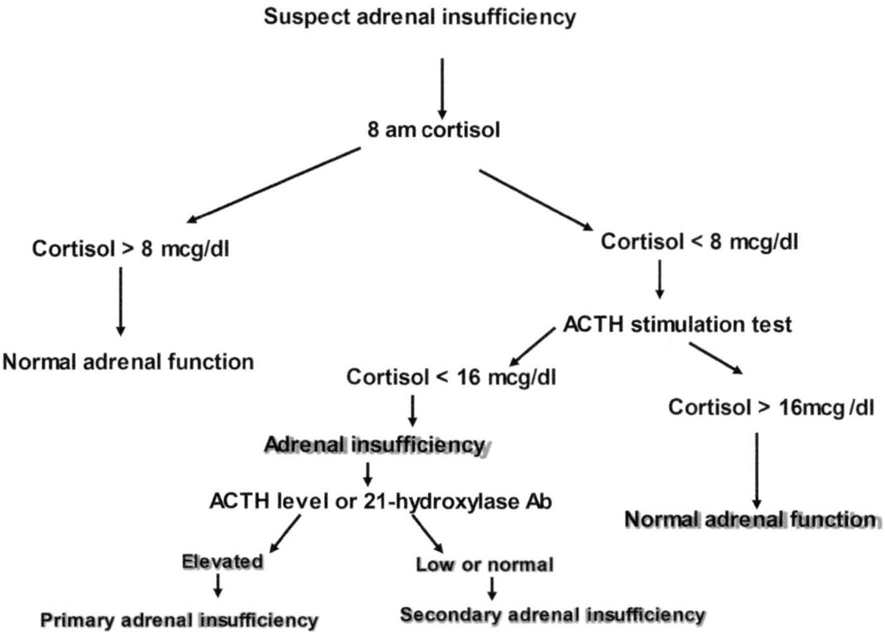

Fig. 13.7 Algorithm for suspected Adrenal Insufficiency Diagnosis

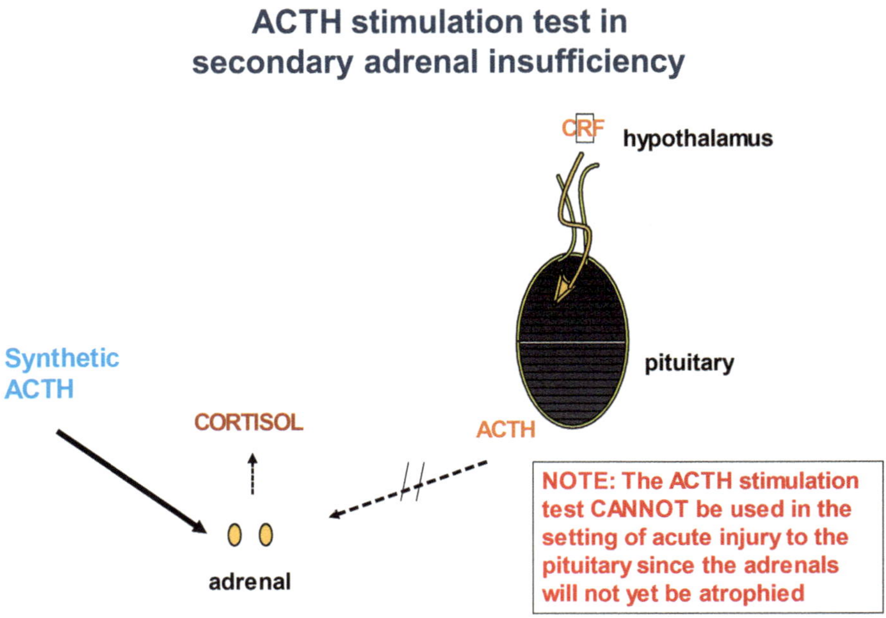

Fig. 13.8 Utility of Cosyntropin Stimulation test in Secondary Adrenal Insufficiency

Labs show TLC 12000, Hb 10, platelet count 400 k. Electrolytes Na 137, potassium 3.8, BUN 30, crt 1.5, Bicarb 26.

In the ICU, AI is suspected. She receives intravenous hydrocortisone. A random cortisol comes back as 2 mcg/dL. A random ACTH level comes back low at 5 pg/mL. With hydrocortisone on board, pressors are weaned off, and she is able to go back to operating room to get the knee replacement.

There are many reasons an HIV-positive individual can have adrenal insufficiency. In his particular case, one is seeing symptoms and signs of both Cushing syndrome (a condition due to excess glucocorticoids in the body) and adrenal insufficiency. This can occur from the use of exogenous steroids. She has been getting intra-articular steroids. Local steroid applications are supposed to have minimal systemic absorption, but they are absorbed to some extent. Steroids are metabolized mostly by cytochrome P450 3A4 enzyme. HIV medications cobicistat and ritonavir are potent CYP3A4 inhibitors. Concomitant use of these HIV medications with steroids increases the systemic concentration of steroids. An increased exogenous plasma concentration of corticosteroids may lead to the development of iatrogenic Cushing's syndrome (ICS), and at supraphysiological concentrations, the suppression of adrenocorticotropic hormone (ACTH), and endogenous corticosteroid secretion, resulting in secondary adrenal insufficiency (SAI). Current evidence shows concurrent use of fluticasone (steroid used for nasal allergies and asthma) with ritonavir increases the plasma concentration of fluticasone by 2500% [8]. Similar effects have been reported with the use of budesonide and mometasone [9]. Of the inhaled steroids, beclomethasone is the safest alternative as it is minimally metabolized by CYP3A4 [10]. None of the intra-articular steroids, i.e., triamcinolone or methylprednisolone, are safe with HIV drugs ritonavir and cobicistat [11, 12]. One should also avoid prolonged use of ocular steroids in these individuals [13].

Recommendations for use of steroid medications for individuals with HIV on ritonavir- and cobicistat-based antiretroviral therapy (Table 13.6).

Keep a high index of suspicion for these individuals for secondary AI especially if they complain of fatigue and have hyponatremia on laboratory testing.

Other reasons for adrenal insufficiency in HIV-positive individuals are opportunistic infections like CMV, *Mycobacterium tuberculosis*, MAC, toxoplasmosis, and fungal infections like histoplasmosis, cryptococcosis, and nocardiosis. Tumors like Kaposi sarcoma and non-Hodgkin's lymphoma can also involve adrenal glands [14]. Infections mostly affect the adrenal gland thus causing primary AI, 90% of adrenal gland needs to be destroyed to lead to primary AI. Infections can be seen as enlarged adrenal glands with necrosis on imaging or adrenal gland atrophy. Biopsy is needed to establish diagnosis. Prior to potent antiretroviral treatment, adrenal involvement was seen in two thirds of cases. Prevalence of these infections is low now.

Also, treatment with antifungal agents like itraconazole and voriconazole can precipitate underlying subclinical adrenal insufficiency as these medications are steroidogenesis inhibitors [8].

Rifampin, a drug used to treat tuberculosis can also precipitate AI. It increases the metabolism of cortisol by stimulating cytochrome P450 enzyme, thus increasing cortisol requirement.

Case 2

A 65-year-old male with primary adrenal insufficiency and diabetes type 1 is admitted to the hospital for right foot ulcer. He has had low-grade fever of up to 100 °F for 7 days and has low appetite. Examination is unremarkable except for an ulcer in the right first metatarsophalangeal joint. Blood tests indicate WBC 15000, neutrophils 70%, hemoglobin 11, elevated ESR and CRP. MRI of the foot shows osteomyelitis. He has started on iv antibiotics and taken to OR on day 2 for debridement. After coming back from OR in the evening, he has fever of up to 102 °F, HR 95, BP 100/60. He is on iv cefazolin, oral hydrocortisone, fludrocortisone, insulin Levemir, insulin aspart. Patient starts to act confused at 10 pm. Fingerstick glucose check shows blood sugar of 54 mg/dL. He is treated for low sugars with 50% dextrose infusion and improves. Electrolytes at the time show Na 132, K+ 4.5, BUN 20, crt

Table 13.6 Recommendations for use of steroid medications for individuals with HIV on ritonavir- and cobicistat-based antiretroviral therapy

Inhaled/Intranasal	Preferred alternative is beclomethasone/Flunisolide
Injectable	Benefits must outweigh the risks
Topical	Steroid sparing alternatives are recommended If steroids are necessary, avoid prolonged use to large areas of the body
Ocular	Steroid sparing alternatives are recommended If steroids are necessary, avoid prolonged use

1.2. His dose of hydrocortisone is changed to intravenous hydrocortisone 25 mg every 8 h. He does well the next day with no fever. By day 3, he is tapered down to home dose of hydrocortisone.

This case highlights the importance of sick day dosing of steroids in individuals with established adrenocortical hypofunction. It is imperative that one increases the dose of steroids in these individuals to help prevent an adrenal crisis [15, 16]. These sick day rules also apply to individuals with secondary AI secondary to chronic steroid use, for example, for autoimmune diseases like sarcoidosis or post-liver, kidney, and heart transplants. Patients with AI should also be taught about sick day rules so that they can advocate for themselves if needed (Table 13.7).

Since exogenous steroid use is the most common cause of adrenal insufficiency, it is good to know the various factors that affect the HPA axis. The degree of suppression is dependent on dose of steroids, kind of steroid, and duration of treatment. Generally, HPA axis suppression is not significant if glucocorticoids are taken for less than 3 weeks [17], if one has taken morning dose of less than prednisone 5 mg daily or its equivalent for any length of time, if one has taken less than prednisone 10 mg every other day or it's equivalent steroid for any length of time. In contrast, patients who are taking prednisone more than 20 mg daily for more than 3 weeks, and anyone who is taking chronic steroid treatment and looks cushingoid can be assumed to have adrenal insufficiency. Individuals who take prednisone 5–20 mg daily for more than 3 weeks may or may not have AI, and they should undergo an ACTH stimulation test to evaluate their axis. Table 13.8 and 13.9 summarize the individuals in whom perioperative steroids are not needed and indicated, respectively. Also, it is important to stop the prednisone for 48 h before testing as prednisolone can be detected in cortisol assays and can give falsely normal results.

Inhaled glucocorticoids can cause a higher degree of HPA axis suppression in children compared to adults. Topical corticosteroids, particularly group 1 (highest potency) agents can cause HPA axis suppression with 2 g/day daily doses for

Table 13.7 Sick Day rules [17]

1	In case of fever >100.4 °F, double the dose of steroids you are taking and stick with that dose till fever lower than 100 °F
2.	In case of fever >102 °F, triple the dose of steroids you are taking and lower the dose to double if fever between 100 and 102 °F
3	If you have vomiting or diarrhea, double or triple the dose depending on severity. If you are unable to keep the pills down, then use the emergency hydrocortisone injection
4.	Call the doctor if fever more than 3 days, lethargy, vomiting, and unable to keep medicines down and persistent diarrhea
5.	Teeth cleanings, minor dental procedures, EGD, colonoscopy, inguinal hernia repair usually do not need dose changes
6.	For moderate surgical stress that is total joint replacement, cholecystectomy, 50 mg just prior to surgery /anesthesia induction and 25 mg every 8 h for 24 h
7.	For major surgical procedures like open heart surgery, gastric bypass, open abdominal surgery, give 100 mg just prior to surgery/anesthesia induction and 50 mg iv 8 h for 24 h and then taper off to maintenance dose

Table 13.8 No need of perioperative corticosteroids in individuals below

1.	Patients who have been taking corticosteroids less than 3 weeks
2.	Patients who have been taking less than the equivalent of 5 mg of prednisone daily
3.	Patients who are undergoing superficial procedures such as cataract extraction, biopsy, dental surgery

Table 13.9 Supplemental perioperative corticosteroids are indicated in individuals below

1	Patient with primary adrenal insufficiency or secondary adrenal insufficiency due to hypopituitarism
2	Patient with clinical Cushing syndrome due corticosteroid exposure
3	Patients taking 5 mg prednisone or more (or equivalent) for more than 3 weeks during past 3 months
4	Patient taking high-dose inhalation glucocorticoid therapy (beclomethasone 1.5 mg/day, fluticasone more than 8 mg/kg daily

Table adapted from Himes et al. Mayo Clin Proc Dec 2020 [18]

Table 13.10 Potency of steroids in HPA axis suppression

Oral steroids	Dexamethasone>prednisone>hydrocortisone
Inhaled steroids	Fluticasone>beclomethasone = budesonide>ciclesonide
Topical steroids	Highest suppression with group 1 agents 0.05% betamethasone, clobetasol, halobetasol, and 0.1% fluocinonide

2 weeks. There are seven groups of topical steroid agents based on potency (Table 13.10). Also, application on highly permeable surfaces like face genitalia, children, and areas of skin breaks can lead to more absorption. Intra-articular and spinal steroids do get absorbed systemically. Higher frequency of injections can lead to more HPA axis suppression.

It may take 1 year to recover HPA axis for individuals who have used long duration high-dose steroid treatment in the past.

Case 3

A 54-year-old woman with history of psoriatic arthritis is admitted to the hospital after bilateral knee arthroplasty. Her operative course was complicated by popliteal artery occlusion for which she underwent urgent thrombectomy. She is started on heparin drip for thromboprophylaxis on postoperative day (POD) 1.

On POD 8, she developed nausea, abdominal pain, tachycardia, and orthostatic hypotension. Laboratory results show leukocytosis (23,000 cells/μL), thrombocytopenia (93,000 /μL), elevated D-dimer (20,000 ng/mL), and fibrinogen (643 mg/dL) levels. A CT scan, done for evaluation of abdominal pain, revealed bilateral hyperdense and enlarged adrenal glands. Adrenal hemorrhage was suspected and she was treated for adrenal insufficiency. Later, a random cortisol drawn before treatment came back as 1.3 mcg/dL.

Adrenal hemorrhage (AH) was classically described as being associated with sepsis from *Neisseria Meningitidis*, commonly known as Waterhouse-Friderichsen syndrome. It can occur with other infections like CMV, parvovirus B19, and bacterial infections. It has also been described in association with antiphospholipid (APLS) syndrome. There have been case reports and reviews on AH after orthopaedic procedures in the setting of heparin-induced thrombocytopenia (HIT), making it important to identify this life-threatening complication in the perioperative setting [19, 20].

HIT has been reported in up to 5% of patients exposed to heparin for more than 4 days. Risk of HIT depends on [21].

- Type of heparin: Bovine unfractionated heparin (UFH) > Porcine UFH > low-molecular-weight heparin (LMWH).
- Higher dosage and longer duration of exposure to heparin.
- Gender: Females > Males.
- Patient population: Surgical > Medical.

Pathophysiology of HIT

Platelet factor-4 (PF4) is a positively charged protein, stored in the alpha granules of platelets and is released upon platelet activation. This protein has a high affinity to heparin and can neutralize it. Heparin on administration to PF4 leads to a conformational change that exposes antigenic epitopes. This may lead to the formation of antibodies (most frequently IgG antibodies) specific to the heparin-PF4 complex. These antibodies then bind to the Fc y receptor 11A on the platelet surface and lead to platelet activation. Platelet activation causes the release of prothrombotic substances and PF4. As more platelets get activated, more PF4 is released into the circulation leading to more heparin-PF4 complexes causing a vicious cycle that can be broken only with heparin discontinuation and appropriate treatment.

The characteristic feature of HIT is thrombocytopenia which results from consumption due to platelet aggregation, thrombus formation and due to macrophage clearance of the IgG-coated platelets.

HIT diagnosis is based on both clinical and serologic findings. It should be suspected in anyone receiving heparin with a sudden and unexplained decrease in platelet count, usually a decrease of 50% or more from baseline along with moderate thrombocytopenia (50–60 × 10^9cells/L). However, the nadir platelet value can range anywhere between 15 × 10^9 and 150 × 10^9cells/L. While the median time of onset is 5–14 days after heparin exposure, it can occasionally happen within 24 h of exposure (rapid-onset HIT) or can be delayed up to 20 days after heparin discontinuation (delayed-onset HIT).

Initial risk stratification is done using the 4 T scoring system, which stands for thrombocytopenia, timing, thrombosis, and the absence of other etiologies for thrombocytopenia (see Table 13.11). The score for each of these characteristics ranges from 0 to 2. The sum of each component yields the total score which is used to determine the pre-test probability [22].

Table 13.11 4Ts score

Thrombocytopenia	
• Platelet decrease >50% and nadir ≥20,000 and no surgery within preceding 3 days	2 points
• Platelet decrease >50% but surgery within preceding 3 days or any combination of platelet fall and nadir that does not fit criteria for 2 or 0 points	1 point
• Platelet decrease <30% or nadir <10,000	0 points
Timing of onset after heparin exposure	
• 5–10 days or 1 day if exposure within past 5 to 30 days	2 points
• Probable 5–10 days or > 10 days or < 1 day if exposure within past 31 to 100 days	1 point
• ≤4 days without exposure within past 100 days	0 points
Thrombosis	
• Confirmed new thrombosis, skin necrosis, anaphylactoid reaction, or adrenal hemorrhage	2 points
• Suspected, progressive, or recurrent thrombosis, skin erythema	1 point
• None	0 points
Other cause for thrombocytopenia	
• None	2 points
• Possible (sepsis)	1 point
• Probable (DIC, medication, within 72 h of surgery)	0 points
Interpretation: – 0 to 3 points—Low probability (<1%) – 4 to 5 points—Intermediate probability (approximately 10%) – 6 to 8 points—High probability (approximately 50%)	

If there is intermediate to high probability of HIT, heparin should be stopped immediately. If they need anticoagulation. One of the following anticoagulants may be selected: argatroban, bivalirudin, danaparoid, fondaparinux, or a direct oral anticoagulant (DOAC). One should not use warfarin immediately in such situations and depletion of protein C and S during hypercoagulable state can lead to skin necrosis and limb gangrene. Diagnosis of HIT can be confirmed by measuring PF4 heparin antibody levels by immunoassays.

Review Questions

1. You are evaluating a patient for knee replacement. He has been a kidney transplant recipient on prednisone 2.5 mg daily for 5 years. Which of the following statements is true?
   (a) Patient does not have secondary AI as he is on only prednisone 2.5 mg daily.
   (b) Patient has AI as he has been on treatment for 6 years.
   (c) It is hard to know if this patient has AI or not. It is better to do ACTH stimulation test to make the determination prior to surgery.
   (d) Since prednisone cannot be stopped in a transplant patient, it is better to assume that patient has AI and presumptively treat him before surgery.

   Answer (a), patient does not have secondary AI as he is only on prednisone 2.5 mg daily.

2. You see a patient for carpal tunnel syndrome, he has history of long-standing adrenal insufficiency because of pituitary tumor resection. Patient is on hydrocortisone for adrenal hormone replacement. What instructions would you give to the patient for the day of surgery?
   (a) Take your normal dose of hydrocortisone in the morning on the day of surgery.
   (b) Take double dose of hydrocortisone in the morning on the day of surgery.
   (c) Skip your morning hydrocortisone on the day of surgery and I will give you intravenous hydrocortisone 50 mg prior to surgery.
   (d) Take your morning hydrocortisone on the day of surgery and I will give you intravenous hydrocortisone prior to surgery.

   Answer (b). Local anesthesia is a minor stress, one will do well with either no jump in baseline hydrocortisone doses or just double dose morning of surgery.
3. Which of the following HIV medications inhibit CYP3A4 and thus decrease steroid metabolism?
   (a) Zidovudine and stavudine.
   (b) Ritonavir and tenofovir.
   (c) Ritonavir and darunavir.
   (d) Ritonavir and cobicistat.

   Answer (d). Ritonavir and cobicistat.

References

1. Feingold KR, Anawalt B, Blackman MR, et al. Endotext. 2000.
2. Fox J, Bessesen D, Cunningham J. Secondary adrenal insufficiency: an insidious consequence of the opioid epidemic? Postgrad Med J. 2021;97(1149):432–3. https://doi.org/10.1136/postgradmedj-2020-137829.
3. Chen H, Hsieh F-N, Yang C-C. Mucocutaneous hyperpigmentation as a clue to diagnose Addison disease—two case reports. Dermatologica Sinica. 2022;40:48–9.
4. Bhake RC, Kluckner V, Stassen H, et al. Continuous free cortisol profiles-circadian rhythms in healthy men. J Clin Endocrinol Metab. 2019;104(12):5935–47. https://doi.org/10.1210/jc.2019-00449.
5. Sbardella E, Isidori AM, Woods CP, et al. Baseline morning cortisol level as a predictor of pituitary-adrenal reserve: a comparison across three assays. Clin Endocrinol. 2017;86(2):177–84. https://doi.org/10.1111/cen.13232.
6. Bornstein SR, Allolio B, Arlt W, et al. Diagnosis and treatment of primary adrenal insufficiency: an Endocrine Society clinical practice guideline. J Clin Endocrinol Metab. 2016;101(2):364–89. https://doi.org/10.1210/jc.2015-1710.
7. El-Farhan N, Pickett A, Ducroq D, et al. Method-specific serum cortisol responses to the adrenocorticotrophin test: comparison of gas chromatography-mass spectrometry and five automated immunoassays. Clin Endocrinol. 2013;78(5):673–80. https://doi.org/10.1111/cen.12039.
8. Duman AK, Fulco PP. Adrenal insufficiency with Voriconazole and inhaled/intranasal corticosteroids:Case Report and Systematic Review. J Pharm Pract. 2017;30(4):459–63. https://doi.org/10.1177/0897190016646510.

9. Saberi P, Phengrasamy T, Nguyen DP. Inhaled corticosteroid use in HIV-positive individuals taking protease inhibitors: a review of pharmacokinetics, case reports and clinical management. HIV Med. 2013;14(9):519–29. https://doi.org/10.1111/hiv.12039.
10. Boyd SD, Hadigan C, McManus M, et al. Influence of low-dose ritonavir with and without darunavir on the pharmacokinetics and pharmacodynamics of inhaled beclomethasone. J Acquir Immune Defic Syndr. 2013;63(3):355–61. https://doi.org/10.1097/QAI.0b013e31829260d6.
11. Elliot ER, Theodoraki A, Jain LR, et al. Iatrogenic Cushing's syndrome due to drug interaction between glucocorticoids and the ritonavir or cobicistat containing HIV therapies. Clin Med (Lond). 2016;16(5):412–8. https://doi.org/10.7861/clinmedicine.16-5-412.
12. Noe S, Jaeger H, Heldwein S. Adrenal insufficiency due to ritonavir-triamcinolone drug-drug interaction without preceding Cushing's syndrome. Int J STD AIDS. 2018;29(11):1136–9. https://doi.org/10.1177/0956462418768689.
13. Molloy A, Matheson NJ, Meyer PA, Chaterjee K, Gkrania-Klotsas E. Cushing's syndrome and adrenal axis suppression in a patient treated with ritonavir and corticosteroid eye drops. AIDS. 2011;25(10):1337–9. https://doi.org/10.1097/QAD.0b013e328347c09c.
14. Mifsud S, Gauci Z, Gruppetta M, Mallia Azzopardi C, Fava S. Adrenal insufficiency in HIV/AIDS: a review. Expert Rev Endocrinol Metab. 2021;16(6):351–62. https://doi.org/10.1080/17446651.2021.1979393.
15. Wass JA, Arlt W. How to avoid precipitating an acute adrenal crisis. BMJ. 2012;345:e6333. https://doi.org/10.1136/bmj.e6333.
16. Hahner S, Loeffler M, Bleicken B, et al. Epidemiology of adrenal crisis in chronic adrenal insufficiency: the need for new prevention strategies. Eur J Endocrinol. 2010;162(3):597–602. https://doi.org/10.1530/EJE-09-0884.
17. Prete A, Bancos I. Glucocorticoid induced adrenal insufficiency. BMJ. 2021;374:n1380. https://doi.org/10.1136/bmj.n1380.
18. Himes CP, Ganesh R, Wight EC, Simha V, Liebow M. Perioperative evaluation and management of endocrine disorders. Mayo Clin Proc. 2020;95(12):2760–74. https://doi.org/10.1016/j.mayocp.2020.05.004.
19. Chow VW, Abnousi F, Huddleston JI, Lin LH. Heparin-induced thrombocytopenia after total knee arthroplasty, with subsequent adrenal hemorrhage. J Arthroplast. 2012;27(7):1413.e15–8. https://doi.org/10.1016/j.arth.2012.01.012.
20. Olevsky OM, Rosove MH. "spontaneous" heparin-induced thrombocytopenia and thrombosis after Total knee arthroplasty: a report of 2 cases. Arthroplast Today. 2021;9:50–2. https://doi.org/10.1016/j.artd.2021.03.005.
21. Warkentin TE, Sheppard JA, Sigouin CS, Kohlmann T, Eichler P, Greinacher A. Gender imbalance and risk factor interactions in heparin-induced thrombocytopenia. Blood. 2006;108(9):2937–41. https://doi.org/10.1182/blood-2005-11-012450.
22. Cuker A, Arepally GM, Chong BH, et al. American Society of Hematology 2018 guidelines for management of venous thromboembolism: heparin-induced thrombocytopenia. Blood Adv. 2018;2(22):3360–92. https://doi.org/10.1182/bloodadvances.2018024489.

Chapter 14
Allergy in Perioperative and Clinical Setting

Wei Zhao

Case Report

A 70-year-old man was evaluated in an allergy clinic following an allergic reaction that occurred during a bilateral femoral endarterectomy. The medications that he received at induction of anesthesia included thiopental, succinylcholine, vecuronium, fentanyl, and midazolam. Following endotracheal general anesthesia, a cystoscopy was performed to dilate the urethral structure in order to insert a urinary catheter. However, during the procedure, the patient developed widespread urticaria and significant swelling of the face, lips, and mouth. There was a transient decrease in his blood pressure to 80 mmHg systolic with stable cardiopulmonary function. The patient responded to treatment with epinephrine, dexamethasone, and diphenhydramine. Bilateral femoral endarterectomy was successfully completed. Further history revealed previous allergic reactions to multiple surgical procedures in the last 8 years in various hospitals. These included hypotension (systolic pressure of 64 mmHg) during total hip arthroplasty; urticaria and hypotension and drop of blood pressure (systolic pressure at low 60 s) while undergoing left carotid stent placement; hives during cystoscopy. He was previously evaluated by skin testing to lidocaine, bupivacaine, and latex that showed negative results to all of them. Tryptase level was not obtained.

Considering that any of the medications used could be potential cause, he was skin tested for fentanyl (50 μg/ml), thiopental (25 mg/ml), succinylcholine (20 mg/ml), vecuronium (1 mg/ml), and midazolam (5 mg/ml) and these were negative. Intradermal testing of above reagents from concentration of 1:100,000 to 1:100–1:10 (based on available data on non-irritating concentration) was also negative. However,

W. Zhao (✉)
Division of Allergy and Immunology, Department of Pediatrics,
Virginia Commonwealth University, Richmond, VA, USA
e-mail: wei.zhao@vcuhealth.org

W. A. Zuelzer, S. Metikala (eds.), *Unusual Conditions That Every Orthopaedic Surgeon Should Know*, https://doi.org/10.1007/978-3-031-58946-1_14

the patient was positive to skin prick testing using 2% chlorhexidine (wheal 8 mm and flare 30 mm). Based on his reaction to previous surgical procedures and the current episode, the patient was diagnosed with chlorhexidine allergy. Tryptase level obtained 6 h after the reaction was 1.27 ng/ml—within normal range.

Six months later, the patient underwent his arthroplasty with strict chlorhexidine avoidance. He received propofol, succinylcholine, fentanyl, and cefazolin. Povidone-iodine (Betadine) was used as topical antiseptic agent. The patient tolerated the surgery well without the development of any allergic signs or symptoms [1].

Questions

1. A 50-year-old male patient previously had multiple lidocaine injections as local anesthetic for his orthopaedic procedures without a problem. Last week, he received lidocaine from a multidose vial. Ten minutes afterwards, he developed itching and hives on his body. He did not have wheezing or trouble breathing. After receiving Benadryl treatment, hives and itch resolved within 60 min. What is the reaction this patient has?
2. A 62-year-old female patient was undergoing hip replacement surgery. During the induction phase, she received Cefazolin, atropine, propofol, and rocuronium. Patient developed hives all over her body within 5 min after receiving the above medications. No drop in her blood pressure. She was treated with IV Benadryl and methylprednisolone. Hives resolved within 10 min and the surgery was completed successfully. How do you evaluate this patient after surgery for her reaction in the operating room?
3. A 52-year-old male patient presented to his primary care with a tick attached to his back and a surrounding rash. He experienced fever, chills, and myalgia. The tick was removed in the clinic. He was found to have classic bull's eye rash with red center surrounded by a clear ring. He was sent home with a 14-day course of oral doxycycline. Labs for Lyme disease were sent that came back with positive IgM antibodies for Lyme disease. His doxycycline course was extended to 28 days total due to her continuous myalgias, severe fatigue, and generalized weakness. After 8 weeks, the patient consumed pork in a picnic. He developed itching on his face, swelling around his lips and some difficulty breathing. He took some Benadryl. Symptoms subsided in 2 h. He saw an allergist 3 weeks later who ordered blood IgE level to alpha-gal that came back positive. He was diagnosed with alpha-gal syndrome. He is scheduled to have right knee surgery in a month. What precautions should be taken during his surgery?

Background

Various medications and substances are used in the setting of outpatient clinic procedures and operating rooms. Local anesthetics are widely used to block pain in surgical procedures. During perioperative period, multiple drugs and substances are introduced to achieve anesthesia and pain control. Just like any other drug, in sensitive patients, such reagents may induce adverse reactions including allergic reactions that are beyond their pharmacological effects. Prompt recognition and proper treatment are essential in managing such patients and facilitating the completion of procedures or surgeries. This chapter will cover allergic reactions caused by local anesthetics, reagents used during anesthesia/operating room, and emerging reactions in patients with α-gal allergy.

Local Anesthetic Allergy

Local anesthetic agents have been widely used in local and regional anesthesia, in the management of chronic pain, and the treatment of cardiac arrhythmia. Lidocaine is used in ventricular arrhythmias. Carl Koller, a Viennese ophthalmologist, first demonstrated local anesthesia effect of cocaine in 1884 [2]. In 1904, Einhorn first described the use of the first synthetic local anesthetic, procaine (marketed as Novocaine) [3]. Local anesthetics are composed of three components, a lipophilic (aromatic) group, an intermediate chain linkage and a hydrophilic (amine) group as shown in Fig. 14.1 [4]. Local anesthetics reversibly bind to the α-subunit of sodium channels of the nerve membrane resulting in blocking of nerve conduction and controlling pain. Based on chemical structure and molecular configuration, local anesthetics can be classified as ester or amide subfamilies. Esters (Table 14.1) include cocaine, procaine, 2-chloroprocaine, tetracaine, and benzocaine. Amides (Table 14.2) include lidocaine, bupivacaine, levobupivacaine, mepivacaine, etidocaine, prilocaine, ropivacaine, and articaine [5].

Esters are degraded by plasma cholinesterases into a metabolite named p-aminobenzoic acid (PABA). PABA is a known allergen that is also present in cosmetics, lotions, and sunscreen. Amide, on the other hand, is metabolized by the liver with renal excretion and does not form PABA metabolites. This explains why allergic reactions to esters are more common than amides. Methylparaben is used as a preservative in multidose vials of local anesthetics. Methylparaben is metabolized into compounds that are similar to PABA and can cause allergic reactions [6]. Single-dose vials do not contain methylparaben.

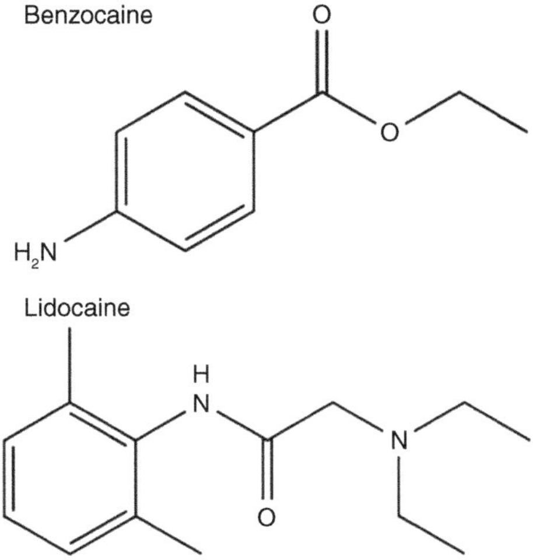

Fig. 14.1 Structure of local anesthetics. Adopted from Thyssen et al. [4]

Table 14.1 Ester local anesthetics

Generic name	Brand name (manufacturer)
Benzocaine	Americane (Fisons), Lanacane (Combe)
Chloroprocaine	Nasacaine (Astra)
Cocaine	Various
Procaine	Novocain (Winthrop)
Propoxycaine	Ravocaine and Novocain (Cook-Waite)
Tetracaine	Pontocaine (Winthrop)

Adopted from Eggleston et al. [2]

Table 14.2 Amide local anesthetics

Generic name	Brand name (manufacturer)
Bupivacaine	Marcaine (Winthrop), Sensorcaine (Astra)
Dibucaine	Nupercainal (Ciba)
Etidocaine	Duranest (Astra)
Lidocaine	Xylocaine (Astra)
Mepivacaine	Carbocaine (Winthrop), Polocaine (Astra)
Prilocaine	Citanest (Astra)

Adopted from Eggleston et al. [2]

Overall, local anesthetics are safe agents. Although about 6 million individuals receive such reagents each day around the world, and adverse reactions are rare [7]. However, they have the potential to cause serious reactions if used without caution. True immunologic reactions to local anesthetics are rare. Many reactions are nonallergic in nature. A survey data from German dental practices of 2731 patients revealed general adverse reaction to local anesthetic to be 4.5% with less than 1% being allergy in nature [8]. This is consistent with the finding from the UK (0.97%) with 75% of cases occurring in patients where more amide agents were used [9].

Toxic reaction: Toxic reactions can occur as a result of overdosing, an inadvertent intravascular injection, in patients with abnormal metabolism of local anesthetics. Local anesthetics can dilate blood vessels, that in turn, enhance their own upload into the central nervous system. Then they can inhibit CNS with diplopia, dizziness, muscle switching, and numbness; in severe cases, tremors and seizures can occur. Toxic concentrations of local anesthetics are associated with bradycardia and decreased cardiac output that may lead to cardiac arrest.

Sympathetic stimulation: Endogenous catecholamines that are released in response to pain may cause tachycardia, hypertension, anxiety, and palpitations. Epinephrine is sometimes added to local anesthetic solutions to reduce local bleeding, prolong local anesthesia, and minimize systemic absorption. In some sensitive patients, epinephrine effect may be observed.

Psychomotor reaction: Psychomotor responses are the most common adverse reaction in patients undergoing dental procedures [10]. It is related to the general anxiety some patients have in anticipating medical procedures. Anxiety can lead to hyperventilation, shortness of breath, and other sympathetic responses such as tachypnea, tachycardia, diaphoresis, and hypertension. Some patients may experience paresthesia of perioral areas and fingers, dizziness, palpitation, and nausea [11].

Vasovagal syncope: Autonomic adverse effects and immediate allergic reactions are difficult to distinguish due to similarity in presentation. Such autonomic-related symptoms include tachycardia, sweating, and syncope in severe cases. They are more often seen in patients who are afraid of injections and in patients with anticipatory problems concerning medical procedures [12]. In contrast to Type 1 immediate allergic reaction, autonomic adverse effects are short-lived with quick resolution of symptoms with minimal supportive treatment.

Although most adverse reactions are nonallergic in nature. Allergic reactions to local anesthetic can occur. Monk first reported the development of contact dermatitis in a dentist repeatedly exposed to apothesin, an ester local anesthetic in 1920 [13]. The development of amide local anesthetics in the 1940s significantly reduced allergic reactions.

Local anesthetics are small molecules that are not big enough to directly trigger host immune responses. Their metabolites may act as hapten that can bind to host protein to trigger allergic reactions. PABA, a metabolite of ester local anesthetics, is a highly antigenic substance [14]. Methylparaben, the preservative agent in both ester and amide local anesthetic preparation, is also known to metabolize PABA to induce allergic reactions. That may explain the cross-reactivity between some ester and amide local anesthetics that contain methylparaben [15].

Two distinct types of allergic reactions to local anesthetics have been described.

Allergic contact dermatitis: This belongs to type 4 hypersensitivity reaction. Typical presentations include popular eczematous, pruritic rash that starts within 72 h at the site of administration. Blisters, vesicles, and weeping may occur as part of the clinical course [16].

Diagnosis is based on the history of receiving local anesthetics, typical rash, and patch testing. Patch testing should be performed by an allergy specialist. Varying concentrations of preservative-free local anesthetic, preservative (methylparaben) are applied to a patient's skin. Patches are removed after 48 h with initial reading. A final reading at 96 h is conducted. Positive responses are scored with 0 = no reaction; 1+ = weak reaction with erythema, infiltration, and possible papules; 2+ = strong reaction with erythema, infiltration, and vesicles; 3+ = extremely severe with blisters formation. Once positive, the agents from the same class should be avoided in the future. If indicated for local anesthetic use, it is recommended to choose an agent from the other chemical group. The commercially available, FDA approved T.R.U.E test panel including caine mix that contains tetracaine hydrochloride, dibucaine hydrochloride, and benzocaine, representing class 1 and 2 local anesthetics. The North American Contact Dermatitis Group LA series includes benzocaine, lidocaine, tetracaine, dibucaine, and prilocaine [17].

Immediate reactions (Urticaria and anaphylaxis): This follows type 1 hypersensitivity reaction. Onset is typically within 1 h after local anesthetic administration. Patients present with pruritus, hives and/or angioedema, sneezing, and running nose. In severe cases, wheezing, shortness of breath, and anaphylaxis can occur.

The mechanism of local anesthetics mediated immediate hypersensitivity reaction has not been fully elucidated. Specific IgE antibodies to local anesthetics have not been identified [18]. Local anesthetics are small molecules with molecular weight of 200–300 DA that are too small to be antigenic. Local anesthetic drugs or their metabolites act as haptens that bind to carrier proteins to form complete antigens. For esters, PABA may be responsible for their hypersensitivity reaction.

Diagnosis is based on detailed history that should include the symptoms and timeline between reaction and local anesthetic administration. Skin test can be conducted to support the diagnosis. Epicutaneous (Prick testing) test is performed with undiluted local anesthetic solution with the application of positive (histamine) and negative (normal saline) controls. Results are read in 15 min. A positive test is considered as wheal size 3 mm larger than negative control. If prick testing is negative, intradermal testing is performed with 1:100 dilution of the medication [19]. However, it carries a relatively high false positive rate between 8% and 15% [20]. Negative skin test may not absolutely exclude IgE-mediated allergic reaction because the allergenic determinants or hapten-carrier complex that are responsible for IgE-mediated allergic reaction to local anesthetics have not been identified. In patients with convincing positive history and negative skin test, challenges can be performed to aid the diagnosis. A three-step incremental subcutaneous challenge was proposed [21] with 0.1 ml, 0.5 ml, and 1 ml of local anesthetic agents in the presence of normal saline control. Challenge is considered positive if patient develops a reaction within 20 min. Of note, such a challenge should be performed ideally in a hospital setting with ready access to emergency management. After completion of the testing, the communication to referring provider should include which local anesthetic drugs were tolerated, at what dose, and whether preservatives were included in the testing formulations.

The mainstay of management of patients with hypersensitivity to local anesthetic is to avoid the culprit agent and choose alternatives for future procedures. For patients with no efficacious or safe alternatives, desensitization may be performed [22].

Perioperative Hypersensitivity (POH) Reactions

In the perioperative setting, patients are introduced to multiple foreign substances such as anesthetics, analgesics, antibiotics, antiseptics, blood products, heparin, and volume expanders. Perioperative hypersensitivity (POH) reactions represent unexpected critical events that occur during a surgical procedure. Such reactions can be allergic or nonallergic in nature. Severity of POH can range from mild skin reaction to anaphylaxis with the possibility of fatality in rare cases. The term hypersensitivity is used to cover all unexpected, but reproducible reactions that are beyond the primary pharmacological actions after exposure to a substance that is tolerated by the general population. Allergic and nonallergic hypersensitivity refer to immune or non-immune underlying mechanisms, respectively. The term anaphylaxis indicates all rapidly developing, life-threatening, generalized, or systemic reactions. IgE-mediated anaphylaxis refers to anaphylactic reaction that is mediated by cross-linking of allergen-specific IgE bound FcεRI on the surface of mast cells and basophils. The terms anaphylactoid and pseudo-allergic should be abandoned as non-specific (IgE-FcεRI independent) hypersensitivity mechanisms such as direct mast cell activation through MRGPRX2 have been identified [23].

Epidemiology: POH has incidence between 1:353 and 1:18,600 procedures [24]. Although most reactions are mild, life-threatening conditions such as anaphylaxis can happen in the context of surgery. The incidence of anaphylaxis is estimated from 1 in 3500 to 1 in 20,000 surgeries [25]. The mortality of POH varies between 1.4% and 4.8% [26]. Multiple medications often are used during general anesthesia that makes as a challenge to identify the culprit agent. Therefore, it often requires close collaboration between allergists and anesthesiologists in managing such patients. Detailed analysis of anesthetic records including clinical manifestations and their association with administration of each drug during the procedure.

Pathogenesis: Perioperative hypersensitivity is mediated by drug-specific IgE in ~60% of cases [1]. The incidence of IgE-mediated reactions during anesthesia is estimated between 1:500 and 1:13,000 [27]. Neuromuscular blocking agents (NMBAs) with quaternary substituted ammonium structures can bind to specific IgE antibodies. In addition to IgE-mediated mechanism, research has demonstrated the ability of allergen-specific cross-linking of IgG/FcγR complexes to activate and induce degranulation of mast cells [28]. However, IgG-mediated anaphylaxis is only demonstrated in animal models and in vitro studies with platelet activation factor (PAF) as mediator that is produced by neutrophils and no IgG-mediated POH has been published. Mast cells and basophils can also be activated by complement through the binding of C3a and C5a to their specific G-protein-coupled receptors (C3aR and C5aR) [29]. Therefore, complement activation may also be involved in POH. In addition to IgE and IgG receptors, mast cells and basophils also express Mas-related G-protein-coupled receptor X2 (MRGPRX2). Off-target occupancy of MRGPRX2 receptor by drugs such as certain antibiotics (fluoroquinolones and vancomycin), opiates/opioids, and some NMBAs [30, 31]. Rocuronium has greater affinity for MRGPRX2 receptors that might explain its higher reaction rate. Animal studies and in vitro models also demonstrated mivacurium and cis-atracurium can directly activate MRGPRX2 in a dose-dependent fashion [32, 33].

Upon activation, mast cells and basophils can release mediators including preformed histamine, and tryptase that can be released immediately, newly synthesized lipids (prostaglandin, leukotrienes, and platelet-activating factor, or PAF) that are released over minutes, and newly de novo synthesized cytokines and chemokines that are released over hours. Histamine, leukotrienes, and PAF can cause vasodilation, capillary leak, and bronchospasm. IgE-mediated mast cell activation that leads to exocytosis of high inflammatory mediators often present with "delayed" but sustained clinical manifestation. In contrast, reactions through MRGPRX2 pathway often lead to rapid but transient release of low content of inflammatory mediators with the "kiss and run" mechanism as described [33].

Clinical presentations: Clinic manifestations vary from mild skin rash to cardiovascular collapse. Skin symptoms include erythema, urticaria, and angioedema that are frequent but less recognized because patients under anesthesia are often covered, sedated, and unable to report pruritus. For the same reason, warning signs such as hoarseness, dysphagia, dizziness, and blurring vision are not recognizable in sedated patients. Perioperative anaphylaxis often presents with flushing, hives and/or angioedema, GI manifestations such as nausea, vomiting, diarrhea, and respiratory manifestations such as cough, wheezing, tachycardia, and hypotension [34].

Currently, severity-based grading system of POH is adopted from Ring and Messmer [35] as shown in Table 14.3. Grade I, cutaneous signs/symptoms only and grade II, non-severe multi-organ involvement (cutaneous signs, bronchial hyperreactivity, tachycardia, hypotension) are not life-threatening and generally not IgE-mediated, i.e., non-specific activation of mast cells and basophils. Grade III, life-threatening multi-organ involvement (cardiovascular collapse, bronchospasm, cardiac arrhythmias) and grade IV, cardiorespiratory arrest are life-threatening and more likely to be IgE-mediated [36]. The main feature of a Grade III reaction is sudden onset hypotension, often associated with tachycardia. However, some patients may present with bradycardia due to hypovolemia secondary to capillary leakage [37]. Bronchospasm is more common in patients with preexisting conditions such as asthma, COPD, and obesity [38]. Grade IV reaction presents cardiac arrest with pulseless electrical activity, often without initial cutaneous signs. Skin symptoms may present once adequate perfusion is restored.

Evaluation: The timing between administration of suspected reagents and the onset of clinical symptoms and signs may provide a clue. Symptoms occurring within 30 min of anesthesia should prompt the suspicion of NMBAs, antibiotics, and hypnotics as potential culprits. When symptoms begin after 30 min of anesthesia, chlorhexidine, latex, plasma expanders, blood products, and IgE-mediated anaphylaxis need to be considered. Early recognition of anaphylaxis is the key to management. Signs of bronchospasm and hypotension should lead to the consideration of anaphylaxis unless there is another clear cause that can explain the symptoms.

Recently, a panel of 25 international multidisciplinary experts developed a scoring system for estimating the likelihood of perioperative immediate hypersensitivity reactions [39]. The likelihood of Immediate Hypersensitivity Reaction (IHR) categories is shown in Table 14.4. Such a scoring system incorporates the severity sign/symptoms of cardiovascular, respiratory, and dermal/mucosal with the timing of onset, as shown in Table 14.5.

Table 14.3 POH grading system

Grade I: Skin or mucosal signs only • Generalized erythema. • Extensive urticaria. • With or without angioedema.
Grade II: Moderate signs from several organ systems • Skin or mucosal signs. • ±hypotension ± tachycardia • ±bronchospasm • ±gastrointestinal signs.
Grade III: Life-threatening signs from one or more organ systems • Cardiovascular collapse (life-threatening hypotension). • Tachycardia or bradycardia ± cardiac dysrhythmia. • ±bronchospasm • ±skin or mucosal signs • ±gastrointestinal signs.
Grade IV: Circulatory and/or respiratory arrest

Adapted from Ring and Messmer [35]

Table 14.4 Likelihood of immediate hypersensitivity reaction (IHR) based on POH scoring system, adapted from Hopkins et al. [39]

Interpretation	Total (net) score
Almost certain to be an IHR	>21
Very likely to be an IHR	15–21
Likely to be an IHR	11–14
Possible IHR	8–10
Unlikely to be an IHR	<8

Table 14.5 POH scoring system, adapted from Hopkins et al. [39]

	Points
1. Cardiovascular (choose hypotension, severe hypotension, or cardiac arrest if appropriate, then any other items that apply)	
Hypotension	4
Severe hypotension	6
Cardiac arrest	9
Tachycardia	2
A poor or unsustained response of hypotension to standard doses of sympathomimertics used treat pharmacological hypotension during anesthesia (e.g. ephedrine, phenylephrine, metaraminol)	2
A point-of-care echocardiogram showing a hyperdynamic and poorlyfilled heart	2
Recurrence or worsening of hypotension after a further dose of a drug given before the initial event	1
Cardiovascular confounders (in the presence of hypotension or cardiac arrest choose any that apply)	
Excessive dose of anesthetic drug or drugs	−2
Surgically induced hypovolaemia or relative hypovolaemia from prolonged fasting/dehydration	−1
Acute illness predisposing to hypotension	−1
Medications affecting cardiovascular responses during anesthesia	−2
Neuraxial regional anesthesia (epidural/spinal)	−1
Onset of hypotension after development of increased peak airway pressure during mechanical ventilation of the lungs	−2
2. Respiratory (choose bronchospasm or severe bronchospasm if appropriate, then any other items that apply)	
Bronchospasm	2
Severe bronchospasm	4
Recurrence or worsening of bronchospasm after a further dose of a drug given before the initial event	1
Bronchospasm occurring before airway instrumentation (having excluded airway obstruction)	2
Respiratory confounders (in the presence of bronchospasm choose any that apply)	
Respiratory disease associated with reactive airways	−1
Prolonged or multiple attempts at tracheal intubation	−1
Inadequate dose of drugs to obtund airway responses before airway instrumentation	−1

(continued)

Table 14.5 (continued)

	Points
3. Dermal/mucosal (choose any items that apply)	
A generalized rash is itchy in the awake patient who has not received epidural/spinal opioids	1
Angioedema	3
Generalized erythema	3
Generalized urticaria	4
Dermal/mucosal confounder	
Angioedema in a patient taking an ACE inhibitor	−3
4. Combinations (choose a maximum of one item)	
CVS >2 and RS >2	5
CVS >2 and D/M >2	5
RS >2 and D/M >2	5
CVS >2 and RS >2 and D/M >2	8
5. Timings (choose a maximum of one item)	
Onset of cardiovascular or respiratory features within 5 min of possible IV trigger	7
Onset of cardiovascular or respiratory features within 15 min of possible IV trigger	3
Onset of cardiovascular or respiratory features within 60 min of possible non-IV trigger	2
Onset of cardiovascular or respiratory features more than 60 min after possible non-IV trigger	−1

Differential diagnosis: Several conditions may present similar manifestations as POH. Table 14.6 lists differential diagnosis of POH. However, they usually involve a single organ/system without the elevation of tryptase.

Identifying causal agents: Patients with perioperative anaphylaxis should be referred to an allergist to identify the drug that led to the reaction. Specific investigation should be conducted 4–6 weeks after the reaction to avoid false negative due to depletion of mast cell mediators during anaphylaxis [41].

Neuromuscular blocking agents (NMBAs): NMBAs can be classified into two forms: depolarizing form (e.g., Succinylcholine) and nondepolarizing form. Nondepolarizing agents can be divided into two categories. Aminosteroids group includes rocuronium, vecuronium, pipercuronium, and pancuronium. Benzylisoquinoliniums group includes atracurium, cis-atracurium, and mivacurium. Figure 14.2 shows the chemical structure of typical NMBAs. NMBAs are the most common cause of POH [42]. Overall incidence of NMBAS reaction is low. However, NMBAs are the most common cause of perioperative anaphylaxis that account for 50–70% of perioperative anaphylaxis [43]. Among them, Succinylcholine and rocuronium are relatively more common than other NMBAs. Reddy and colleagues reported more than ten-fold anaphylactic risk of patients exposed to rocuronium and succinylcholine than atracurium (1 in 2499 for rocuronium, 1 in 2080 for succinylcholine, 1 in 22,451 for atracurium) [44]. Cross-sensitivity among NMBAs is often

Table 14.6 Differential diagnoses of perioperative hypersensitivity reactions

Isolated hypotension without tryptase increase • Relative overdose of anesthetic agents. • Vasodilatory effect of neuraxial blockade. • Bone cement implantation syndrome. • Amniotic fluid embolism. • Pulmonary embolism. • Treatments with tricyclic antidepressants. • Uncontrolled bleeding. • Other types of shock.
Isolated bronchospasm without tryptase increase • Undiagnosed and/or uncontrolled asthma/COPD. • Airway hyperreactivity (predisposing factors such as asthma, smoking or viral infection). • Inadequate depth of anesthesia. • Endotracheal tube malposition. • Aspiration.
Isolated angioedema or pharyngeal/laryngeal angioedema without tryptase increase • Soft tissue swelling/edema due to manipulation of the airway during laryngeal mask insertion or handling of difficult intubation. • ACE inhibitor-elicited angioedema (onset 1–8 h after surgery). • Inherited or acquired angioedema.
Isolated skin symptoms or combined skin symptoms, hypotension and tachycardia without tryptase increase • Nonspecific histamine release. • Exacerbation of existing chronic urticaria/angioedema. • Relative overdose of oxytocin. • Mesenteric traction syndrome.
Others • Clonal or nonclonal mast cell disorders.

Adapted from Garvey et al. [40]

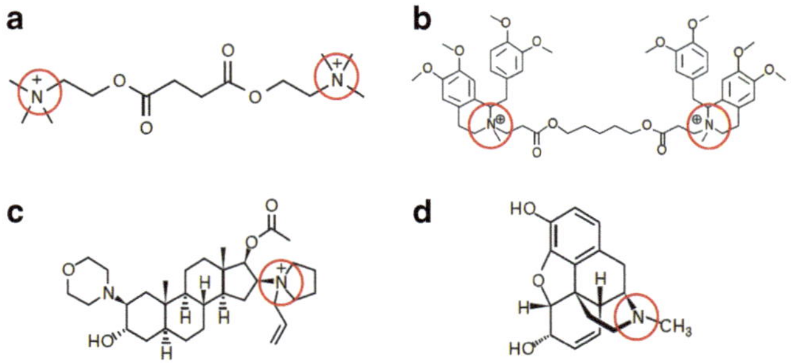

Fig. 14.2 Chemical structures of common neuromuscular blocking agents comparing to morphine. (**a**) Succinylcholine; (**b**) Atracurium; (**c**) Recuronium; (**d**) Morphine. Quaternary ammonium compounds are circled in red. Adopted from Dejoux et al. [51]

reported within the same category (36–70%) [43, 45]. However, interclass cross-reactivity is low. Sadleir et al. reported 5% cross-reactivity between aminosteroids and benzylisoquinoliniums [43]. NMBAs can activate mast cells through IgE-dependent mechanism or by direct mast cell activation through MRGPRX2 receptors. It is estimated that the incidence of IgE-mediated reaction is 184 per million anesthetics [46]. Although not used in the USA, pholcodine, often as component of antitussive agent, is thought to explain the fact that some patients can react on first exposure to NMBAs due to cross-hypersensitivity [47]. Studies have shown that the tertiary and quaternary substituted ammonium as major epitope for IgE-mediated reaction [48]. Some over-the-counter drugs, food products, cosmetics, or disinfectants also contain tertiary substituted or quaternary substituted ammonium group that may be an alternative explanation of reaction to NMBAs without previous exposure. This may also help explain the three-fold higher risk in females than males [49].

Skin tests are used to investigate NMBA anaphylaxis. Serum IgE to quaternary ammonium ions can be performed. Drug-specific IgE is limited to suxamethonium with relatively poor sensitivity [50].

Latex: Natural rubber latex (NRL) from *Hevea brasiliensis* has been used in medical devices and procedures since mid-nineteenth century when Goodyear and Hayward discovered the vulcanization process. Stern and Grimm reported the first case of allergy to NRL in 1927 while Turjanmaa and colleagues described the first case of perioperative anaphylaxis due to NRL in 1989 [52]. In 1990, Moneret-Vautrin reported increased risk of allergy to latex in patients with spina bifida due to IgE-mediated reaction [53]. Latex allergy incidence increased rapidly from 1980s to reach peak in the 1990s, probably due to the increased use of latex gloves. High-risk populations include children with spina bifida, patients with history of multiple surgeries, and healthcare (including dental) workers [54]. Latex is generally considered to induce IgE-mediated allergic reaction in sensitive patients with primary cutaneous exposure through gloves, tourniquets, and bandages. Patients may present with urticaria and angioedema. Severe allergic reactions can be induced by latex contacting mucosal and/or endothelial surfaces via invasive procedures. Airborne exposure such as inhalation of latex powder during anesthesia may trigger bronchospasm. Latex was previously the leading cause of POH. Studies done on patients between 1997 and 2004 showed incidence of NRL-related perioperative IgE-mediated reaction to be 59.1 reactions per 1 million anesthetics [46]. However, over the last couple of decades, identification of high-risk patients, and reduction in powdered glove use in the OR have markedly decreased the incidence of latex allergy as POH. Habre and colleagues reported one in 31,000 pediatric anesthetic procedures in Europe from patients between 2014 and 2015 [55]. The diagnosis of latex hypersensitivity is based on positive history and positive skin test and/or measurement of specific IgE [56].

Antibiotics: Antibiotics are often used for perioperative prophylaxis and are the leading cause of POH in countries like the UK and the United States [42]. β-lactams such as Amoxicillin and Cefazolin are the most common antibiotics that induce POH. Skin test to Penicillin is more standardized than other types of antibiotics. Non-specific binding of IgE antibodies in solid phase assay to β-lactams has been reported due to the effect of elevated total IgE titers or specific IgE to phenylethylamine. Therefore, specific IgE antibodies to β-lactams have very limited utility in diagnosing or excluding immediate hypersensitivity reactions to such antibiotics [57]. Details regarding the presentation and workup on antibiotics, specifically β-lactams, are discussed in Chap. 16 of this book.

Disinfectants: In many countries, Chlorhexidine (CHX) is the most common disinfectant used in operating rooms. Chlorhexidine is used in surgical settings for skin preparation to clean the skin before insertion of central venous lines, arterial lines, and epidural catheters. Urinary catheters are often passed using chlorhexidine gel. Okano et al. reported the first case of chlorhexidine-induced anaphylaxis in 1989 [58]. Since then, numerous cases have been reported in surgical settings. The incidence of CHX caused POH is about 9% in the UK and other European countries [59, 60]. Such an increase is due to the increased use of chlorhexidine in medical products and its disinfectant use in surgical procedures [61]. In addition, chlorhexidine is found in non-medical environments such as mouthwashes, antiseptic creams, toothpaste, and plasters. Initial presentation of chlorhexidine reaction may be mild such as itch and urticaria. Chlorhexidine skin test and *in vitro*-specific IgE test are available in supporting the diagnosis of suspected patients [60]. However, more severe reactions following additional exposure can happen [62]. Povidone-iodine-mediated reaction is extremely rare as only a few cases of anaphylaxis have been reported [63]. Such cases are usually due to the topical application of povidone-iodine to skin or mucosa [64]. Of note, povidone-iodine can be safely used in shellfish allergic patients. The main allergic component of shellfish is tropomyosin [36].

Anesthetic agents: Propofol contains two isopropyl groups that are considered as antigenic epitopes to induce allergic reactions. It contains 10% soybean oil, 2.25% glycerol, and 1.2% egg lecithin. Propofol has been associated with anaphylactic reactions in surgical setting. Of note, the lecithin found in propofol is a highly purified egg yolk protein, not a common egg-allergy epitope as most egg allergic patients have IgE specific to egg white. The soybean oil in propofol formulation is highly refined and is unlikely antigenic. Therefore, there is no solid evidence to support the relationship between egg and soy allergy and increased risk of anaphylaxis to propofol. It was suggested that propofol is safe to use in patients with peanut, soy, or egg allergy [65]. Reactions to ketamine and etomidate are extremely rare. Therefore, it is considered safe to use them in perioperative settings. Currently, there are no reports of allergy to inhaled volatile anesthetics [66].

Opioids: Opioids include three categories: naturally occurring opiate alkaloids such as morphine and codeine; semisynthetic opioids such as pholcodine, hydrocodone, hydromorphone, and diamorphine; synthetic compounds that are chemically not related to opiates such as methadone, pethidine, fentanyl, and tramadol. There has been no evidence of IgE-mediated reaction to opioids [67, 68] despite positive skin testing of patients to opioids. That is because opioids can trigger non-IgE-mediated reaction due to direct mast cell activation through off-target occupation of the MRGPRX2 receptor rather than from binding with opioid μ-receptor [67]. Cross-reactivity between morphine and codeine has been reported. However, there is no evidence of cross-reactivity among different opioid subclasses [50, 69]. The incidence of reaction to opioids is 1:100,000 to 1:200,000 procedures.

Dyes: There have been increasingly recognized reactions to dyes in the perioperative settings. Harper and colleagues reported patent blue dye as the fourth most common reagent in perioperative anaphylaxis behind antibiotics, neuromuscular blockers, and chlorhexidine [59]. Patent blue V and isosulfan blue are the most used dyes with high cross-reactivity due to structural similarity. They are used in identifying lymph nodes in melanoma and breast cancer [70]. Methylene blue, structurally different from patent blue and isosulfan blue, is also used in surgical settings.

Colloids: Colloids such as albumin, dextran, hetastarch, and gelatin are commonly used in the operating room. Gelatins and dextrans are more likely to cause allergic reactions than others [71]. Evaluation of gelatin allergy includes demonstrating specific IgE antibody and positive skin test [72].

Investigation: Investigation is aimed at identifying a culprit drug and safe alternative, therefore ensuring the safety of future anesthesia. Medications patients receive prior to the onset of reaction need to be thoroughly documented. Documentation should include anesthetic records, medication charts, anesthetist's notes, and details of perioperative exposures such as disinfectants, local anesthetics, dyes, cements, and procedure details. Usually, it is much less productive to plan investigations based on a referral letter from surgical team. Although multiple drugs are administered during perioperative duration, focus should be centered on meds that are given immediately prior to the onset of reaction. Some centers limit the drugs that are given 1 h IV and 2 h orally before the reaction [60, 73]. Certainly, drugs that are safely administered after the event are not considered culprits. All drugs of suspicion should be tested as in some patients as more than one drug can be the culprit. It is generally recommended that testing takes place 1–4 months post-event, ideally with 4–6 weeks after the event to avoid false negatives [74].

Diagnostic Testing

Skin test: Skin test is the cornerstone in evaluating patients with perioperative hypersensitivity. It is generally recommended that testing takes place 4–6 weeks after the event to avoid false negatives. However, patients should ideally be evaluated within 1–2 months after POH to increase the chance of detecting causative reagent as previous data suggested a decline of drug-specific IgE antibody over time [75]. Epicutaneous (skin prick) test and intradermal skin test are used in POH investigation. Skin prick test should be performed first on forearm with proper negative and positive controls. A wheal size ≥3 mm is considered positive. When skin prick test is negative, intradermal skin test is performed. A 0.02 ml volume of testing reagent is injected to achieve a bleb of 3–5 mm. Again, wheal size ≥3 mm increase compared to the original bleb is considered positive. Recommended non-irritant concentrations of common perioperative drugs are listed in Table 14.7. Skin test negative reagent is generally safe to be used in future procedures of a patient with history of reaction to another NMBA. However, a break through reaction has been reported in 4–7.5% of patients. Based on such residual risk, some authors suggest repeating intradermal testing prior to future procedures [76].

IgE Testing: Skin test is often considered the primary diagnostic test in the evaluation of POH reactions. However, for many compounds, skin tests have not been thoroughly validated with less ideal predictive values. In addition, skin tests cannot distinguish IgE-mediated reaction from off-target occupation of the MRGPRX2 receptor caused reaction. *In vitro* tests, therefore, can help facilitate the diagnosis of POH. Serum-specific IgE testing is available for succinylcholine, rocuronium, and atracurium with a sensitivity of 40–90% and a specificity of 85%. Such testing is not

Table 14.7 Recommended concentrations of perioperative drugs

Drug	Maximum nonirritative concentration skin prick test	Maximum nonirritative concentration Intradermal test	Drug	Maximum nonirritative concentration skin prick test	Maximum nonirritative concentration Intradermal test
Neuromuscular blocking agents			*IV anesthetic agents*		
Atracurium	SPT 1 mg/ml	IDT 0.01 mg/ml	Propofol	SPT 10 mg/ml	IDT 1 mg/ml
Cisatracurium	SPT 2 mg/ml	IDT 0.02 mg/ml	Etomidate	SPT 2 mg/ml	IDT 0.2 mg/ml
Mivacurium	SPT 0.2 mg/ml	IDT 0.002 mg/ml	Ketamine	SPT 100 mg/ml	IDT 0.1 mg/ml
Rocuronium	SPT 10 mg/ml	IDT 0.05 mg/ml	S-ketamine	SPT 25 mg/ml	IDT 0.25 mg/ml
Vecuronium	SPT 4 mg/ml	IDT 0.04 mg/ml	Thiopental	SPT 25 mg/ml	IDT 2.5 mg/ml
Pancuronium	SPT 2 mg/ml	IDT 0.02 mg/ml	Midazolam	SPT 5 mg/ml	IDT 0.05 mg/ml
Suxamethonium	SPT 10 mg/ml	IDT 0.1 mg/ml			
Reversal agents			*Local anesthetics*		
Sugammadex	SPT 100 mg/ml	IDT 10 mg/ml	Lidocaine	SPT 10 mg/ml	IDT 1 mg/ml
Opiates			Articaine	SPT 20 mg/ml	IDT 2 mg/ml
Fentanyl	SPT 0.05 mg/ml	IDT 0.005 mg/ml	Prilocaine	SPT 20 mg/ml	IDT 2 mg/ml
Alfentanil	SPT 0.5 mg/ml	IDT 0.05 mg/ml	Bupivacaine	SPT 2.5 mg/ml	IDT 0.25 mg/ml
Sufentanil	SPT 0.005 mg/ml	IDT 0.0005 mg/ml	Levobupivacaine	SPT 7.5 mg/ml	IDT 0.75 mg/ml
Remifentanil	SPT 0.05 mg/ml	IDT 0.005 mg/ml	Mepivacaine	SPT 20 mg/ml	IDT 2 mg/ml
Morphine	SPT 1 mg/ml	IDT 0.005 mg/ml	Ropivacaine	SPT 10 mg/ml	IDT 1 mg/ml
Antiseptics			*Ester derivative*		
Providone iodine	SPT 100 mg/ml	No IDT	Chloroprocaine	SPT 10 mg/ml	IDT 1 mg/ml
Chlorhexidine	SPT 5 mg/ml	IDT 0.002 mg/ml			

Table 14.7 (continued)

Drug	Maximum nonirritative concentration skin prick test	Maximum nonirritative concentration Intradermal test	Drug	Maximum nonirritative concentration skin prick test	Maximum nonirritative concentration Intradermal test
Plasma expanders			*Additives*		
Dextran	No skin test, IgG mediated mechanism		PEG/macrogol 300 3000 6000	SPT undiluted SPT 50% w/v SPT 50% w/v	High risk of systemic reactions on IDT
Hydroxyethyl starch	SPT 60 mg/ml	IDT 6 mg/ml	Polysorbate 80 Poloxamer 407	SPT 20% w/v SPT 10% w/v	
Sentinel node dyes			Carboxymethl cellulose	SPT 1% w/v	
Methylene blue	SPT 10 mg/ml	IDT 0.1 mg/ml			
Patent blue	SPT 25 mg/ml	IDT 0.25 mg/ml			

Adapted from Garvey et al. [40]

reliable to detect benzylisoquinolines-mediated reaction, indicating non-IgE-mediated mast cell activation [77].

Serum tryptase: Immediate hypersensitivity reactions, such as POH, are mediated by activation of mast cells and basophils, resulting in the release of inflammatory mediators [25]. Demonstrating the presence of such inflammatory mediators in circulation is the biochemical basis to support the diagnosis of POH. Diagnosis of anaphylaxis is based on history and clinical presentations. Serum tryptase levels can be used to support the diagnosis. With a half-life of 2 h, blood samples should be collected 1–4 h after the onset of reaction. Since basophils only contribute <1% of the serum tryptase levels compared to mast cells, an increase in serum tryptase concentration is considered an indication of mast cell activation [78]. If possible, a baseline level should also be obtained around 2 days after resolution of symptoms. An increase of serum tryptase of 2 + 1.2x baseline level is suggestive of mast cell activation [79]. This formula has been validated for POH with sensitivity, specificity, positive predictive value, and negative predictive value of 78%, 91%, 98%, and 44%, respectively [80]. A French study demonstrated 75% sensitivity for perioperative anaphylaxis using the above tryptase cutoff, as compared with 53% sensitivity using an acute tryptase level >11.4 ng/ml. Other measures that are used in mast cell activation syndrome, but not studied in perioperative hypersensitivity include urine n-methyl histamine, 2,3 β-prostaglandin F2a, leukotriene E4.

Basophil activation test (BAT): Although the foundation of the current flow cytometry-based basophil activation test was laid 25 years ago, the technique has recently received greater attention that was transitioned from research based to commercially available testing [81]. Typical basophil activation tests are based on the detecting of degranulation markers (CD203c, CD63) on basophil surface by flow cytometry analysis [82]. BAT is used to evaluate patients where skin tests are not practical. It has comparable sensitivity (50–90%) and specificity (90%) as skin test [83]. Since basophils do not express MRGPPRX2, BAT cannot be used to detect such receptor-mediated mechanisms.

Drug provocation testing: Recently, some centers introduced the concept of low-dose provocation tests to NMBAs as part of the clinical evaluation of patients with history of reaction to NMBAs but negative skin test [84]. Typically, a 3–4 step approach with 10% therapeutic dose is used. It should be performed in highly specialized centers with full monitoring and resuscitation facilities [66]. Small studies done in Danish conclude that provocation with low-dose NMBA is safe with only a few side effects. However, it requires further validation with large cohorts.

Diagnostic algorithm for POH has been developed by Ebo et al. [83] as seen in Fig. 14.3.

Treatment

The first step in the treatment of POH is to withdraw the drug that is likely the cause of reaction. Once POH is suspected, treatment should start immediately. For mild non-anaphylaxis reactions with only skin involvement, patients can be managed with antihistamines such as IV diphenhydramine.

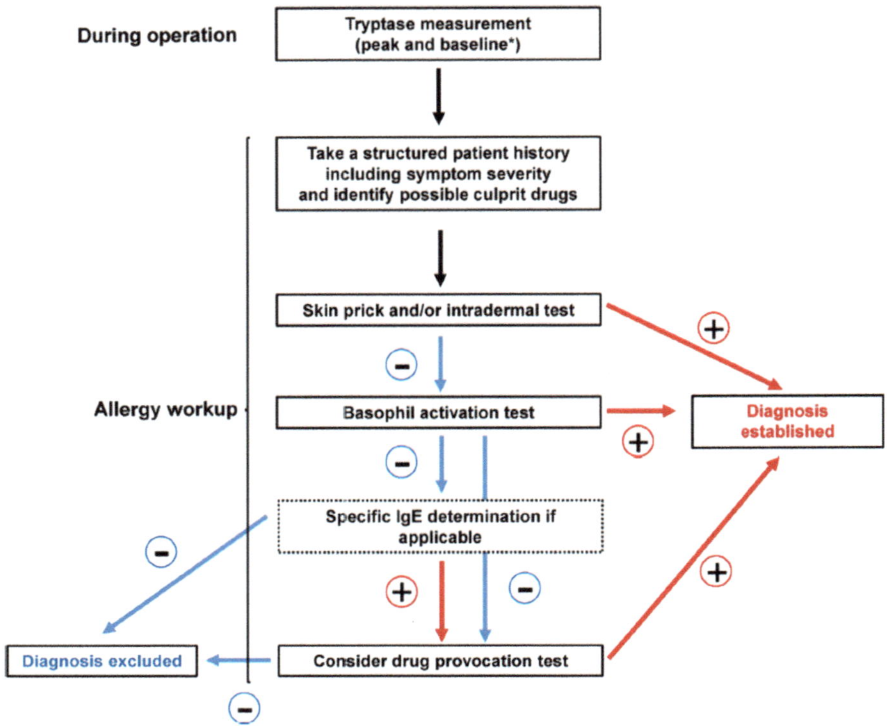

Fig. 14.3 Diagnostic algorithm of perioperative hypersensitivity. Adapted from Ebo et al. [83]

Treatment of ≥grade II perioperative anaphylaxis include early epinephrine administration, volume expansion, and securing the airway. The recommended epinephrine dose for grade II anaphylaxis is 10–20 μg and 50–100 μg for more life-threatening reactions [85]. It is also essential to assess the airway, breathing, and circulation (ABC). Any anesthetic agents that can cause vasodilation should also be decreased in dosage or discontinued. Airway support such as 100% oxygen should be started as well as intravenous volume replacement. β2-adrenergic agonists such as albuterol can be used in treating bronchospasm. European guidelines suggest the use of corticosteroids. NAP6 reports no evidence of harm from steroid use. However, no studies proved its benefit [86]. In refractory anaphylaxis cases, epinephrine doses can be doubled followed by epinephrine drip to maintain blood pressure. i.v. glucagon at 1–2 mg may be given to patients who are taking beta-adrenergic receptor blockers. Alternative vasopressors such as vasopressin, norepinephrine, metaraminol, or phenylephrine are also considered in refractory cases [86].

Once the patient is treated and stabilized, a decision needs to be made whether to continue or abort the procedure. This will depend on the type of surgery (elective vs emergency), the indication (trauma vs cosmetic surgery), and the grade of POH. For Grade I-III cases, outcomes were similar whether abort or continue surgery.

However, it is generally agreed that surgery should be abandoned for Grade IV patients due to the high rate of complications [87].

Prevention

For patients who had a history of previous perioperative reaction, a comprehensive review of previous perioperative history is essential. A referral to allergy evaluation is necessary to help identify the culprit drug or substance. Careful review of anesthesia records including exact timeline of medications, substances, and symptom development should be performed. Proper skin test and/or specific IgE test to all medications, and substances should be administered. If positive to NMBA, skin tests to other NMBAs should be conducted to aid future use. Once identified, such reagent(s) should be clearly documented in the patient's allergy section of medical record and avoided during future surgical procedures.

Perioperative Alpha-Gal Allergies

A newly emerged allergy named "Alpha Gal Syndrome" (AGS) was discovered in 2007. This allergy was first described in oncologic patients receiving monoclonal antibody, cetuximab to treat solid tumors [88]. Some of those patients developed anaphylaxis following cetuximab. Further studies revealed IgE antibody-mediated reaction to cetuximab is specific to galactose-α-1,3 galactose oligosaccharide (α-Gal) [89]. Based on this concept, patients who ingested mammalian products (red meat) containing α-Gal displayed IgE-mediated anaphylaxis due to AGS [90]. Further research discovered that such patients can be sensitized through tick bites. The primary tick that triggers the initial sensitization is the Lone Star tick (*Amblyomma americanum*) [91].

There have been emerging literature describing the association of AGS with perioperative exposure to α-Gal containing substances in surgical settings. This includes inactive ingredients in medications and implants such as gelatin, monoclonal antibodies, heparin, bovine extracts, animal-derived glycerol and -valves and/or implants. Table 14.8 lists some inactive ingredients and common examples of medicines used in perioperative period that contain α-Gal. Many capsulated medicines and vaccines contain gelatin as a stabilizer.

The onset of AGS in patients is usually delayed at 2–6 h after ingestion of trigging meat (beef, lamb, and pork) [92]. Symptoms include urticaria, gastrointestinal symptoms, and in rare cases, anaphylaxis. However, parental exposure to α-Gal containing medications may present immediate symptoms within 1 h [93]. Diagnosis of AGS is based on detailed history such as tick bites, delayed symptoms, and the presence of specific IgE to α-Gal [92].

Table 14.8 Concise list of perioperative drugs and devices

Drug or device	Potential to contain alpha-gal (where the alpha-gal exposure is found)
Induction agents	
Propofol	Yes (check inactive ingredients)
Etomidate, ketamine, Fospropofol, Barbitutates	No
Anesthetic agents	
Volatile	No
Analgesics	
Opioid tablet/capsule	Yes (check inactive ingredients)
Acetaminophen	Yes (check inactive ingredients)
Gabapentinoid tablet/capsule	Yes (check inactive ingredients)
Muscle relaxants	Yes (check inactive ingredients)
Miscellaneous	
Intralipid	Yes (check inactive ingredients)
Anticoagulants	
Heparin	Yes (active ingredient)
Enoxaparin	Yes (active ingredient), less commonly than heparin
Fondaparinux	No
Devices	
Mechanical heart valve	No
Surgical foams containing gelatin	Yes (active ingredient)
Xenotransplant tissues from mammals	Yes (active ingredient)
Gore-TEXThrombin glues	No Yes (active ingredient)

Adapted from Nourian et al. [95]

Presurgical screening is done in some medical centers. Prior to surgery, a detailed medical history including meat allergy or history of reaction to certain medications that may contain inactive ingredients such as gelatin is collected. If there is suspicion of AGS in preoperative visit, an α-Gal-specific IgE test should be ordered, and referral should be made to allergy service. If confirmed, such patients should go through anesthesia and surgery in an α-Gal-free environment. Prior to surgery, the surgical team should discuss avoiding surgical products that contain mammalian products. Unfractionated heparin that is derived from porcine intestine and/or bovine lung should be avoided [94]. Heparin alternatives such as bivalirudin and argatroban are available. Medical decision is based on patient's risk of α-Gal allergy (low when IgE < 8 U/ml, moderate 8–50 U/ml, and high >50 U/ml). For high-risk patients, if heparin is indicated, heparin desensitization or alternative anticoagulant should be used. For low and moderate risk patients, premedication with antihistamine and steroid is recommended. If needed, low dose of IV heparin challenge can be performed in the operating room with careful monitoring. A typical dose of 10 U/kg IV heparin is used in such an event [95]. Reaction to low molecular weight (LMW) heparin is very rare and is generally considered safe to use in AGS patients

[94]. Some authors advocate a heparin skin test in AGS patients who will undergo surgery [94]. Large-scale studies are needed to further explore such an approach.

Answers and Discussion of Review Questions

1. A 50-year-old male patient previously had multiple lidocaine injections as local anesthetic for his orthopaedic procedures without a problem. Last week, he received lidocaine from a multidose vial. Ten minutes afterwards, he developed itching and hives on his body. He did not have wheezing or trouble breathing. After receiving Benadryl treatment, hives and itch resolved within 60 min. What is the reaction this patient has?
   Lidocaine comes in preservative-free (single-dose vial) and with preservative. The typical preservative is methylparaben. Methylparaben has a structure similar to PABA (p-aminobenzoic acid). PABA is able to induce IgE-mediated allergic reaction. In this patient, the reaction is caused by preservative instead of lidocaine itself. Switching back to single-dose, preservative-free lidocaine should prevent his future reaction.
2. A 62-year-old female patient was undergoing hip replacement surgery. During the induction phase, she received Cefazolin, atropine, propofol, and rocuronium. Patient developed hives all over her body within 5 min after receiving the above medications. No drop in her blood pressure. She was treated with IV Benadryl and methylprednisolone. Hives resolved within 10 min and the surgery was completed successfully. How do you evaluate this patient after surgery for her reaction in the operating room?
   This patient developed typical symptoms of perioperative hypersensitivity (POH) reaction. Since multiple medications were administered, she underwent allergy evaluation with skin test 4 weeks after discharge from hospital. Prick testing to Cefazolin, atropine, propofol, and rocuronium was negative. Intradermal skin testing was performed using 1:100 and 1:10 dilution of stock solution. Patient was found to be positive to rocuronium (1:100 dilution) and atropine (1:10 dilution). She was negative to Cefazolin, propofol. Therefore, she was diagnosed with immediate allergic reaction to rocuronium and atropine. Recommendation was made to avoid those two agents in future procedures.
3. A 52-year-old male patient presented to his primary care with a tick attached to his back and a surrounding rash. He experienced fever, chills, and myalgia. The tick was removed in the clinic. He was found to have classic bull's eye rash with red center surrounded by a clear ring. He was sent home with a 14-day course of oral doxycycline. Labs for Lyme disease were sent that came back with positive IgM antibodies for Lyme disease. His doxycycline course was extended to 28 days total due to her continuous myalgias, severe fatigue, and generalized weakness. After 8 weeks, the patient consumed pork in a picnic. He developed itching on his face, swelling around his lips and some difficulty breathing. He took some Benadryl. Symptoms subsided in 2 h. He saw an allergist 3 weeks later who ordered blood IgE level to alpha-gal that came back positive. He was diagnosed with alpha-gal syndrome. He is scheduled to have right knee surgery in a month. What precautions should be taken during his surgery?

Some medications and surgical materials used in the operating room may contain alpha-gal. The list includes, but not limited to, mammalian-derived valves/implants, some monoclonal antibodies, heparin, and bovine extracts. Alpha-gal syndrome patients should avoid such exposure during surgical process. If necessary, alternative devices or medications should be considered, i.e., low molecular weight heparin, Bivalirudin, and Argatroban as alternatives for unfractionated heparin.

Summary

1. In real-world practice, allergic reactions to local anesthetics are extremely rare. Most patients, after careful evaluation, can receive such reagents in dental and surgical settings. In rare cases when patient is tested positive to local anesthetics, reagents from separate family should be chosen for future procedures.
2. Antibiotics, neuromuscular blockers, chlorhexidine, and dye are the leading reagents responsible for perioperative hypersensitivity. Mechanisms include IgE-mediated activation of mast cells and basophils and direct activation of mast cells through MRGPRX2 receptor. Skin test, serum IgE, and tryptase levels are used to identify culprit reagents. Once identified, the culprit drug(s) should be avoided in future operations.
3. A recently recognized α-Gal allergy has surgical implications since some medications, and surgical devices containing mammalian components may trigger allergic reaction in this patient population. It is advised to include α-Gal allergy as part of the presurgical screening process.

References

1. Volcheck GW, Hepner DL. Identification and management of perioperative anaphylaxis. J Allergy Clin Immunol Pract. 2019;7(7):2134–42. https://doi.org/10.1016/j.jaip.2019.05.033. Epub 2019 May 31
2. Eggleston ST, Lush LW. Understanding allergic reactions to local anesthetics. Ann Pharmacother. 1996;30(7-8):851–7. https://doi.org/10.1177/106002809603000724.
3. Boren E, Teuber SS, Naguwa SM, Gershwin ME. A critical review of local anesthetic sensitivity. Clin Rev Allergy Immunol. 2007;32(1):119–28. https://doi.org/10.1007/BF02686088.
4. Thyssen JP, Menné T, Elberling J, Plaschke P, Johansen JD. Hypersensitivity to local anaesthetics--update and proposal of evaluation algorithm. Contact Derm. 2008;59(2):69–78. https://doi.org/10.1111/j.1600-0536.2008.01366.x.
5. McLure HA, Rubin AP. Review of local anaesthetic agents. Minerva Anestesiol. 2005;71(3):59–74.
6. Phillips JF, Yates AB, Deshazo RD. Approach to patients with suspected hypersensitivity to local anesthetics. Am J Med Sci. 2007;334(3):190–6. https://doi.org/10.1097/MAJ.0b013e3181406001.
7. Milgrom P, Fiset L. Local anaesthetic adverse effects and other emergency problems in general dental practice. Int Dent J. 1986;36(2):71–6.

8. Daubländer M, Müller R, Lipp MD. The incidence of complications associated with local anesthesia in dentistry. Anesth Prog. 1997;44(4):132–41. PMID: 9481957; PMCID: PMC2148940
9. Bhole MV, Manson AL, Seneviratne SL, Misbah SA. IgE-mediated allergy to local anaesthetics: separating fact from perception: a UK perspective. Br J Anaesth. 2012;108(6):903–11. https://doi.org/10.1093/bja/aes162. Erratum in: Br J Anaesth 2012 Oct;109(4):669
10. Sindel LJ, de Shazo RD. Accidents resulting from local anesthetics. True or false allergy? Clin Rev Allergy. 1991;9(3–4):379–95. https://doi.org/10.1007/BF02802315.
11. Dower JS Jr. A review of paresthesia in association with administration of local anesthesia. Dent Today. 2003;22(2):64–9.
12. Levy SM, Baker KA. Considerations in differential diagnosis of adverse reactions to local anesthetic: report of case. J Am Dent Assoc. 1986;113(2):271–3. https://doi.org/10.14219/jada.archive.1986.0171.
13. Monk W. Skin reactions to apothesin and quinine (sic) in susceptible persons. Arch Derrmatol. 1920;1:651–5.
14. Doyle KA, Goepferd SJ. An allergy to local anesthetics? The consequences of a misdiagnosis. ASDC J Dent Child. 1989;56(2):103–6.
15. Canfield DW, Gage TW. A guideline to local anesthetic allergy testing. Anesth Prog. 1987;34(5):157–63. PMID: 3318567; PMCID: PMC2148541
16. Melamed J, Beaucher WN. Delayed-type hypersensitivity (type IV) reactions in dental anesthesia. Allergy Asthma Proc. 2007;28(4):477–9. https://doi.org/10.2500/aap.2007.28.3020.
17. Mackley CL, Marks JG Jr. Lidocaine hydrochloride. Am J Contact Dermat. 2003;14(4):221–3.
18. Gall H, Kaufmann R, Kalveram CM. Adverse reactions to local anesthetics: analysis of 197 cases. J Allergy Clin Immunol. 1996;97(4):933–7. https://doi.org/10.1016/s0091-6749(96)80067-4.
19. Trautmann A, Goebeler M, Stoevesandt J. Twenty years' experience with anaphylaxis-like reactions to local anesthetics: genuine allergy is rare. J Allergy Clin Immunol Pract. 2018;6(6):2051–2058.e1. https://doi.org/10.1016/j.jaip.2018.04.005. Epub 2018 Apr 12, 2051
20. Chandler MJ, Grammer LC, Patterson R. Provocative challenge with local anesthetics in patients with a prior history of reaction. J Allergy Clin Immunol. 1987;79(6):883–6. https://doi.org/10.1016/0091-6749(87)90236-3.
21. Schatz M. Skin testing and incremental challenge in the evaluation of adverse reactions to local anesthetics. J Allergy Clin Immunol. 1984;74(4 Pt 2):606–16. https://doi.org/10.1016/0091-6749(84)90114-3.
22. McGarry DP, Kim YM, Casselman J, Wenz R, Jhaveri D, Tcheurekdjian H, Hostoffer RW. Ocular desensitization in the face of local anesthetic hypersensitivity. J Allergy Clin Immunol Pract. 2017;5(3):819–20. https://doi.org/10.1016/j.jaip.2016.09.040. Epub 2016 Nov 9
23. Jimenez-Rodriguez TW, Garcia-Neuer M, Alenazy LA, Castells M. Anaphylaxis in the 21st century: phenotypes, endotypes, and biomarkers. J Asthma Allergy. 2018;(11):121–42. https://doi.org/10.2147/JAA.S159411. PMID: 29950872; PMCID: PMC6016596
24. Mertes PM, Volcheck GW, Garvey LH, Takazawa T, Platt PR, Guttormsen AB, Tacquard C. Epidemiology of perioperative anaphylaxis. Presse Med. 2016;45(9):758–67. https://doi.org/10.1016/j.lpm.2016.02.024. Epub 2016 May 12
25. Mertes PM, Malinovsky JM, Jouffroy L, Working Group of the SFAR and SFA, Aberer W, Terreehorst I, Brockow K, Demoly P, ENDA, EAACI interest group on drug allergy. Reducing the risk of anaphylaxis during anesthesia: 2011 updated guidelines for clinical practice. J Investig Allergol Clin Immunol. 2011;21(6):442–53.
26. Melchiors BLB, Garvey LH. Investigation of perioperative hypersensitivity reactions: an update. Curr Opin Allergy Clin Immunol. 2020;20(4):338–45. https://doi.org/10.1097/ACI.0000000000000654.
27. Fisher MM, More DG. The epidemiology and clinical features of anaphylactic reactions in anaesthesia. Anaesth Intensive Care. 1981;9(3):226–34. https://doi.org/10.1177/0310057X8100900304.
28. Zhao W, Kepley CL, Morel PA, Okumoto LM, Fukuoka Y, Schwartz LB. Fc gamma RIIa, not fc gamma RIIb, is constitutively and functionally expressed on skin-derived human mast

cells. J Immunol. 2006;177(1):694–701. https://doi.org/10.4049/jimmunol.177.1.694. PMID: 16785568; PMCID: PMC2176083
29. Arroyave CM, Tan EM. Mechanism of complement activation by radiographic contrast media. Clin Exp Immunol. 1977;29(1):89–94. PMID: 891038; PMCID: PMC1541049
30. Navinés-Ferrer A, Serrano-Candelas E, Lafuente A, Muñoz-Cano R, Martín M, Gastaminza G. MRGPRX2-mediated mast cell response to drugs used in perioperative procedures and anaesthesia. Sci Rep. 2018;8(1):11628. https://doi.org/10.1038/s41598-018-29965-8. Erratum in: Sci Rep 2021 Jun 8;11(1):12449. PMID: 30072729; PMCID: PMC6072780
31. Lansu K, Karpiak J, Liu J, Huang XP, McCorvy JD, Kroeze WK, Che T, Nagase H, Carroll FI, Jin J, Shoichet BK, Roth BL. In silico design of novel probes for the atypical opioid receptor MRGPRX2. Nat Chem Biol. 2017;13(5):529–36. https://doi.org/10.1038/nchembio.2334. Epub 2017 Mar 13. PMID: 28288109; PMCID: PMC5391270
32. Che D, Wang J, Ding Y, Liu R, Cao J, Zhang Y, Hou Y, An H, Gao Z, Zhang T. Mivacurium induce mast cell activation and pseudo-allergic reactions via MAS-related G protein coupled receptor-X2. Cell Immunol. 2018;332:121–8. https://doi.org/10.1016/j.cellimm.2018.08.005. Epub 2018 Aug 10
33. Gaudenzio N, Sibilano R, Marichal T, Starkl P, Reber LL, Cenac N, McNeil BD, Dong X, Hernandez JD, Sagi-Eisenberg R, Hammel I, Roers A, Valitutti S, Tsai M, Espinosa E, Galli SJ. Different activation signals induce distinct mast cell degranulation strategies. J Clin Invest. 2016;126(10):3981–98. https://doi.org/10.1172/JCI85538. Epub 2016 Sep 19. PMID: 27643442; PMCID: PMC5096814
34. Harper NJ, Dixon T, Dugué P, Edgar DM, Fay A, Gooi HC, Herriot R, Hopkins P, Hunter JM, Mirakian R, Pumphrey RS, Seneviratne SL, Walls AF, Williams P, Wildsmith JA, Wood P, Nasser AS, Powell RK, Mirakhur R, Soar J, Working Party of the Association of Anaesthetists of Great Britain and Ireland. Suspected anaphylactic reactions associated with anaesthesia. Anaesthesia. 2009;64(2):199–211. https://doi.org/10.1111/j.1365-2044.2008.05733.x. PMID: 19143700; PMCID: PMC3082210
35. Ring J, Messmer K. Incidence and severity of anaphylactoid reactions to colloid volume substitutes. Lancet. 1977;1(8009):466–9. https://doi.org/10.1016/s0140-6736(77)91953-5.
36. Dewachter P, Mouton-Faivre C, Hepner DL. Perioperative anaphylaxis: what should be known? Curr Allergy Asthma Rep. 2015;15(5):21. https://doi.org/10.1007/s11882-015-0522-4.
37. Barriot P, Riou B. Hemorrhagic shock with paradoxical bradycardia. Intensive Care Med. 1987;13(3):203–7. https://doi.org/10.1007/BF00254705.
38. Dewachter P, Mouton-Faivre C, Emala CW, Beloucif S. Case scenario: bronchospasm during anesthetic induction. Anesthesiology. 2011;114(5):1200–10. https://doi.org/10.1097/ALN.0b013e3182172cd3.
39. Hopkins PM, Cooke PJ, Clarke RC, Guttormsen AB, Platt PR, Dewachter P, Ebo DG, Garcez T, Garvey LH, Hepner DL, Khan DA, Kolawole H, Kopac P, Krøigaard M, Laguna JJ, Marshall SD, Mertes PM, Rose MA, Sabato V, Savic LC, Savic S, Takazawa T, Volcheck GW, Voltolini S, Sadleir PHM. Consensus clinical scoring for suspected perioperative immediate hypersensitivity reactions. Br J Anaesth. 2019;123(1):e29–37. https://doi.org/10.1016/j.bja.2019.02.029. Epub 2019 Apr 24
40. Garvey LH, Ebo DG, Mertes PM, Dewachter P, Garcez T, Kopac P, Laguna JJ, Chiriac AM, Terreehorst I, Voltolini S, Scherer K. An EAACI position paper on the investigation of perioperative immediate hypersensitivity reactions. Allergy. 2019;74(10):1872–84. https://doi.org/10.1111/all.13820. Epub 2019 Jun 18
41. Soetens F, Rose M, Fisher M. Timing of skin testing after a suspected anaphylactic reaction during anaesthesia. Acta Anaesthesiol Scand. 2012;56(8):1042–6. https://doi.org/10.1111/j.1399-6576.2011.02643.x. Epub 2012 Feb 7
42. Gurrieri C, Weingarten TN, Martin DP, Babovic N, Narr BJ, Sprung J, Volcheck GW. Allergic reactions during anesthesia at a large United States referral center. Anesth Analg. 2011;113(5):1202–12. https://doi.org/10.1213/ANE.0b013e31822d45ac. Epub 2011 Aug 24
43. Sadleir PH, Clarke RC, Bunning DL, Platt PR. Anaphylaxis to neuromuscular blocking drugs: incidence and cross-reactivity in Western Australia from 2002 to 2011. Br J Anaesth. 2013;110(6):981–7. https://doi.org/10.1093/bja/aes506. Epub 2013 Jan 18

44. Reddy JI, Cooke PJ, van Schalkwyk JM, Hannam JA, Fitzharris P, Mitchell SJ. Anaphylaxis is more common with rocuronium and succinylcholine than with atracurium. Anesthesiology. 2015;122(1):39–45. https://doi.org/10.1097/ALN.0000000000000512.
45. Dewachter P, Chollet-Martin S, Mouton-Faivre C, de Chaisemartin L, Nicaise-Roland P. Comparison of basophil activation test and skin testing performances in NMBA allergy. J Allergy Clin Immunol Pract. 2018;6(5):1681–9. https://doi.org/10.1016/j.jaip.2017.12.037. Epub 2018 Feb 22
46. Mertes PM, Alla F, Tréchot P, Auroy Y, Jougla E. Groupe d'Etudes des Réactions Anaphylactoïdes Peranesthésiques. Anaphylaxis during anesthesia in France: an 8-year national survey. J Allergy Clin Immunol. 2011;128(2):366–73. https://doi.org/10.1016/j.jaci.2011.03.003. Epub 2011 Apr 17
47. Florvaag E, Johansson SG. The pholcodine story. Immunol Allergy Clin N Am. 2009;29(3):419–27. https://doi.org/10.1016/j.iac.2009.04.002.
48. Baldo BA, Fisher MM, Pham NH. On the origin and specificity of antibodies to neuromuscular blocking (muscle relaxant) drugs: an immunochemical perspective. Clin Exp Allergy. 2009;39(3):325–44. https://doi.org/10.1111/j.1365-2222.2008.03171.x.
49. Light KP, Lovell AT, Butt H, Fauvel NJ, Holdcroft A. Adverse effects of neuromuscular blocking agents based on yellow card reporting in the U.K.: are there differences between males and females? Pharmacoepidemiol Drug Saf. 2006;15(3):151–60. https://doi.org/10.1002/pds.1196.
50. Ebo DG, Fisher MM, Hagendorens MM, Bridts CH, Stevens WJ. Anaphylaxis during anaesthesia: diagnostic approach. Allergy. 2007;62(5):471–87. https://doi.org/10.1111/j.1398-9995.2007.01347.x.
51. Dejoux A, de Chaisemartin L, Bruhns P, Longrois D, Gouel-Chéron A. Neuromuscular blocking agent induced hypersensitivity reaction exploration: an update. Eur J Anaesthesiol. 2023;40(2):95–104. https://doi.org/10.1097/EJA.0000000000001765. Epub 2022 Oct 18
52. Turjanmaa K, Reunala T, Tuimala R, Kärkkäinen T. Allergy to latex gloves: unusual complication during delivery. BMJ. 1988;297(6655):1029. https://doi.org/10.1136/bmj.297.6655.1029. PMID: 3142599; PMCID: PMC1834797
53. Moneret-Vautrin DA, Mata E, Gueant JL, Turgeman D, Laxenaire MC. High risk of anaphylactic shock during surgery for spina bifida. Lancet. 1990;335(8693):865–6. https://doi.org/10.1016/0140-6736(90)90989-i.
54. Bousquet J, Flahault A, Vandenplas O, Ameille J, Duron JJ, Pecquet C, Chevrie K, Annesi-Maesano I. Natural rubber latex allergy among health care workers: a systematic review of the evidence. J Allergy Clin Immunol. 2006;118(2):447–54. https://doi.org/10.1016/j.jaci.2006.03.048. Epub 2006 Jul 3
55. Habre W, Disma N, Virag K, Becke K, Hansen TG, Jöhr M, Leva B, Morton NS, Vermeulen PM, Zielinska M, Boda K, Veyckemans F, APRICOT Group of the European Society of Anaesthesiology clinical trial network. Incidence of severe critical events in paediatric anaesthesia (APRICOT): a prospective multicentre observational study in 261 hospitals in Europe. Lancet Respir Med. 2017;5(5):412–25. https://doi.org/10.1016/S2213-2600(17)30116-9. Epub 2017 Mar 28. Erratum in: Lancet Respir Med 2017 May;5(5):e19. Erratum in: Lancet Respir Med. 2017 Jun;5(6):e22
56. Ebo DG, Stevens WJ, Bridts CH, De Clerck LS. Latex-specific IgE, skin testing, and lymphocyte transformation to latex in latex allergy. J Allergy Clin Immunol. 1997;100(5):618–23. https://doi.org/10.1016/s0091-6749(97)70165-9.
57. Johansson SG, Adédoyin J, van Hage M, Grönneberg R, Nopp A. False-positive penicillin immunoassay: an unnoticed common problem. J Allergy Clin Immunol. 2013;132(1):235–7. https://doi.org/10.1016/j.jaci.2012.11.017. Epub 2012 Dec 25
58. Okano M, Nomura M, Hata S, Okada N, Sato K, Kitano Y, Tashiro M, Yoshimoto Y, Hama R, Aoki T. Anaphylactic symptoms due to chlorhexidine gluconate. Arch Dermatol. 1989;125(1):50–2.
59. Harper NJN, Cook TM, Garcez T, Farmer L, Floss K, Marinho S, Torevell H, Warner A, Ferguson K, Hitchman J, Egner W, Kemp H, Thomas M, Lucas DN, Nasser S, Karanam S, Kong KL, Farooque S, Bellamy M, McGuire N. Anaesthesia, surgery, and life-threatening allergic reactions: epidemiology and clinical features of perioperative anaphylaxis in the 6th

National Audit Project (NAP6). Br J Anaesth. 2018;121(1):159–71. https://doi.org/10.1016/j.bja.2018.04.014. Epub 2018 May 21
60. Opstrup MS, Malling HJ, Krøigaard M, Mosbech H, Skov PS, Poulsen LK, Garvey LH. Standardized testing with chlorhexidine in perioperative allergy--a large single-centre evaluation. Allergy. 2014;69(10):1390–6. https://doi.org/10.1111/all.12466. Epub 2014 Aug 13
61. Odedra KM, Farooque S. Chlorhexidine: an unrecognised cause of anaphylaxis. Postgrad Med J. 2014;90(1070):709–14. https://doi.org/10.1136/postgradmedj-2013-132291. Epub 2014 Oct 28
62. Opstrup MS, Jemec GBE, Garvey LH. Chlorhexidine allergy: on the rise and often overlooked. Curr Allergy Asthma Rep. 2019;19(5):23. https://doi.org/10.1007/s11882-019-0858-2.
63. Le Pabic F, Sainte-Laudy J, Blanchard N, Moneret-Vautrin DA. First case of anaphylaxis to iodinated povidone. Allergy. 2003;58(8):826–7. https://doi.org/10.1034/j.1398-9995.2003.00254.x.
64. Caballero MR, Lukawska J, Dugué P. A hidden cause of perioperative anaphylaxis. J Investig Allergol Clin Immunol. 2010;20(4):353–4.
65. Harper NJ. Propofol and food allergy. Br J Anaesth. 2016;116(1):11–3. https://doi.org/10.1093/bja/aev401.
66. Laguna JJ, Archilla J, Doña I, Corominas M, Gastaminza G, Mayorga C, Berjes-Gimeno P, Tornero P, Martin S, Planas A, Moreno E, Torres MJ. Practical guidelines for perioperative hypersensitivity reactions. J Investig Allergol Clin Immunol. 2018;28(4):216–32. https://doi.org/10.18176/jiaci.0236. Epub 2018 Feb 7
67. Baldo BA, Pham NH. Histamine-releasing and allergenic properties of opioid analgesic drugs: resolving the two. Anaesth Intensive Care. 2012;40(2):216–35. https://doi.org/10.1177/0310057X1204000204.
68. Swerts S, Van Gasse A, Leysen J, Faber M, Sabato V, Bridts CH, Jorens PG, De Clerck LS, Ebo DG. Allergy to illicit drugs and narcotics. Clin Exp Allergy. 2014;44(3):307–18. https://doi.org/10.1111/cea.12177.
69. Garvey LH. Old, new and hidden causes of perioperative hypersensitivity. Curr Pharm Des. 2016;22(45):6814–24. https://doi.org/10.2174/1381612822666161004125143.
70. Scherer K, Studer W, Figueiredo V, Bircher AJ. Anaphylaxis to isosulfan blue and cross-reactivity to patent blue V: case report and review of the nomenclature of vital blue dyes. Ann Allergy Asthma Immunol. 2006;96(3):497–500. https://doi.org/10.1016/S1081-1206(10)60921-0.
71. Barron ME, Wilkes MM, Navickis RJ. A systematic review of the comparative safety of colloids. Arch Surg. 2004;139(5):552–63. https://doi.org/10.1001/archsurg.139.5.552.
72. Mertes PM, Ebo DG, Garcez T, Rose M, Sabato V, Takazawa T, Cooke PJ, Clarke RC, Dewachter P, Garvey LH, Guttormsen AB, Hepner DL, Hopkins PM, Khan DA, Kolawole H, Kopac P, Krøigaard M, Laguna JJ, Marshall SD, Platt PR, Sadleir PHM, Savic LC, Savic S, Volcheck GW, Voltolini S. Comparative epidemiology of suspected perioperative hypersensitivity reactions. Br J Anaesth. 2019;123(1):e16–28. https://doi.org/10.1016/j.bja.2019.01.027. Epub 2019 Mar 4
73. Christiansen IS, Krøigaard M, Mosbech H, Skov PS, Poulsen LK, Garvey LH. Clinical and diagnostic features of perioperative hypersensitivity to cefuroxime. Clin Exp Allergy. 2015;45(4):807–14. https://doi.org/10.1111/cea.12455.
74. Opstrup MS, Poulsen LK, Malling HJ, Jensen BM, Garvey LH. Dynamics of plasma levels of specific IgE in chlorhexidine allergic patients with and without accidental re-exposure. Clin Exp Allergy. 2016;46(8):1090–8. https://doi.org/10.1111/cea.12743. Epub 2016 May 11
75. Lafuente A, Javaloyes G, Berroa F, Goikoetxea MJ, Moncada R, Núñez-Córdoba JM, Cabrera-Freitag P, D'Amelio C, Sanz ML, Gastaminza G. Early skin testing is effective for diagnosis of hypersensitivity reactions occurring during anesthesia. Allergy. 2013;68(6):820–2. https://doi.org/10.1111/all.12154. Epub 2013 May 6
76. Miller J, Clough SB, Pollard RC, Misbah SA. Outcome of repeat anaesthesia after investigation for perioperative anaphylaxis. Br J Anaesth. 2018;120(6):1195–201. https://doi.org/10.1016/j.bja.2018.02.033. Epub 2018 Apr 10

77. Rose MA, Anderson J, Green SL, Yun J, Fernando SL. Morphine and pholcodine-specific IgE have limited utility in the diagnosis of anaphylaxis to benzylisoquinolines. Acta Anaesthesiol Scand. 2018;62(5):628–34. https://doi.org/10.1111/aas.13077. Epub 2018 Jan 24
78. Schwartz LB. Diagnostic value of tryptase in anaphylaxis and mastocytosis. Immunol Allergy Clin N Am. 2006;26(3):451–63. https://doi.org/10.1016/j.iac.2006.05.010.
79. Vitte J, Amadei L, Gouitaa M, Mezouar S, Zieleskiewicz L, Albanese J, Bruder N, Lagier D, Mertès PM, Mège JL, Schwartz LB, Leone M. Paired acute-baseline serum tryptase levels in perioperative anaphylaxis: an observational study. Allergy. 2019;74(6):1157–65. https://doi.org/10.1111/all.13752. Epub 2019 Mar 21
80. Baretto RL, Beck S, Heslegrave J, Melchior C, Mohamed O, Ekbote A, Huissoon AP, Krishna MT. Validation of international consensus equation for acute serum total tryptase in mast cell activation: a perioperative perspective. Allergy. 2017;72(12):2031–4. https://doi.org/10.1111/all.13226. Epub 2017 Jul 12
81. Knol EF, Koenderman L, Mul FP, Verhoeven AJ, Roos D. Differential activation of human basophils by anti-IgE and formyl-methionyl-leucyl-phenylalanine. Indications for protein kinase C-dependent and -independent activation pathways. Eur J Immunol. 1991;21(4):881–5. https://doi.org/10.1002/eji.1830210404.
82. Bridts CH, Sabato V, Mertens C, Hagendorens MM, De Clerck LS, Ebo DG. Flow cytometric allergy diagnosis: basophil activation techniques. Methods Mol Biol. 2020;2163:183–95. https://doi.org/10.1007/978-1-0716-0696-4_15.
83. Ebo DG, Faber M, Elst J, Van Gasse AL, Bridts CH, Mertens C, De Clerck LS, Hagendorens MM, Sabato V. In vitro diagnosis of immediate drug hypersensitivity during anesthesia: a review of the literature. J Allergy Clin Immunol Pract. 2018;6(4):1176–84. https://doi.org/10.1016/j.jaip.2018.01.004. Epub 2018 Feb 14, 1176
84. Garvey LH, Ebo DG, Krøigaard M, Savic S, Clarke R, Cooke P, Dewachter P, Garcez T, Guttormsen AB, Hopkins PM, Hepner DL, Khan DA, Kolawole H, Kopac P, Marshall S, Mertes PM, Platt P, Rose M, Sabato V, Sadleir P, Savic L, Scherer K, Takazawa T, Volcheck GW, Voltolini S, Laguna JJ. The use of drug provocation testing in the investigation of suspected immediate perioperative allergic reactions: current status. Br J Anaesth. 2019;123(1):e126–34. https://doi.org/10.1016/j.bja.2019.03.018. Epub 2019 Apr 23
85. Brown JC, Simons E, Rudders SA. Epinephrine in the management of anaphylaxis. J Allergy Clin Immunol Pract. 2020;8(4):1186–95. https://doi.org/10.1016/j.jaip.2019.12.015. Erratum in: J Allergy Clin Immunol Pract 2021 Jan;9(1):604
86. Garvey LH, Dewachter P, Hepner DL, Mertes PM, Voltolini S, Clarke R, Cooke P, Garcez T, Guttormsen AB, Ebo DG, Hopkins PM, Khan DA, Kopac P, Krøigaard M, Laguna JJ, Marshall S, Platt P, Rose M, Sabato V, Sadleir P, Savic L, Savic S, Scherer K, Takazawa T, Volcheck GW, Kolawole H. Management of suspected immediate perioperative allergic reactions: an international overview and consensus recommendations. Br J Anaesth. 2019;123(1):e50–64. https://doi.org/10.1016/j.bja.2019.04.044. Epub 2019 May 24
87. Sadleir PHM, Clarke RC, Bozic B, Platt PR. Consequences of proceeding with surgery after resuscitation from intra-operative anaphylaxis. Anaesthesia. 2018;73(1):32–9. https://doi.org/10.1111/anae.14106. Epub 2017 Nov 2
88. Chung CH, Mirakhur B, Chan E, Le QT, Berlin J, Morse M, Murphy BA, Satinover SM, Hosen J, Mauro D, Slebos RJ, Zhou Q, Gold D, Hatley T, Hicklin DJ, Platts-Mills TA. Cetuximab-induced anaphylaxis and IgE specific for galactose-alpha-1,3-galactose. N Engl J Med. 2008;358(11):1109–17. https://doi.org/10.1056/NEJMoa074943. PMID: 18337601; PMCID: PMC2361129
89. Koike C, Uddin M, Wildman DE, Gray EA, Trucco M, Starzl TE, Goodman M. Functionally important glycosyltransferase gain and loss during catarrhine primate emergence. Proc Natl Acad Sci U S A. 2007;104(2):559–64. https://doi.org/10.1073/pnas.0610012104. Epub 2006 Dec 28. PMID: 17194757; PMCID: PMC1766424
90. Vaz-Rodrigues R, Mazuecos L, de la Fuente J. Current and future strategies for the diagnosis and treatment of the alpha-gal syndrome (AGS). J Asthma Allergy. 2022;18(15):957–70. https://doi.org/10.2147/JAA.S265660. PMID: 35879928; PMCID: PMC9307871

91. Young I, Prematunge C, Pussegoda K, Corrin T, Waddell L. Tick exposures and alpha-gal syndrome: a systematic review of the evidence. Ticks Tick Borne Dis. 2021;12(3):101674. https://doi.org/10.1016/j.ttbdis.2021.101674. Epub 2021 Jan 27
92. Platts-Mills TAE, Li RC, Keshavarz B, Smith AR, Wilson JM. Diagnosis and management of patients with the α-gal syndrome. J Allergy Clin Immunol Pract. 2020;8(1):15–23.e1. https://doi.org/10.1016/j.jaip.2019.09.017. Epub 2019 Sep 28. PMID: 31568928; PMCID: PMC6980324
93. Stone CA Jr, Commins SP, Choudhary S, Vethody C, Heavrin JL, Wingerter J, Hemler JA, Babe K, Phillips EJ, Norton AE. Anaphylaxis after vaccination in a pediatric patient: further implicating alpha-gal allergy. J Allergy Clin Immunol Pract. 2019;7(1):322–324.e2. https://doi.org/10.1016/j.jaip.2018.06.005. Epub 2018 Jun 15. PMID: 29913263; PMCID: PMC6295282
94. Koo G, Plager J, Fahrenholz JM, Phillips E, Stone C Jr. Reactivity to heparin in patients with alpha-gal allergy: a potential role for skin testing? Ann Allergy Asthma Immunol. 2022;129(4):515–7. https://doi.org/10.1016/j.anai.2022.07.010. Epub 2022 Jul 21
95. Nourian MM, Stone CA Jr, Siegrist KK, Riess ML. Perioperative implications of patients with alpha gal allergies. J Clin Anesth. 2023;86:111056. https://doi.org/10.1016/j.jclinane.2023.111056. Epub 2023 Jan 20

Chapter 15
Alpha-Gal Syndrome

Nidhi Desai, Shilen Thakrar, Mark Maas, Sergio Navarrete, Ezoza Rajabaliev, Lawrence Schwartz, and Wilhelm A. Zuelzer

Clinical Case

A 62-year-old male is assessed preoperatively to undergo an elective left total knee replacement. He has class I obesity and hypertension which is well-controlled on amlodipine. He is physically active and plays golf three times a week and swims twice a week. He has been vegan for more than 20 years. He takes vegan appropriate iron, vitamin D, and daily multivitamin supplements. He reports no drug allergies, and there were no anesthetic complications during an inguinal hernia repair performed under general anesthesia 8 years ago.

Prior to the surgical procedure, he underwent spinal anesthesia with moderate to deep propofol sedation without any hemodynamic complications. During the surgical procedure, 10 min following administration of bovine-derived topical thrombin, the patient had generalized urticaria followed by severe hypoxemia,

N. Desai · S. Thakrar (✉) · S. Navarrete · E. Rajabaliev
Department of Anesthesiology, Virginia Commonwealth University, Richmond, VA, USA
e-mail: desain4@vcu.edu; shilen.thakrar@vcuhealth.org; sergio.navarrete1@vcuhealth.org; ezoza.rajabaliev@vcuhealth.org

M. Maas
Department of Pharmacy Services, VCU Health System, Richmond, VA, USA
e-mail: mark.maas@vcuhealth.org

L. Schwartz
Department of Internal Medicine, Virginia Commonwealth University, Richmond, VA, USA
e-mail: lawrence.schwartz@vcuhealth.org

W. A. Zuelzer
Orthopaedic Surgery, Virginia Commonwealth University Medical School, Richmond, VA, USA
e-mail: wilhelm.zuelzer@vcuhealth.org

W. A. Zuelzer, S. Metikala (eds.), *Unusual Conditions That Every Orthopaedic Surgeon Should Know*, https://doi.org/10.1007/978-3-031-58946-1_15

hypotension, and tachycardia. Emergent intubation followed by administration of epinephrine, diphenhydramine, and methylprednisolone occurred. The patient rapidly stabilized. Postoperatively, the patient was transferred to the surgical intensive care unit where continued support with epinephrine infusion was required. Serum tryptase levels were drawn 15 min and 2 h after symptom onset. Approximately 12 h after onset, the patient was weaned from epinephrine and was extubated. On the second postoperative day, an additional serum tryptase level was obtained and the patient was discharged with instructions to follow-up with an allergist.

Questions

1. What are the critical questions required to identify a patient at risk for alpha-gal syndrome?
2. If a patient has a history consistent with alpha-gal syndrome, what perioperative changes should be made?
3. In the event of a significant event including hypotension in the operating room, what diagnostic test/s are required to confirm that the event occurred as a result of an anaphylactic reaction?

Background

Although the immune system is critical for protecting against microbial invasions, in certain circumstances, the same system can lead to significant adverse outcomes due to immune inflammatory responses known as hypersensitivity reactions. Type I hypersensitivity involves IgE-mediated release of antibodies against an antigen such as a foreign protein or carbohydrate which may result in release of histamine and other vasoactive mediators when antigen cross-links IgE bound to the surfaces of both mast cells and/or basophils, classically within 30 min of exposure to the antigen. However, depending on the antigen's route, source, and nature, the onset of clinical symptoms can be delayed for 2–10 h. This hypersensitivity reaction may result in rash, hives, erythema, pruritus, edema, flushing, bronchospasm, wheezing, rhinitis, hypotension, diarrhea, or abdominal cramping. The presence of wheal and flare reactions are hallmarks of mast cell activation in the skin. In more severe reactions, anaphylaxis may result in orthostatic hypotension, loss of consciousness, nausea, vomiting, diarrhea, angioedema, hypotension, tachycardia, tachypnea, and death. It is estimated that anaphylaxis has skin involvement in 80–90%, respiratory involvement in up to 70%, gastrointestinal tract involvement in up to 45%, cardiovascular involvement in up to 45%, and central nervous system (CNS) manifestations in up to 15% of patients (see Table 15.1) [1]. It is estimated that 2% of adults will experience anaphylaxis in their lifetime [2].

Table 15.1 Symptoms and signs of anaphylaxis [1]

Cutaneous/subcutaneous/mucosal tissue
Flushing, pruritus, hives (urticaria), swelling, morbilliform rash, piloerection
Pruritus, erythema and swelling, conjunctival erythema, tearing
Pruritus and swelling of lips, tongue, uvula/palate
Pruritus in the external auditory canals
Pruritus of genitalia, palms, soles
Respiratory
Nose: Pruritus, congestion, rhinorrhea, sneezing
Larynx: Pruritus and tightness in the throat, dysphonia and hoarseness, dry staccato (repetitive but clearly separated) cough, stridor, dysphagia
Lung: Shortness of breath, chest tightness, deep cough, wheezing/bronchospasm (decreased peak expiratory flow)
Cyanosis
Gastrointestinal
Nausea, cramping abdominal pain, vomiting (stringy mucus), diarrhea
Cardiovascular
Chest pain, palpitations, tachycardia, bradycardia, angina [3] or dysrhythmia
Feeling faint, altered mental status, hypotension, loss of sphincter control, shock, cardiac arrest
CNS
Aura of impending doom, uneasiness, throbbing headache, dizziness, confusion, tunnel vision; in infants and children, sudden behavioral changes, such as irritability, cessation of play, and clinging to parent
Other
Metallic taste in the mouth
Dysphagia
Uterine contractions in post-pubertal female patients

Anaphylaxis is likely when any of the three criteria are fulfilled [1, 4]:

1. Acute onset of illness minutes to hours with involvement of skin mucosal tissue such as hives, generalized itching, flushing, swollen lips, tongue, uvula, and airway compromise such as dyspnea, wheezing, bronchospasm, stridor or reduced blood pressure, or associated symptoms such as hypotonia and syncope.
2. Two or more of the following after exposure to known allergen for the patient in minutes to hours, with a history of severe allergic reactions, skin mucosal tissue with hives, itching, flushing, swollen lips, airway compromise, reduced blood pressure or associated symptoms such as hypotonia and syncope and in suspected food allergies such as GI symptoms, crampy abdominal pain, and vomiting.
3. Hypotension minutes to hours after exposure to known allergens; for instance, a greater than 30% drop in systolic blood pressure in infants and children or an adult with systolic blood pressure less than 100 mmHg or 30% drop from the baseline.

All living animals are made up of glycans, also called polysaccharides, which are sugar-based polymers that coat cells and join with proteins to form glycoproteins. They are essential for maintenance of tissue structure, porosity, and integrity, and they shield underlying polypeptide from recognition by proteases or antibodies [5].

Scientific Name	Common Name(s)[a]	Geographic Range[a]
Amblyomma americanum	Lone Star Tick	North America (Southeastern US, Canada, Mexico)
Amblyomma cajennense	Cayenne Tick	North and Central America
Amblyomma hebraeum[b]	South African Bont Tick	South Africa
Amblyomma sculptum	N/A	South America (Brazil)
Amblyomma testudinarium	N/A	South Asia (India, Sri Lanka) and East Asia (including Japan)
Amblyomma variegatum[b]	Tropical Bont Tick	Southeast Asia, Africa
Haemaphysalis longicornis	Asian Longhorned Tick, Bush Tick	Japan
Ixodes australiensis	N/A	Australia
Ixodes holocyclus	Paralysis Tick	Australia, Southern Asia
Ixodes nipponensis[b]	Cattle Tick	Asia (including Korea, Japan)
Ixodes ricinus	Sheep Tick, Wood Tick, Deer Tick, Castor Bean Tick	North America, Europe and Northern Asia, Africa
Ixodes scapularis	Blacklegged Tick	Middle America, North America
Rhipicephalus spp (including *R. microplus; R. evertsi*)[b]	Asian Blue Tick, Australian Cattle Tick, Southern Cattle Tick, Cuban Tick, Madagascar Blue Tick, Puerto Rican Tick	Southern Asia, South America, North America, Caribbean, Australia, Africa

Chart 15.1 Species of ticks [13]. [a]Common name and Geographic Range reported in Integrated Taxonomic Information System. [b]Suspected link, but not definitive association of tick with the development of alpha-gal syndrome

The critical issue in alpha-gal syndrome is that fish, reptiles, birds, and humans do not have a certain glycan, galactose-α-1,3-galactose, in their system. However, pigs, cows, rabbits, and sheep do have this glycan in their system. Alpha-gal syndrome (AGS) is characterized by sensitivity to galactose-α-1,3-galactose (alpha-gal) [6–10]. Sensitivity to alpha-gal initially may develop following a tick bite, after which alpha-Gal-specific IgE is produced. In the United States, the Lone Star tick (*Amblyomma americanum*) is primarily responsible and is distributed in the southeastern states. North Carolina, Kentucky, and Tennessee have the highest prevalence of AGS in the United States [11]. AGS in other countries may correspond to sensitization by other species of ticks (See Chart 15.1). Commins estimated that the percentage of individuals living in endemic tick areas that have been sensitized to alpha-gal range from 15 to 30% [12]. After sensitization, subsequent bites by this tick might boost IgE production against alpha-gal, but they do not cause systemic reactions, presumably because this antigen is not present as a multivalent antigen and/or in a high enough amount. The mechanism as to why a tick bite specifically initiates sensitization to alpha-gal is not well understood, but the onset suggests the presence of an adjuvant (a substance that enhances the body's immune response to an antigen) that enhances immunogenicity [13–16]. Subsequent exposure to alpha-gal on proteins or glycolipids in medical therapeutics can manifest as an immediate anaphylaxis, which is of particular concern in the perioperative setting [13], whereas ingestion of foods containing alpha-gal can result in delayed anaphylaxis, starting 2–6 h after ingestion.

Unlike protein antigens, alpha-gal is a unique antigen that is not denatured by high cooking temperatures [17]. In the Southeastern United States, alpha-gal syndrome is a leading cause of anaphylaxis among adults and adolescents. [18] Furthermore, patients who present with a history of urticaria (severely itching skin with wheal or angioedema or both) or anaphylaxis, have a significant chance of having elevated serum alpha-gal IgE [19]. The orthopaedic surgeon must be aware of this condition and ask appropriate questions to identify this type of patient. Certain routine medications and xenotransplants place the patient with alpha-gal syndrome at risk for anaphylaxis. The number of patients with meat allergies appears to be increasing, further emphasizing the importance of this allergy.

Epidemiology

Alpha-gal has been reported on all continents except Antarctica. In 2007, van Nunen and colleagues described 25 cases of adults who developed red meat allergy after tick bites in Eastern Australia [20]. IgE-mediated hypersensitivity reactions to alpha-gal were first reported in 2008 in southeastern United States. Cases of immediate anaphylaxis, some fatal, beginning during or shortly after cetuximab i.v. infusions, were observed, and associated with pre-existing IgE antibodies to alpha-gal, which is expressed on cetuximab because this mAb is produced by the murine SP2/0 hybridoma [9, 11, 21]. AGS was then identified in 2009, when cases of delayed anaphylaxis after ingestion of mammalian meat were also associated with IgE antibodies to alpha-gal but not to protein epitopes [6]. The Centers for Disease Control and Prevention (CDC) recently reported that nearly half a million Americans could be living with AGS [22]. Given the variable presentations of signs and symptoms as well as presence of asymptomatic but sensitized individuals, sensitization is necessary but not sufficient for these IgE-dependent reactions, and thus the prevalence of disease is less than the prevalence of sensitization. The prevalence of alpha-gal sensitization varies across the country, is higher in the southeastern United States, where the lone star tick is endemic (Fig. 15.1) [13, 23–25]. A retrospective study investigated positivity trends from 2010 to 2018 and found the highest sensitization prevalence rates ($\geq$2.35 per 100,000 persons) were in Arkansas, Virginia, Kentucky, Oklahoma, and Missouri [26]. While *A. americanum* (lone star tick) is the main tick species linked to the condition in North America, other species such as *Ixodes holocyclus*, *Ixodes ricinus*, and *Haemaphysalis longicornis* have been linked to sensitization in Australia, Europe, and Asia, respectively [11, 13, 27]. Ascaris lumbricoides also has been reported to sensitize some individuals [28]. Of interest is that when alpha-gal sensitized individuals are bitten by such ticks, alpha-gal IgE titers are boosted, but immediate or delayed allergic reactions do not typically occur, perhaps because multivalent alpha-gal antigens are lacking and/or the total amounts of alpha-gal-haptenized protein or lipid entities transferred with a tick bite are low.

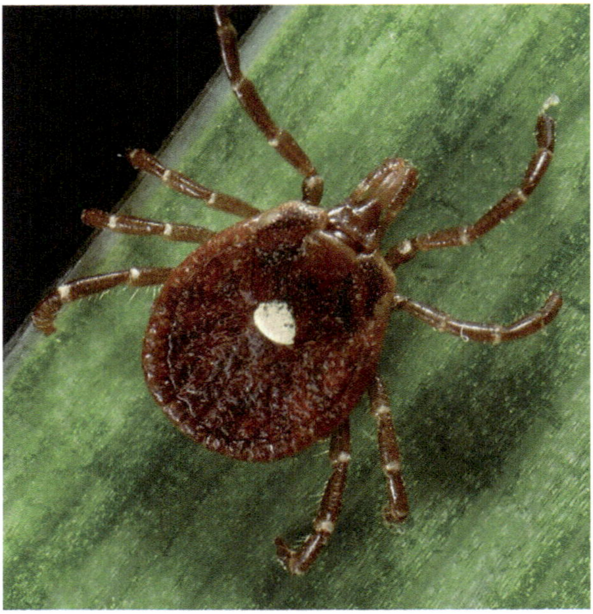

Fig. 15.1 Lone Star tick—Adapted from CDC.gov [29]

Clinical Presentation

The clinical presentation of alpha-gal syndrome is variable, ranging from multiple organ-system involvement to an asymptomatic carrier state. Following consumption of mammalian meat, there is usually a delay in the presentation by 3–6 h and signs and symptoms generally include urticaria, angioedema, and/or pruritus [6, 23]. Non-classical symptoms mainly involve the gastrointestinal system. Interestingly, the prevalence of stand-alone GI symptoms, including abdominal pain, reflux, diarrhea, or cramping, have been reported in up to 20% of AGS patients [30]. After intravenous or mucosal administration of some medications, including cetuximab, unfractionated heparin, or bovine-derived topical thrombin, reactions are often more severe and acute, including anaphylaxis. In addition to dermatologic and gastrointestinal symptoms, upper airway symptoms such as throat constriction due to angioedema, and itching may occur [13, 31] (see Table 15.2). Variability in signs, symptoms, and severity may contribute to the underdiagnosis of this condition, which underscores the challenge associated with identification of alpha-gal sensitization and prompt intervention in the perioperative setting.

Commonly identified meats in the high-risk category for triggering AGS reactions include beef, pork, deer, and lamb. The risk for dairy and gelatin-containing foods (such as Gummies, Marshmallows, Jell-O), or collagen (Catgut sutures, Collagen-derived contact lenses, Shampoo, Tattoo ink) in triggering such reactions is lower [32, 33]. Those with symptoms elicited after ingestion of dairy products were more likely to have gastrointestinal symptoms [34]. Non-food products such

Table 15.2 Common symptoms and symptom distribution [13]

Organ System	Presentation	Percentage (Number Out of 15)
Cutaneous	Urticaria (hives), pruritus, angioedema	93% (14)
Gastrointestinal	Emesis, diarrhea, gastroesophageal reflux, abdominal pain, abdominal bloating,	73% (11)
Respiratory	Respiratory distress, dyspnea, coughing, chest tightness, wheeze, hypoxia	33% (5)
Oropharyngeal	Throat itching, throat constriction, neck tightness, mouth/throat swelling	26% (4)
Cardiovascular	Syncope, pre-syncope	13% (2)

Notes: [a]Adapted from Iweala OI, Choudhary SK, Addison CT, Commins SP. T and B Lymphocyte Transcriptional States Differentiate between Sensitized and Unsensitized Individuals in Alpha-Gal Syndrome. *Int J Mol Sci.* 2021;22(6).[27]

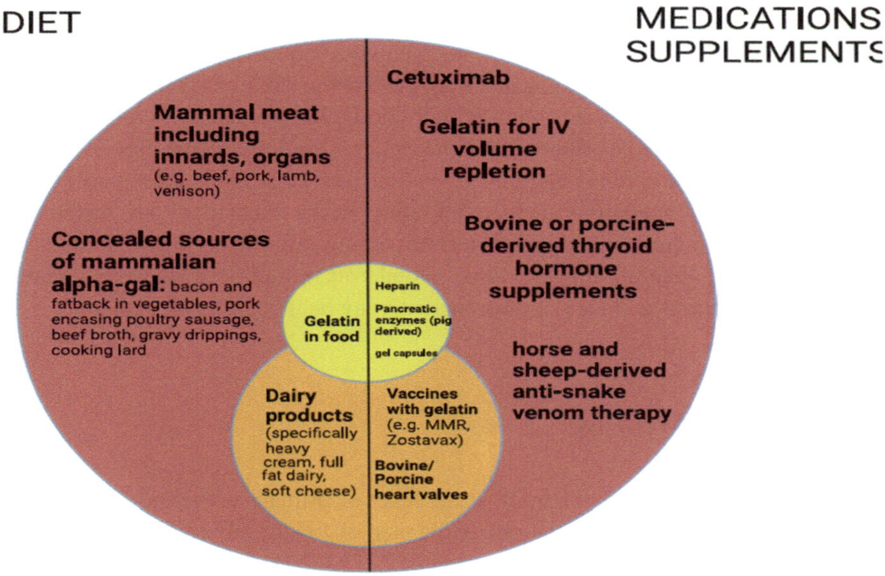

Fig. 15.2 Variety of products that can induce AGS [13]

as medications and therapeutics that are considered high risk for inducing AGS include, but are not limited to, cetuximab, bovine/porcine heart valves, gelatin-containing medical products, unfractionated heparin, antivenom, and pancreatic enzyme replacement [9–11, 32, 35, 36] (see Fig. 15.2). Alpha-gal may be found in various vaccines, antivenom, acetaminophen, oxycodone, lisinopril, and oxycontin. Carrageenan, an ingredient made from red algae, may contain alpha-gal and is used in beer, condiments, infant formulas, and salad dressings. A critical problem is that many manufacturers of drugs do not report the source of inactive ingredients nor test for alpha-gal content of their drugs.

The *Medications and Surgical Products* section below contains a more complete list of medications.

Diagnosis

A recent survey revealed a significant percentage of healthcare providers had limited familiarity with AGS; furthermore, those that were familiar were uncertain on how to diagnose it [22]. Moreover, among clinicians who were aware of the syndrome, AGS is a clinical diagnosis largely based on patient clinical history in combination with detection of alpha-gal-specific IgE antibodies [13, 32]. Important factors to consider include history of tick bites in endemic settings, history of atopy, and established constellation of symptoms consistent with delayed meat allergy reactions or immediate reactions to animal-derived biologic therapies. Diagnosis often begins at the primary care level, where suspicious patient history prompts further workup. Laboratory workup to support the diagnosis includes immunoassays that detect IgE antibodies against galactose-alpha-1-3-galactose, with IgE levels >2 IU/mL or a percentage of total IgE >2% indicating a high likelihood of diagnosis [11, 26, 32]. In suspected cases of food allergy, an oral food challenge test can also be used [12, 54]. However, food challenges require a cautious approach as they can lead to severe symptoms and may be delayed. Skin prick and intradermal skin tests have also been used to investigate food allergies, but their reliability for predicting AGS induced by mammalian meats is not well established [6, 54]. Next-generation testing research is ongoing given that current methods are suboptimal in terms of sensitivity, specificity, and patient safety. At the molecular level, histamine-release assays and mast cell activation tests are being explored as potential diagnostic methods [25]. Overall, this condition is underdiagnosed because of its variable clinical presentations and lack of awareness among healthcare professionals.

Management Overview

Management of AGS begins largely at the level of primary prevention. Following the identification of AGS in a patient, avoidance of foods and products that induce the syndrome is the established treatment [12, 13, 23] (see Table 15.3). Patients should be given proper education and guidance on avoidance of tick bites, especially in endemic settings, including treatment of clothing with permethrin and skin with an insect repellant such as DEET. Some patients are able to regain tolerance to meat and products containing alpha-gal with long-term avoidance of tick bites [12, 25] and might be able to resume eating mammalian meats. However, sensitivity may return after subsequent tick or chigger bites. Avoidance of alpha-gal-containing foods is associated with reductions in levels of IgE antibodies in most individuals [7, 55]. Thus, diet modifications and proper nutrition counseling are important components of management. When severe cases of alpha-gal-triggered anaphylaxis occur, emergent interventions can include supine positioning to prevent hypotensive sequelae and administration of intramuscular epinephrine to treat angioedema and hypotension. Other pharmacological treatments, such as antihistamines and corticosteroids, are of little value for the acute treatment of anaphylaxis.

Table 15.3 Frequently used medications containing alpha-gal with potential contraindications for patients with alpha-gal syndrome sensitized by ticks [53]

Medications and products	Alpha-gal-containing ingredient
Medication	
Acetaminophen	Magnesium stearate
Alvimopan	Gelatin, bovine and porcine
Aminocaproic acid	Magnesium stearate and stearic acid
Baclofen	Magnesium stearate
Carbidopa-levodopa	Magnesium stearate
Celecoxib	Gelatin, bovine and porcine
Clonidine	Magnesium stearate
Gabapentin	Gelatin, bovine and porcine
Haloperidol	Lactic acid
Heparin	Porcine
Hydrocodone	Magnesium stearate
Hydromorphone	Lactic acid
Ibuprofen	Glycerin
Levothyroxine	Magnesium stearate
Lidocaine patch	Gelatin
Liothyronine	Magnesium stearate
Lisinopril	Magnesium stearate
Metoclopramide	Magnesium stearate
Naproxen	Magnesium stearate
Oxycodone	Stearic acid
Oxycontin	Magnesium stearate
Synthetic triiodothyronine	Magnesium stearate
Synthetic thyroxine	Magnesium stearate
Devices and products	
Bioprosthetic valves	Porcine or bovine derived
Catgut sutures	Mammalian derived

While there is no cure for AGS, research in the realm of immunotherapy is ongoing. One proposed treatment is oral immunotherapy, which requires slow and incremental exposures to alpha-gal containing foods in order to achieve clinical tolerance [25]. Anti-IgE therapies are also in the exploration phase, as they may help to reduce the severity of anaphylactic reaction [25]. Ultimately, further understanding of the mechanism behind alpha-gal sensitization is needed to develop targeted therapeutic interventions.

Perioperative Anesthetic Considerations and Management

Alpha-gal syndrome presents an interesting challenge in the realm of anesthetic management of patients. Preoperative management largely focuses on identification of the condition and proper planning of the procedure. If alpha-gal syndrome is suspected at a preoperative clinic visit based on patient history, providers should order α-Gal specific-IgE and total IgE blood tests and refer the patient to an allergy specialist [24].

Important history to obtain includes inquiring whether a patient has a history of allergic responses to red meat or medications and surgical products implicated in AGS (e.g., cetuximab) [9, 10, 35, 36, 56]. In addition, the timing and characteristics of symptoms should also be explored. Once appropriate screening and diagnostic testing has been performed, it is imperative that a patient's chart is updated, and a tailored plan is developed prior to the procedure. Hospital systems should also maintain a record of common perioperative materials and their alpha-gal content to allow for cross-referencing of patient allergies with their procedure plan and anticipated medications. Awareness of the condition and proper documentation are needed for the operative teams to modify a procedure accordingly and be prepared for complications [21, 56].

Management of Anaphylactic Reactions

An anaphylactic reaction to alpha-gal is a life-threatening medical emergency, requiring acute intervention in the perioperative setting. Anaphylaxis can be confirmed with an elevated acute serum tryptase (AST) level (drawn 1–2 h after the onset of signs or symptoms) compared to the baseline serum tryptase (BST) level (obtained from blood drawn prior to the procedure or at least 24 h after all signs and symptoms have completely resolved) [56–63]. It should be noted that these test results will not be available during the acute event. AST > 2 + 1.2xBST is considered clinically significant and is thus diagnostic of an allergic reaction [64]. It should be emphasized that a significant hypotensive event without the AST increase makes an anaphylactic reaction as the cause very unlikely. Acute intervention of alpha-gal allergy involves stabilization methods similar to those generally implemented in any anaphylactic hypersensitivity reactions. Specifically, stabilization may be achieved via epinephrine, bronchodilators, supine positioning, intravenous fluids and/or oxygen [21, 65]. Following acute management, patients should be appropriately advised on avoidance of allergen triggers for prevention. The main goal in postoperative care for AGS patients is to ensure that medications, such as those for pain or DVT prophylaxis, do not contain alpha-gal or other allergens to which the patient may be sensitive [24]. Follow up with appropriate healthcare providers, such as an allergy specialist, may be warranted [64].

Medications and Surgical Products

In the operative setting, various medication and surgical product allergies have been implicated in induction of immune responses to alpha-gal [11, 32]. Careful screening of patient medical records along with all medications and products used in the perioperative period is essential. Screening of medications should take place even if the patient's allergy status is unconfirmed, as allergic reactions can be severe from injections compared with the patient's historical intolerance to alpha-gal-containing foods. Alpha-gal reactions to injectable or mucosal medications occur rapidly, often within 15 min of exposure. Table 15.4 describes the active and inactive ingredients

Table 15.4 Medications and inactive ingredients associated with alpha-gal allergic reactions [9, 24, 32, 37–52]

Medication	Comments
Active ingredients in the perioperative setting	
Unfractionated heparin	Heparin is derived from porcine intestinal mucosa, which may contain protein impurities with alpha-gal, though impurity levels may vary from lot to lot. All formulations of heparin carry risk, including heparin injections, heparinized syringes with other active ingredients, and heparin intravenous flush syringes. Low-molecular weight heparins (e.g., enoxaparin) are associated with a low risk of having protein impurities, while non-heparin-based anticoagulants (e.g., argatroban) are associated with the lowest risk.
Topical hemostatic agents: Bovine-derived thrombin, collagen-based dry matrices, or gelatin-based dry matrices	Various topical hemostatic agents, including combination products, may contain animal-derived gelatin, collagen, or thrombin. Presently available cellulose-based agents, recombinant topical thrombin agents, or future agents derived from an alpha-gal-free animal may be suitable alternatives.
Inactive ingredients	
Ingredient	Comments
Gelatin	Gelatin is commonly derived from mammalian animal bone. It is one of the most common inactive ingredients in oral capsules. Gelatin is always animal derived and is the most likely inactive ingredient to be implicated in an alpha-gal reaction.
Collagen	Collagen is derived from mammalian animal connective tissue. It is an unusual inactive ingredient in pharmaceuticals, but it may be present in some topical gels, particularly in herbal products.
Stearates (e.g., magnesium stearate, stearic acid)[a]	Stearates may be animal or plant derived. They are very commonly used in oral tablets as lubricating agents, but are less likely to have protein impurities with alpha-gal.
Glycerin[a]	Glycerin is a sweetener and emollient that may be derived from animal fats, and it is unlikely to have protein impurities with alpha-gal. It is commonly used in topical medications and oral solutions. It is an inactive ingredient in propofol, a commonly used anesthetic. It is also present in clevidipine injection.
Lactose[a]	Lactose is potentially derived from bovine sources and is commonly used in dry-powder inhalers or as a tablet diluent and is unlikely to have protein impurities with alpha-gal.
Lanolin[a]	Lanolin is derived from oil glands of sheep and may be used as an emulsifying agent or ointment base.
Other notable active ingredients	
Antivenom agents (e.g., crotalidae immune $F(ab')_2$)	
Cetuximab	
Pancreatic enzyme replacements (porcine-derived)	
Thyroid supplements (porcine-derived)	
Vaccines: Measles/mumps/rubella, live-attenuated herpes zoster, tetanus/diphtheria/acellular pertussis, yellow fever	

[a] Manufacturing processes make alpha-gal reactions unlikely with these ingredients, but reactions are possible

most implicated in alpha-gal reactions in the perioperative setting [9, 24, 32, 37–40, 42–52, 66].

Unfractionated heparin is a commonly used anticoagulant in the perioperative setting and is derived from porcine intestine mucosa [21, 24, 38, 65]. The purification process of unfractionated heparin largely filters out alpha-gal proteins, but unfractionated heparin has nonetheless been implicated in alpha-gal reactions, likely due to glycoprotein impurities [67, 68]. Low-molecular-weight heparins, such as enoxaparin, appear to carry a low risk of reactions, likely due to a more extensive filtration process that removes larger molecules. Patients may require unfractionated heparin as a bridge for oral therapies or for treatment of new thrombi. Non-heparin-based anticoagulants, such as argatroban, may be suitable for therapeutic anticoagulation. However, certain cardiac and vascular surgery procedures require systemic forms of anticoagulation that provide easy reversibility (i.e., unfractionated heparin anticoagulation that is rapidly reversed with protamine). Therefore, risks and benefits should be considered regarding alpha-gal allergy versus rapid reversibility of anticoagulation. A recent review article on alpha-gal syndrome in the perioperative setting suggested a risk stratification algorithm for determining choice of anticoagulation in procedures though data verifying its efficacy is lacking [24]. In the event that a patient with a known alpha-gal allergy is in need for systemic anticoagulation during the perioperative period of an elective surgery, coordination with Allergy Immunology specialists for desensitization therapy may be necessary. Otherwise, development of an alternative anticoagulation plan with inpatient pharmacists and hematology specialists would be warranted [69].

Topical hemostatic agents are used to control intraoperative bleeding after a variety of standard surgical techniques [41–43, 70]. Many hemostatic agents are animal derived, and care should be taken to ensure only non-animal derived products are used in alpha-gal patients. Products to avoid include gelatin-based dry matrices, collagen-based dry matrices, bovine-derived topical thrombin, and bovine albumin-glutaraldehyde tissue adhesive. Combination products containing one or more of these ingredients are also available and should be avoided. Non-animal derived examples include cellulose-based agents or recombinant topical thrombin [71, 72]. In the future, such animal-derived products might be derived from animals for whom the alpha-gal producing enzyme is genetically removed, and such agents would be safe to use in AGS patients.

Active pharmaceutical ingredients are often accompanied by inactive ingredients, and these inactive ingredients may be derived from mammalian sources [21, 24, 37, 65, 73]. The most common reaction-inducing inactive ingredients derived from mammalian animals are gelatin and collagen. Other inactive ingredients are derived from animals, but reactions in patients with AGS have not been observed. These other inactive ingredients include lanolin, stearates, glycerin, and lactose [12, 37]. These agents are all used in a variety of oral medications, and some may be present in other dosage forms, such as dry-powder inhalers. Gelatin may be especially problematic, as many oral capsules utilize gelatin-based coating. Additionally, gelatin is always derived from mammals and is present in a higher quantity per dose than the other mammalian-derived inactive ingredients. Stearates are present in many different oral tablets, including commonplace analgesics such as oxycodone, and may be animal derived. The other inactive ingredients described in Table 15.4 are often present in lower quantities, are uncommonly used, or carry a lower risk of alpha-gal contamination. Overall, oral drugs contain a low enough quantity of alpha-gal excipients that they might not be problematic in the perioperative setting, but additional research is needed in this area.

Inactive ingredients in injectable medications are not usually derived from animals, as these agents typically only contain small quantities of buffer chemicals. One notable exception is propofol, which is suspended in a soybean oil emulsion that also contains glycerin [24, 51]. While glycerin carries low overall risk of alpha-gal contamination, caution is warranted, and alternative anesthetics (e.g., ketamine) should be considered in patients with severe allergies. Finally, biologics produced by the murine SP2/0 hybridoma should be avoided because it places alpha-gal haptens on the mAb, including cetuximab, which was one of the first medications identified to induce alpha-gal allergic reactions [9]. However, biologics are not typically utilized in the perioperative setting.

Prior to surgical procedures, all medical products that could potentially contain an allergen should be discussed among the medical team and patient. In cardiac surgeries, common products that may contain alpha-gal include bovine and porcine heart valves, which may induce hypersensitivity reactions in the perioperative time period or cause premature degeneration of the valve in an AGS patient [10, 11, 35, 36]. Alternative approaches for valve replacement include use of mechanical valves or minimization of the immune response via decellularization processes [11, 24, 74].

Recommended Practical Steps for a Patient with Alpha-Gal Syndrome

Mitigation of risk from AGS may be achieved through leverage of the electronic health record (EHR) and through multidisciplinary collaboration. Patients with AGS are often identified via preoperative screening at outpatient visits. Several practical steps should be taken as soon as AGS is identified or suspected in the patient, and these steps reduce the risk of perioperative complications. EHR systems often have a framework for allergy documentation (See Table 15.5), and users may be notified if an ordered medication is cross-reactive with the patient's documented allergies. In the case of AGS, several different substances and drugs are potentially problematic and may need to be documented individually.

Because galactose-alpha-1,3-galactose is a newly identified allergen, simple documentation of "alpha-gal" as a patient allergy may be insufficient to fully describe the extent of a patient's AGS. Clearly stated allergies to the most problematic agents, such as unfractionated heparin and cetuximab, decrease the chance that these drugs are accidentally ordered, particularly if users are unfamiliar with AGS. Additionally, adding "beef allergy" and "pork allergy" as patient allergies (See Table 15.5) will educate other providers on AGS and will ensure that agents

Table 15.5 Example AGS documentation in the electronic health record (EHR)

Allergen	Reaction	Severity	Date noted	Documentation
Beef and/or pork allergy	Anaphylaxis	High	01/22/2023	Due to alpha-gal allergy: Includes beef, pork, venison, goat, bison, or lamb. Eggs, poultry, and fish do not trigger allergic reactions
Cetuximab	Anaphylaxis	High	01/22/2023	Due to alpha-gal allergy
Collagen	Anaphylaxis	High	01/22/2023	Due to alpha-gal allergy
Gelatin	Anaphylaxis	High	01/22/2023	Due to alpha-gal allergy: Includes gelatin-containing foods (e.g., gummy bears, marshmallows)
Unfractionated heparin	Anaphylaxis	High	01/22/2023	Due to alpha-gal allergy; LMWH (enoxaparin) is preferred

such as bovine-derived thrombin are flagged consistently. The allergies should be labeled as high severity until proven otherwise; this is to ensure patients do not experience a severe reaction from direct exposure outside of the gastrointestinal tract, irrespective of the previous reaction severity from alpha-gal foods.

History of red meat allergies, which can be elucidated with a patient interview, requires follow-up beyond allergy documentation. Patients should be scheduled with an allergy specialist, ideally before the day of surgery. Allergy documentation should be added, and "Allergy to meat" should be added to the patient's problem list until AGS can be ruled out or confirmed. Preoperative personnel should notify the relevant surgery, anesthesiology, and pharmacy staff of the patient's allergy and the date of the procedure.

On the day of surgery, pharmacy personnel should be engaged in screening of medications for possible alpha-gal content, as appropriate. Because generic drugs often have multiple different manufacturers, screening of the dispensed medication for problematic inactive ingredients may be necessary. For example, acetaminophen from manufacturer 1 may be free of alpha-gal excipients, but the pharmacy may have acetaminophen from manufacturer 2 in stock, and this product may contain excipients such as gelatin or stearates. Identification of inactive ingredients is typically accomplished using publicly available resources, such as DailyMed or the manufacturer's prescribing information. If it is unclear whether a medication could be contaminated with alpha-gal, the manufacturer should be contacted directly to ensure the drug is not animal derived. When possible, providers in the operating room should ensure that medications used in the perioperative setting are consistently documented before administration to ensure the EHR database screens for allergy potential.

Conclusion

Alpha-gal syndrome, an IgE-mediated hypersensitivity reaction to galactose-alpha-1,3-galactose in mammalian meat and meat-derived products, presents a rising global challenge in the realm of food allergies. Sensitization and development

Table 15.6 Holistic guidance for patients with AGS [12]

Guidance for all patients at initial AGS diagnosis
FOOD
Avoid mammalian meats
Be cautious with high fat dairy & large amounts of butter
Educate regarding co-factors (esp., alcohol and activity) in setting of alpha-gal food exposure
Eating out can be challenging – inquire about fry oil, gravies, sauces and stocks. Some fast food restaurants add lard or suet to fryer (including French fries)
If tolerating dairy, full avoidance of this exposure may not be necessary
Equally, if dairy is tolerated then gelatin and carrageenan are often not issues
Cross-contamination during home cooking is typically ok (e.g., sharing spatulas)
Consider emu and duck as sources of meat to supplement chicken, turkey, seafood
Reminder about sausage casing as potential source of alpha-gal exposure
Consider referral to nutritionist if concern about safe and healthy forms of protein
ENVIRONMENT
Discuss tick bite prevention; refer to CDC website
Additional tick bites can increase sensitivity to various exposures (often transiently)
Having pets is fine but educate that pet dander can contain alpha-gal
Fumes from cooking mammalian meats are reported as an issue for some patients – consider educating in advance (although avoidance is not typically necessary)
Educate that bee, wasp, hornet stings may also lead to increased alpha-gal IgE
MEDICATIONS
Educate about heparin as possible iatrogenic exposure
Gelatin-based capsules are commonly not an issue
Lactose, microcrystalline cellulose and magnesium stearate may contain alpha-gal but are frequently not an issue
Should not receive vaccines with gelatin, if possible
Guidance for patients with continued reactivity despite avoidance diet
FOODS
Remove dairy in all forms, including butter
Remove gelatin and carrageenan
Read labels to avoid 'natural' flavoring as this often means pork or beef
ENVIRONMENT
Consider monthly washing of pets
Avoid fumes of mammalian meats being cooked
MEDICATION
Consider starting a daily oral anti-histamine
Switch to tablet formulations, consider opening capsules and taking with foods, if appropriate (e.g., medication is not time-release), or consider compounding pharmacy that will use plant-based gelatin capsule.
PERSONAL PRODUCTS
Switch to natural toothpaste
Avoid creams or lotions with lanolin

of IgE antibodies is thought to occur following exposure to tick bites, most notably the lone star tick (*A. americanum*) in the United States. Re-exposure to the alpha-gal allergen in ingested meats triggers a delayed anaphylactic reaction, which may manifest with cutaneous allergy symptoms, gastrointestinal disturbances, and potentially life-threatening shock, whereas exposure to alpha-gal proteins administered parenterally or on mucosal surfaces can produce immediate anaphylactic reactions. Diagnosis is established via detection of serum IgE antibodies to alpha-gal. Long-term management largely relies on avoidance of ticks and tick bites as well as medications and foods containing alpha-gal (see Table 15.6). Given the diverse presentation of symptoms and new emerging information on diagnosis and management, alpha-gal syndrome presents a unique challenge in the perioperative setting. The optimal algorithm for evaluating and managing such patients in the preoperative phase to limit reactions during surgery is a work in progress.

Chapter Summary

What are the critical questions required to identify a patient at risk for alpha gal syndrome?	•History of tick bites in endemic area? •History of delayed meat allergy reactions? •History of atopy (genetic tendency to develop allergic diseases such as allergic rhinitis, asthma, and eczema and association with heightened immune responses to allergen)?
If a patient has a history consistent with alpha gal syndrome, what perioperative changes should be made?	•Review of patient history and documentation in procedure plan •Avoidance of medications and surgical products implicated in inducing allergic reaction to alpha-gal •Contigency plans ready for potential anaphylactic reactions
In the event of a significant event including hypotension in the operating room, what diagnostic tests are required to confirm that the event occurred as a result of an anaphylactic reaction?	•Acute serum tryptase level (sAT), measured 30min to 120min after symptom onset, is higher compared to serum baseline level (sBT) by the calculation: sAT > 1.2 x sBT + 2

References

1. Simons FER. Anaphylaxis. J Allergy Clin Immunol. 2010;125(2):S161–81. https://doi.org/10.1016/j.jaci.2009.12.981.
2. Lieberman P, Camargo CA, Bohlke K, et al. Epidemiology of anaphylaxis: findings of the American College of Allergy, Asthma and Immunology Epidemiology of Anaphylaxis Working Group. Ann Allergy Asthma Immunol. 2006;97(5):596–602. https://doi.org/10.1016/S1081-1206(10)61086-1.
3. Liping Z, Bin H, Qiming F. An extraordinary case associated with an allergic reaction to Clopidogrel: coronary artery spasm or Kounis syndrome? Heart Lung Circ. 2015;24(11):e180–3. https://doi.org/10.1016/j.hlc.2015.04.183.
4. Sampson HA, Muñoz-Furlong A, Campbell RL, et al. Second symposium on the definition and management of anaphylaxis: summary report--Second National Institute of Allergy and Infectious Disease/Food Allergy and Anaphylaxis Network symposium. J Allergy Clin Immunol. 2006;117(2):391–7. https://doi.org/10.1016/j.jaci.2005.12.1303.

5. Varki A, Kornfeld S. Historical background and overview. In: Varki A, Cummings RD, Esko JD, et al., editors. Essentials of glycobiology. 4th ed. Cold Spring Harbor Laboratory Press; 2022. Accessed 1 Sep 2023. http://www.ncbi.nlm.nih.gov/books/NBK579927/.
6. Commins SP, Satinover SM, Hosen J, et al. Delayed anaphylaxis, angioedema, or urticaria after consumption of red meat in patients with IgE antibodies specific for galactose-α-1,3-galactose. J Allergy Clin Immunol. 2009;123(2):426–33. https://doi.org/10.1016/j.jaci.2008.10.052.
7. Commins SP, James HR, Kelly EA, et al. The relevance of tick bites to the production of IgE antibodies to the mammalian oligosaccharide galactose-α-1,3-galactose. J Allergy Clin Immunol. 2011;127(5):1286–1293.e6. https://doi.org/10.1016/j.jaci.2011.02.019.
8. Commins SP, Platts-Mills TAE. Delayed anaphylaxis to red meat in patients with IgE specific for galactose alpha-1,3-galactose (alpha-gal). Curr Allergy Asthma Rep. 2013;13(1):72–7. https://doi.org/10.1007/s11882-012-0315-y.
9. Chung CH, Mirakhur B, Chan E, et al. Cetuximab-induced anaphylaxis and IgE specific for galactose-α-1,3-galactose. N Engl J Med. 2008;358(11):1109–17. https://doi.org/10.1056/NEJMoa074943.
10. Hawkins RB, Frischtak HL, Kron IL, Ghanta RK. Premature bioprosthetic aortic valve degeneration associated with allergy to galactose-Alpha-1,3-galactose. J Card Surg. 2016;31(7):446–8. https://doi.org/10.1111/jocs.12764.
11. Kuravi KV, Sorrells LT, Nellis JR, et al. Allergic response to medical products in patients with alpha-gal syndrome. J Thorac Cardiovasc Surg. 2022;164(6):e411–24. https://doi.org/10.1016/j.jtcvs.2021.03.100.
12. Commins SP. Diagnosis & management of alpha-gal syndrome:lessons from 2,500 patients. Expert Rev Clin Immunol. 2020;16(7):667–77. https://doi.org/10.1080/1744666X.2020.1782745.
13. Macdougall JD, Thomas KO, Iweala OI. The meat of the matter: understanding and managing Alpha-gal syndrome. ImmunoTargets Ther. 2022;11:37–54. https://doi.org/10.2147/ITT.S276872.
14. Crispell G, Commins SP, Archer-Hartman SA, et al. Discovery of Alpha-gal-containing antigens in north American tick species believed to induce red meat allergy. Front Immunol. 2019;10:1056. https://doi.org/10.3389/fimmu.2019.01056.
15. Choudhary SK, Karim S, Iweala OI, et al. Tick salivary gland extract induces alpha-gal syndrome in alpha-gal deficient mice. Immun Inflamm Dis. 2021;9(3):984–90. https://doi.org/10.1002/iid3.457.
16. Park Y, Kim D, Boorgula GD, et al. Alpha-gal and cross-reactive carbohydrate determinants in the N-Glycans of salivary glands in the lone star tick, *Amblyomma americanum*. Vaccine. 2020;8(1):18. https://doi.org/10.3390/vaccines8010018.
17. Apostolovic D, Tran TAT, Hamsten C, Starkhammar M, Cirkovic Velickovic T, van Hage M. Immunoproteomics of processed beef proteins reveal novel galactose-α-1,3-galactose-containing allergens. Allergy. 2014;69(10):1308–15. https://doi.org/10.1111/all.12462.
18. Pattanaik D, Lieberman P, Lieberman J, Pongdee T, Keene AT. The changing face of anaphylaxis in adults and adolescents. Ann Allergy Asthma Immunol. 2018;121(5):594–7. https://doi.org/10.1016/j.anai.2018.07.017.
19. Zurbano-Azqueta L, Antón-Casas E, Duque-Gómez S, Jiménez-Gómez I, Fernández-Pellón L, López-Gutiérrez J. Alpha-gal syndrome. Allergy to red meat and gelatin. Rev Clin Esp. 2022;222(7):401–5. https://doi.org/10.1016/j.rceng.2021.06.005.
20. Van Nunen SA, O'Connor KS, Clarke LR, Boyle RX, Fernando SL. An association between tick bite reactions and red meat allergy in humans. Med J Aust. 2009;190(9):510–1. https://doi.org/10.5694/j.1326-5377.2009.tb02533.x.
21. Dunkman WJ, Rycek W, Manning MW. What does a red meat allergy have to do with anesthesia? Perioperative management of alpha-gal syndrome. Anesth Analg. 2019;129(5):1242–8. https://doi.org/10.1213/ANE.0000000000003460.

22. Anthes E. A half-million Americans may have tick-linked meat allergy, C.D.C. Says. The New York Times. https://wwwnytimescom/2023/07/27/health/alpha-gal-ticks-meat-allergyhtml Published July 27, 2023. Accessed 30 Aug 2023.
23. Platts-Mills TAE, Commins SP, Biedermann T, et al. On the cause and consequences of IgE to galactose-α−1,3-galactose: a report from the National Institute of allergy and infectious disease workshop on understanding IgE-mediated mammalian meat allergy. J Allergy Clin Immunol. 2020;145(4):1061–71. https://doi.org/10.1016/j.jaci.2020.01.047.
24. Nourian MM, Stone CA, Siegrist KK, Riess ML. Perioperative implications of patients with alpha gal allergies. J Clin Anesth. 2023;86:111056. https://doi.org/10.1016/j.jclinane.2023.111056.
25. Vaz-Rodrigues R, Mazuecos L, de la Fuente J. Current and future strategies for the diagnosis and treatment of the Alpha-gal syndrome (AGS). J Asthma Allergy. 2022;15:957–70. https://doi.org/10.2147/JAA.S265660.
26. Binder AM, Commins SP, Altrich ML, et al. Diagnostic testing for galactose-alpha-1,3-galactose, United States, 2010 to 2018. Ann Allergy Asthma Immunol. 2021;126(4):411–416.e1. https://doi.org/10.1016/j.anai.2020.12.019.
27. Carson AS, Gardner A, Iweala OI. Where's the beef?: Understanding allergic responses to red meat in Alpha-gal syndrome. J Immunol Baltim Md 1950. 2022;208(2):267–277. doi: https://doi.org/10.4049/jimmunol.2100712.
28. Murangi T, Prakash P, Moreira BP, et al. Ascaris lumbricoides and ticks associated with sensitization to galactose α1,3-galactose and elicitation of the alpha-gal syndrome. J Allergy Clin Immunol. 2022;149(2):698–707.e3. https://doi.org/10.1016/j.jaci.2021.07.018.
29. Tick-Borne Diseases: Resources | NIOSH | CDC. Published September 15, 2021. Accessed 30 Aug 2023. https://www.cdc.gov/niosh/topics/tick-borne/resources.html
30. Mabelane T, Basera W, Botha M, Thomas HF, Ramjith J, Levin ME. Predictive values of alpha-gal IgE levels and alpha-gal IgE: Total IgE ratio and oral food challenge-proven meat allergy in a population with a high prevalence of reported red meat allergy. Pediatr Allergy Immunol. 2018;29(8):841–9. https://doi.org/10.1111/pai.12969.
31. Iweala OI, Choudhary SK, Addison CT, Commins SP. T and B lymphocyte transcriptional states differentiate between sensitized and Unsensitized individuals in Alpha-gal syndrome. Int J Mol Sci. 2021;22(6):3185. https://doi.org/10.3390/ijms22063185.
32. Platts-Mills T, Li R, Keshavarz B, Smith A, Wilson J. Diagnosis and management of patients with the α-gal syndrome. J Allergy Clin Immunol Pract. 2020;8(1):15–23.e1. https://doi.org/10.1016/j.jaip.2019.09.017.
33. Commins SP, James HR, Stevens W, et al. Delayed clinical and ex vivo response to mammalian meat in patients with IgE to galactose-alpha-1,3-galactose. J Allergy Clin Immunol. 2014;134(1):108–115.e11. https://doi.org/10.1016/j.jaci.2014.01.024.
34. Binder AM, Cherry-Brown D, Biggerstaff BJ, et al. Clinical and laboratory features of patients diagnosed with alpha-gal syndrome—2010–2019. Allergy. 2023;78(2):477–87. https://doi.org/10.1111/all.15539.
35. Mangold A, Szerafin T, Hoetzenecker K, et al. Alpha-gal specific IgG immune response after implantation of bioprostheses. Thorac Cardiovasc Surg. 2009;57(4):191–5. https://doi.org/10.1055/s-0029-1185395.
36. Mozzicato SM, Tripathi A, Posthumus JB, Platts-Mills TAE, Commins SP. Porcine or bovine valve replacement in three patients with IgE antibodies to the mammalian oligosaccharide galactose-alpha-1,3-galactose. J Allergy Clin Immunol Pract. 2014;2(5):637–8. https://doi.org/10.1016/j.jaip.2014.04.016.
37. Rowe RC, Sheskey PJ, Quinn ME. Handbook of pharmaceutical excipients. 5th ed. Pharmaceutical Press; 2006.
38. Heparin sodium injection (single- and multi-dose vials) [prescribing information]. Lake Zurich, IL: Fesenius Kabi; 2023.
39. Lovenox (enoxaparin) [prescribing information]. Bridgewater, NJ: Sanofi-Aventis US LLC; 2022.

40. Argatroban injection [prescribing information]. Schaumburg, IL: Sagent Pharmaceuticals; 2021.
41. Thrombin-JMI (thrombin) [prescribing information]. New York, NY: Pfizer Inc; 2022.
42. Gelfoam (gelatin [absorbable]) sponge [prescribing information]. New York, NY: Pfizer Inc; 2022.
43. Avitene (microfibrillar collagen hemostat) [prescribing information]. Franklin Lakes, NJ: Becton, Dickinson and Company; 2023.
44. Erbitux (cetuximab) [prescribing information]. Indianapolis, IN: Eli Lilly and Company; 2021.
45. Creon (pancrelipase) [prescribing information]. North Chicago, IL: AbbVie Inc; 2022.
46. Armour thyroid (thyroid tablet) [prescribing information]. Madison, NJ: Allergan; 2018.
47. M-M-R II (measles, mumps, and rubella virus vaccine live) [prescribing information]. Whitehouse Station, NJ: Merck Sharp & Dohme Corp; 2023.
48. Zostavax (zoster vaccine live) [prescribing information]. Whitehouse Station, NJ: Merck Sharp & Dohme Corp; 2019.
49. Boostrix (tetanus toxoid, reduced diphtheria toxoid and acellular pertussis vaccine, adsorbed) [prescribing information]. Durham, NC: GlaxoSmithKline; 2022.
50. YF-VAX (yellow fever vaccine) [prescribing information]. Swiftwater, PA: Sanofi Pasteur Inc; 2020.
51. Diprivan (propofol) [Prescribing information]. Lake Zurich, IL: Fresenius Kabi; 2022.
52. Cleviprex (clevidipine) [prescribing information]. Cary, NC: Chiesi USA Inc; 2022.
53. Shah R, Schwartz RA. Meat allergy: a ticking time bomb. Am J Clin Dermatol. 2022;23(4):515–21. https://doi.org/10.1007/s40257-022-00696-x.
54. Calvani M, Bianchi A, Reginelli C, Peresso M, Testa A. Oral food challenge. Medicina (Mex). 2019;55(10):651. https://doi.org/10.3390/medicina55100651.
55. Kim M, Straesser MD, Keshavarz B, et al. IgE to galactose-α-1, 3-galactose wanes over time in patients who avoid tick bites. J Allergy Clin Immunol Pract. 2020;8(1):364–367.e2. https://doi.org/10.1016/j.jaip.2019.08.045.
56. Wolaver W, Thakrar S, Thomas K, et al. Demystifying α-gal syndrome: identification and risk management in the perioperative setting. Curr Opin Anaesthesiol. 2021;34(6):761–5. https://doi.org/10.1097/ACO.0000000000001066.
57. Payne V, Kam PCA. Mast cell tryptase: a review of its physiology and clinical significance. Anaesthesia. 2004;59(7):695–703. https://doi.org/10.1111/j.1365-2044.2004.03757.x.
58. Valent P, Akin C, Bonadonna P, et al. Proposed diagnostic algorithm for patients with suspected mast cell activation syndrome (MCAS). J Allergy Clin Immunol Pract. 2019;7(4):1125–1133.e1. https://doi.org/10.1016/j.jaip.2019.01.006.
59. Baretto RL, Beck S, Heslegrave J, et al. Validation of international consensus equation for acute serum total tryptase in mast cell activation: a perioperative perspective. Allergy. 2017;72(12):2031–4. https://doi.org/10.1111/all.13226.
60. Vitte J, Amadei L, Gouitaa M, et al. Paired acute-baseline serum tryptase levels in perioperative anaphylaxis: an observational study. Allergy. 2019;74(6):1157–65. https://doi.org/10.1111/all.13752.
61. Laroche D, Gomis P, Gallimidi E, Malinovsky JM, Mertes PM. Diagnostic value of histamine and tryptase concentrations in severe anaphylaxis with shock or cardiac arrest during anesthesia. Anesthesiology. 2014;121(2):272–9. https://doi.org/10.1097/ALN.0000000000000276.
62. Guyer AC, Saff RR, Conroy M, et al. Comprehensive allergy evaluation is useful in the subsequent care of patients with drug hypersensitivity reactions during anesthesia. J Allergy Clin Immunol Pract. 2015;3(1):94–100. https://doi.org/10.1016/j.jaip.2014.11.011.
63. Mertes PM, Alla F, Tréchot P, Auroy Y, Jougla E. Groupe d'Etudes des Réactions Anaphylactoïdes Peranesthésiques. Anaphylaxis during anesthesia in France: an 8-year national survey. J Allergy Clin Immunol. 2011;128(2):366–73. https://doi.org/10.1016/j.jaci.2011.03.003.
64. van Klei WA, Szabo MD, Hesterberg PE. Case 22-2023: a 59-year-old woman with hypotension and electrocardiographic changes. N Engl J Med. 2023;389(3):263–72. https://doi.org/10.1056/NEJMcpc2300898.

65. Wolfe RC, Blunt J. Perioperative considerations for the emerging Alpha-gal allergy. J Perianesth Nurs. 2021;36(4):435–7. https://doi.org/10.1016/j.jopan.2021.05.002.
66. ANAVIP (Crotalidae Immune F[ab']2 [Equine]) [prescribing information]. Franklin, TN: Rare Disease Therapeutics Inc; 2022.
67. Nwamara U, Kaplan MC, Mason N, Ingemi AI. A retrospective evaluation of heparin product reactions in patients with alpha-gal allergies. Ticks Tick-Borne Dis. 2022;13(1):101869. https://doi.org/10.1016/j.ttbdis.2021.101869.
68. Hawkins RB, Wilson JM, Mehaffey JH, Platts-Mills TAE, Ailawadi G. Safety of intravenous heparin for cardiac surgery in patients with Alpha-gal syndrome. Ann Thorac Surg. 2021;111(6):1991–7. https://doi.org/10.1016/j.athoracsur.2020.07.050.
69. McRae AS, Tidwell WP, Patel S, Lombard FW. Heparin desensitisation prior to cardiopulmonary bypass in a patient with alpha-gal allergy. Anaesth Rep. 2022;10(2):e12203. https://doi.org/10.1002/anr3.12203.
70. Summary of Safety and Effectiveness: CryoLife, Inc., BioGlue Surgical Adhesive. U.S. Food & Drug Administration website. Accessed 18 Apr 2023. https://www.accessdata.fda.gov/cdrh_docs/pdf/p010003b.pdf.
71. Surgicel Original, Nu-Knit, and Fibrillar (oxidized regenerated cellulose) [prescribing information]. Somerville, NJ: Ethicon US LLC; 2018.
72. Recothrom (thrombin) [prescribing information]. Deerfield, IL: Baxter Healthcare Corp; 2020.
73. D'Ercole FJ, Dhandha VH, Levi ML, Todd AB, Kumar PA. Perioperative challenges in patients with Alpha-gal allergy. J Clin Anesth Pain Manag. 2019;3(1) Accessed 5 Jul 2023. https://scholars.direct/Articles/anesthesia-and-pain-management/jcapm-3-016.php?jid=anesthesia-and-pain-management
74. Lim HG, Kim GB, Jeong S, Kim YJ. Development of a next-generation tissue valve using a glutaraldehyde-fixed porcine aortic valve treated with decellularization, α-galactosidase, space filler, organic solvent and detoxification. Eur J Cardio-Thorac Surg Off J Eur Assoc Cardio-Thorac Surg. 2015;48(1):104–13. https://doi.org/10.1093/ejcts/ezu385.

Chapter 16
Penicillin and Beta-Lactam Drug Allergy

Wei Zhao

Case Report

Case 1

A 25-year-old woman in her first trimester of pregnancy was seen in OB clinic for her routine prenatal screening. Serologic testing was positive for syphilis. After consulting an infectious disease specialist, late latent syphilis was diagnosed. Infectious disease service recommended three weekly intramuscular injections of penicillin G benzathine. However, the patient reports that she had allergic reaction to Amoxicillin when she was a young child based on what her mother told her. The details of the reaction are not available since it happened many years ago.

The patient was referred to an allergist for drug allergy evaluation. Skin test was performed with pre-pen and penicillin G that showed negative. She then received one dose of Amoxicillin as a drug challenge. The patient tolerated the challenge. She was then treated with intramuscular penicillin G benzathine for her late latent syphilis without any adverse reaction. Her allergy history was updated in her medical chart to indicate no allergy to penicillin [1].

Case 2

A 58-year-old man with medical history of left anterior cruciate ligament repair was admitted for work-up of acute-onset polyarthralgia, intense pruritus of hands and feet, and fever for 4 days.

Patient was prescribed 10-day course of amoxicillin/clavulanic for the treatment of right-hand cellulitis resulting from biting of blue crabs. His cellulitis symptoms were completely resolved after 4 days of treatment. However, 5 days after

W. Zhao (✉)
Division of Allergy and Immunology, Department of Pediatrics, Virginia Commonwealth University, Richmond, VA, USA
e-mail: wei.zhao@vcuhealth.org

W. A. Zuelzer, S. Metikala (eds.), *Unusual Conditions That Every Orthopaedic Surgeon Should Know*, https://doi.org/10.1007/978-3-031-58946-1_16

completion of his antibiotic course, the patient developed joint swelling of his right hand, accompanied by fever, chills, and malaise. He then presented to the local emergency department and later on was admitted to internal medicine service. Laboratory findings included leukocytosis without left shift, mild elevation of LFT, CRP of 16.9 mg/dl. C3 and C4 were within normal range. UA revealed trace proteinuria. A diagnosis of serum sickness-like reaction was made. Patient was started on non-steroidal anti-inflammatories. Three days after admission, patient reported dramatic improvement in pain and range of motion. Physical examination showed minimal residual swelling and full range of motion of all joints except right wrist. Patient was discharged home with follow-up with PCP [2].

Case 3

One year after a left total knee replacement (TKR), a 69-year-old woman developed joint infection. She was treated with antibiotics. Revision of the implant was performed including insertion of an articulated spacer with antibiotic-loaded bone cement containing 1.0 g of gentamicin, 3.0 g of vancomycin, and 4.5 g of Tazocin per 40 g package of cement (previous skin test to each antibiotic was negative). On the 15th postoperative day, she developed moderate pain in the left knee without swelling and generalized erythematous changes accompanied by rigor. Lab testing showed WBC $3.8 \times 10^3/mm^3$, ESR 81 mm/h, eosinophils 11.2%, and CRP 6.1 mg/dl. Her left knee was hot and tender, but not swollen. She developed fever (38.6 °C), tachypnea, hypertension, and tachycardia with maculopapular skin eruptions on the neck, face, and both arms with itching. Left knee aspirate testing was not consistent with infection. The patient underwent intravenous provocation challenge using low doses of gentamycin, vancomycin, Tazocin, and first generation of cephalosporin, respectively. Seven hours after intravenous injection of a half dose of piperacillin/tazobactam, rigors with a fever >38 °C developed, lasting for 2 days accompanied by a reddish skin rash and an itching sensation over the entire body. Laboratory findings showed an increase in WBC, CRP, and ESR. Patient reported no previous exposure to piperacillin/tazobactam. It was concluded that the reaction was due to piperacillin/tazobactam in the bone cement. The cement spacer and all the beads were removed and a second-stage revision TKR with vancomycin-loaded bone cement was performed. All symptoms resolved thereafter and laboratory findings returned to normal 1 month after the second revision. Six months later, she had no pain on walking or exercise and a range of movement at the knee from 5° of extension to 100° of flexion [3].

Review Questions

1. A 60-year-old man presents with osteomyelitis. Infectious disease consultation recommends the use of Zosyn as treatment. Patient revealed that his mother told him that he developed rash after Amoxicillin treatment for ear infection when he was toddler. The characteristic of rash is not clear since his mother passed away 5 years ago. He has not received Penicillin or Amoxicillin because he was labeled as penicillin allergic. What is the best approach regarding antibiotic treatment for his osteomyelitis?

2. A 30-year-old man developed wound infection after laceration on his right thumb. Urgent care facility placed him on Augmentin treatment. He previously tolerated Amoxicillin for bronchitis. The patient developed hives after 3 days of Augmentin treatment. Hives appeared first on face, then spread to trunk, arms, and legs within 12 h. By this time, wound culture grows Streptococcus. Sensitivity test shows sensitive to Ampicillin, Cephalexin, and Bactrim. His primary doctor stopped his Augmentin due to concern of Augmentin allergy. Patient reported that he developed skin rash after Bactrim when he was in college. In this case, can Cephalexin be used in this patient for wound treatment even if it is part of the β-lactam antibiotic category?
3. A 45-year-old woman presents to the emergency department for fever, malaise, and a diffuse rash that almost completely covers her body. She reports that the symptoms started 4 weeks after she began to take Amoxicillin for strep throat. Your examination shows a diffuse, erythematous, maculopapular eruption, and facial swelling. There are no mucosal findings. Associated cervical lymphadenopathy and hepatomegaly are noted. Laboratory testing reveals peripheral eosinophilia. What is your diagnosis?

Background

WHO defines adverse drug reactions (ADRs) as any noxious, unintended, and undesired effect of a drug that occurs at doses used for prevention, diagnosis, or treatment. ADRs can be divided into two subtypes. Type A reaction is predictable, dose-dependent, related to the pharmacologic action of the drug, and accounts for about 80% of ADRs. Type A reaction can be subdivided into overdosing, side effects, secondary effects, and drug interactions. Type B reaction, on the other hand, is unpredictable, unrelated to the pharmacologic action of the drug, less dose-dependent, and occurs only in 20% of ADRs individuals who are susceptible to such drug. Type B reaction includes drug intolerance, drug allergy, and nonallergic reactions with immunologic manifestations (previously referred to as pseudoallergic reaction) through direct release of mediators from mast cells and basophils without the involvement of IgE antibodies. About 15–20% patients experience ADRS with 6.7% being severe and 0.32% fatal, making ADRs the fourth to sixth leading cause of death in hospital setting [4].

Most drugs (except biologics) are small molecules that will not act as allergen to directly induce immune response. The hapten-prohapten model and the pharmacologic-interaction model are popular theories that explain the immunomechanism of drug allergy. A hapten is defined as small molecules such as drugs or drug metabolites that are too small to elicit a specific immune response. Such hapten can covalently bind to host protein on cell surfaces and in plasma to form hapten-protein complex (complete antigen) that can induce T- and B-cell responses. Typically, penicillin and its metabolites are considered as hapten. Some drugs such as sulfonamides are considered as pro-haptens that gain their ability to covalently bind to protein only after being metabolized [5]. Hapten theory can explain IgE-mediated drug reaction such as anaphylaxis. However, severe skin-related reactions such as fixed drug rash, Stevens-Johnson Syndrome, and Toxic Epidermal Necrolysis are mainly T cell-mediated processes. An alternative model based on pharmacologic interaction with immune receptors (p-i) concept was developed to explain such non-IgE-mediated drug allergic reaction. Herein, some drugs that are unable to covalently bind to protein can form noncovalent bonds directly to T cell receptors and/or major histocompatibility complex (MHC) protein on antigen-presenting cells. Such binding leads to T cell-mediated reaction [5].

Based on Gell and Coombs classification, drug allergy can be classified into four types according to immune mediators involved. Types 1 to 3 are mainly antibody-dependent reactions. Type 4 reaction, the T cell-mediated delayed hypersensitivity, has recently been classified into four subtypes. Type 1 hypersensitivity reactions, also known as immediate reaction, usually occur within minutes to hours after repeated exposure to the antigen (drug). In Type 1 reaction, upon initial exposure, antigen-presenting cells such as dendritic cells can process penicillin-carrier protein complex to present to CD4+ T cell. The latter then develops into penicillin-specific Helper T cells. Such Th2 cells in turn, induce B cells to produce penicillin-specific IgE. Those IgE molecules bind to IgE receptors on the surface of mast cells. After further exposure, penicillin-protein career binds to specific IgE and cross-link IgE receptors and activate mast cells. Mast cells undergo degranulation and release inflammatory mediators such as histamine, prostaglandins, and leukotrienes, leading to the clinical manifestations of anaphylaxis, angioedema, urticaria, and bronchospasm. Type 2 hypersensitivity reactions occur within days to weeks after medication exposure. They are mediated by IgM or IgG type of antibodies specific to drug antigen. Such a reaction is cytotoxic. Clinical presentations include leukocytosis, thrombocytopenia, hemolytic anemia. Type 3 hypersensitivity reactions are mediated by immune-complex formed by drug antigen and antibodies (IgG or IgM). Such a reaction also happens within days to weeks after exposure to the drug. Serum sickness and drug fever are the prototypes of type 3 reaction with presentations including fever, rash, and joint pain. Delayed reactions, also known as Type 4 hypersensitivity reactions, where activated T cells mediate cascade of inflammation that leads to drug rash, in rare cases, systemic involvement such as SJS-TEN, DRESS, and AGEP. In Type 4a reactions, Th1 cells secrete IFN-γ that in turn activates macrophages and CD8 T cell responses with prototype of contact dermatitis. Type 4b reactions are triggered by Th2 cells that produce IL-4, IL-5, and IL-13, leading to response of B cells, mast cells, and eosinophils. A typical example of type 4b is DRESS. Type 4c reaction is mediated by cytotoxic T cells that release mediators such as granulysin, perforin, and granzyme B that cause cell death, resulting in disorders like SJS and TEN. Type 4d results from T cell producing chemokine CXCL8 and GM-CSF. Those mediators recruit neutrophils that lead to sterile inflammation such as AGEP and Behcet disease [6] (Table 16.1).

About 10% of patients report a history of allergic reaction to penicillin family antibiotics. Such patients often need to receive alternative, maybe less effective, often more expensive, potentially more toxic, antibiotics such as vancomycin, cephalosporins, clindamycin, and fluoroquinolones for the treatment of their infection or

Table 16.1 Classification of hypersensitivity reaction

Extended coombs and gell classification[a]	Type of immune response[b]	Pathologic characteristics	Clinical symptoms[b]	Covalent and noncovalent drug Binding[c]	Cell type
Type I	IgE[d]	Mast-cell degranulation	Urticaria, anaphylaxis	Covalent drug binding	B cells/Ig
Type II	IgG and FcR[d]	FcR–dependent cell destruction	Blood cell dyscrasia	Covalent drug binding	B cells/Ig
Type III	IgG and complement or FcR[d]	Immunocomplex deposition	Vasculitis	Covalent drug binding	B cells/Ig
Type IVa	Th 1 (IFN-γ)	Monocyte activation	Eczema	Covalent and noncovalent drug binding	T cells
Type IVb	Th 2 (IL-5 and IL-4)	Eosinophilic inflammation	Maculopapular exanthema, bullous exanthema	Covalent and noncovalent drug binding	T cells
Type IVc	CTL (perforin and granzyme B)	CD4- or CD8-mediated killing of cells (i.e., keratinocyte)	Maculopapular exanthema, eczema, bullous exanthema, pustular exanthema	Covalent and noncovalent drug binding	T cells
Type IVd	T cells (IL-8)	Neutrophil recruitment and activation	Pustular exanthema	Covalent and noncovalent drug binding	T cells

Adapted from Werner J Pichler. Delayed drug hypersensitivity reactions. [6]

[a]Modified from original Gell and Coombs Classification [6]

[b]Only dominant reaction is shown. Multiple types of reactions can occur together

[c]Covalent binding can elicit both T- and B-cell mediated reactions, while noncovalent binding may only elicit T-cell reaction

[d]γ T-cell help for Ig (IL-4, IL-5, and IFN- γ

perioperative prophylaxis [7–9]. Such practice is associated with increased risk of postoperative complications including surgical site infection (SSI) [10]. After reviewing over 8000 penicillin allergic patients with half of them having orthopaedic conditions, Blumenthal and colleagues revealed 50% increased odds of surgical site infection from penicillin allergy patients who had to be put on alternative antibiotics [11]. Niu et al. recently reported increased SSI (1.06%, 18 /1704) in penicillin allergy patients than non-penicillin allergic patients (0.51%, 93/18,318) who underwent orthopaedic surgeries [12]. However, after proper evaluation, over 90% of those Penicillin allergic patients can tolerate penicillins [13]. The use of alternative antibiotics is also associated with increased healthcare-associated infections such as 23% increased odds of *Clostridium difficile*, a 14% increased odds of methicillin-resistant *Staphylococcus aureus*, and 30% increased odds of vancomycin-resistant Enterococcus [14–16].

Reasons for such discrepancy are losing of penicillin-specific IgE, underlying infection-related rash, mislabeling non-immunologic symptoms as allergic. Therefore, clinicians should make an effort to delabel penicillin allergy in outpatient as well as perioperative settings.

Topic

In 1928, Alexander Flemming discovered penicillin, the active component of penicillium fungus that could kill bacteria in laboratory. In 1942, penicillin was widely used in the treatment of staphylococcal and streptococcal bacterial infections. Fleming, Florey, and Chain jointly received the 1945 Nobel Prize in Physiology or Medicine due to their discovery of penicillin and its impact in treating various infectious diseases [17].

The first penicillin allergy case was reported in 1945. Penicillin family antibiotics share the same core β-lactam and thiazolidine ring structures. However, they differ in their side chains. The ring structure is metabolized into penicilloyl (major determinates) and Penicillin, penicilloate, and penilloate (minor determinates). Both major and minor determinates are considered as hapten. They need to bind to host protein to form hapten-carrier complex. Such hapten-protein model applies to immediate or antibody-mediated penicillin hypersensitivity (Gell-Coombs type I, II, and III reactions) [18].

IgE-mediated reaction: IgE-mediated allergic reaction to β-lactam antibiotics follows the typical mast-cell and basophil degranulation through IgE-crosslinking of high-affinity IgE receptors. It usually has quick onset (<1 h) but can be considered within 6 h of exposure. Urticaria and angioedema are the most common presentations, followed by bronchospasm, drop of blood pressure, and GI symptoms such as vomiting and diarrhea. Any organ and system can be involved. Severe cases present with anaphylaxis. Diagnosis is based on thorough history to demonstrate the association of symptoms with the introduction of penicillin, physical examination, in conjunction with penicillin skin test. In patients suspected anaphylaxis, serum tryptase levels measured between 30 min and 1.5 h after reaction is recommended.

Treatment of acute IgE-mediated reaction to penicillin family of antibiotics: Patients with acute anaphylaxis should receive immediate treatment of IM epinephrine 0.3–0.5 mg. Other therapies include H1 and H2 antihistamines such as diphenhydramine 25–50 mg IV and famotidine 40 mg IV. Patients who are refractory to treatment should receive Epinephrine drip at 1 mcg/kg/min. Albuterol at 2.5 mg should be used for patients who experience bronchospasm. All patients who present with acute anaphylaxis should be placed on telemetry monitoring and receive IV normal saline bolus (1–2 L) [19].

Penicillin skin testing is used to evaluate IgE-mediated penicillin allergy by board-certified allergist. This is done by skin-prick testing with major and minor determinants followed by intradermal testing. A wheal size of at least 3 mm above negative control is considered as positive. Such testing has a positive predictive value of 30.7% and negative predictive value over 96.8% [20–22]. Of course, the test should not be performed in patients with severe non-IgE-mediated reaction.

When skin test is negative, a graded-dose challenge can then be performed. Patient will receive 1/100 (history of anaphylaxis) or 1/10 (nonanaphylactic reaction) of a dose followed by 30 min observation. If no reaction, the patient will then receive a full treatment dose followed by a period of observation. Recent recommendation is to perform direct, one dose amoxicillin challenge without penicillin skin test in patients with history of mild cutaneous reactions. The graded-challenge is contraindicated in patients with history of severe non-IgE-mediated reaction such as Stevens-Johnson syndrome (SJS) or toxic epidermal necrolysis (TEN).

In patients with low-risk reaction history, one-step challenge (full strength dose) or two-step challenge (1/10 followed by full dose in 30–60 min interval) is indicated.

Desensitization: For patients with proved Type 1 IgE-mediated penicillin allergy, alternative antibiotics should be used for treatment. If no equally efficacious antibiotic is available and penicillin is the first-line therapy, the patient should undergo drug desensitization [23]. Protocols using intramuscular, intravenous, and oral desensitization have been developed and validated. A typical 14-step oral desensitization protocol is listed below. Penicillin doses are doubled every 15–30 min until therapeutic dosage is reached. Mild symptoms are treated with antihistamines. Anaphylaxis is rare, occuring in <1% of patients [24]. Of note, desensitization only has temporary effects. It lasts for up to two dosing intervals of the medication. If lapsed, desensitization needs to be repeated (Table 16.2).

Skin test procedures for delayed reaction to penicillins such as patch, delayed prick, and intradermal testing are not standardized [25].

Cross-reactivity: Historically, it was considered 10% cross-reactivity between penicillin and cephalosporin. Such notion is mainly based on some early studies from 1970s [26, 27]. Such concept had led to the notion that Cephalosporin "should not be used in patients with documented or presumed IgE-mediated penicillin allergy" as recommended by surgical guidelines for antimicrobial prophylaxis [28]. Later on, it was understood that cephalosporins introduced before 1980 had contamination of trace amount of penicillin [29]. This may explain a much lower true cross-reactivity between penicillin and cephalosporin. Although both penicillin and cephalosporins share a core β-lactam ring, penicillin has a five-membered thiazolidine ring while cephalosporins have a six-membered dihydrothiazine ring [30]. After metabolism, penicillin retains its thiazolidine ring while cephalosporins degrade both their β-lactam and dihydrothiazine rings. Such difference in breakdown products and predominant R-1 based allergy may explain the very low cross-reactivity between penicillin and cephalosporin (1–2%). Table 16.3 lists β-lactam antibiotics that share identical R1-group side chains. Typical examples are: Amoxicillin shares R1 structure with Cefadroxil and Cefprozil. Ampicillin shares with Cefaclor and Cephalexin. Aztreonam shares with Ceftazidime. The current drug allergy practice parameter recommends cephalosporin to be routinely administered without testing on patients with history of unverified nonanaphylactic penicillin allergy. For patients with history of anaphylaxis to penicillin, a

Table 16.2 Penicillin desensitization protocol

Step	Concentration of drug (mg/mL)	Amount (mL)	Dose given (mg)	Cumulative dose (mg)
1	0.5	0.1	0.05	0.05
2	0.5	0.2	0.10	0.15
3	0.5	0.4	0.20	0.35
4	0.5	0.8	0.40	0.75
5	0.5	1.6	0.80	1.55
6	0.5	3.2	1.60	3.15
7	0.5	6.4	3.20	6.35
8	5.0	1.2	6.00	12.35
9	5.0	2.4	12.00	24.35
10	5.0	4.8	24.00	48.35
11	50.0	1.0	50.00	98.35
12	50.0	2.0	100.00	198.35
13	50.0	4.0	200.00	398.35
14	50.0	8.0	400.00	798.35
Observe patient for 30 min, and then administer 1 g of same agent intravenously				

Adapted from β Yates AB. Management of patients with a history of allergy to β-lactam antibiotics [24]

Table 16.3 β-lactam antibiotics that share the same R1-group

Amoxicillin	Ampicillin	Ceftriaxone	Cefoxitin	Cefamandole	Ceftazidime
Cefadroxil	Cefaclor	Cefotaxime	Cephaloridine	Cefonicid	Aztreonam
Cefprozil	Cephalexin	Cefpodoxime	Cephalothin		
Cefatrizine	Cephradine	Cefditoren			
	Cephaloglycin	Ceftizoxime			
	Loracarbef	Cefmenoxime			

Adapted from Khan. Drug Allergy: an updated practice parameter [31]

non-cross-reactive cephalosporin (different R1 structure such as Cefazolin) can be administered routinely without prior testing. Kurcz and colleagues reported their experience from 2451 total joint arthroplasty patients. Only one patient with a documented penicillin allergy who received cefazolin had mild allergic reaction. No difference was observed in the rate of allergic reaction between patients with and without a history of penicillin allergy [32]. Bhathal et al. reported Cephalosporin prophylactic use in 597 surgeries of 544 patients with history of penicillin allergy. None of the patients experienced allergic reaction; data supported the use of cephalosporin surgical prophylaxis in patients with documented penicillin allergy [33].

For patients with demonstrated allergy to cephalosporin, a similar principle should be followed, i.e., for patients with a history of unverified nonanaphylactic cephalosporin allergy, penicillin can be administered without testing. For patients with history of anaphylaxis to cephalosporin, penicillin skin testing and drug challenge should be performed prior to administration of penicillin (Figs. 16.1, 16.2).

For patients with a history of penicillin or cephalosporin allergy, carbapenem may be administered without testing. For monobactams, patients with a history of penicillin or cephalosporin allergy can be administered without prior testing except ceftazidime (aztreonam and ceftazidime sharing identical R1 side chain).

Serum Sickness and Serum Sickness-Like Reaction: Serum sickness was first described by von Pirquet and Schick in 1905 that is a clinical syndrome triggered by equine serum serving as antitoxin [35]. Classic serum sickness results from antigen-antibody complex formation with foreign protein (serum) as antigen. Typical symptoms include fever, skin rash, edema, arthralgias, and lymphadenopathy. True serum sickness is rare in modern days due to the decline in need for foreign antisera. However, serum sickness-like reaction has been recognized due to reaction to non-protein drugs such as penicillins, cephalosporins sulfonamides, phenylbutazone, and thiazide. Generally, serum sickness-like reaction occurs 1 to 3 weeks after the start of administration of the medication. In previously sensitized patients, the reaction can begin as early as 12–36 h after exposure. Fever is the earliest and most common sign of serum sickness. Cutaneous eruptions such as urticaria and morbilliform rash are present in most affected patients. Arthralgia or arthritis is present in one third of the patients. Affected joints include knees, ankles, shoulders, elbows, wrists, low thoracic and cervical spine, and metacarpophalangeal, and temporomandibular joint. Lymphadenopathy, a typical presentation of serum sickness, is not noticed in response to oral penicillin. Other symptoms and signs including GI presentation (vomiting, diarrhea), splenomegaly, and rarely, hepatomegaly, may also be noted. The diagnosis of serum sickness-like reaction is made clinically with the constellation of symptoms and the relationship with non-protein drug within the

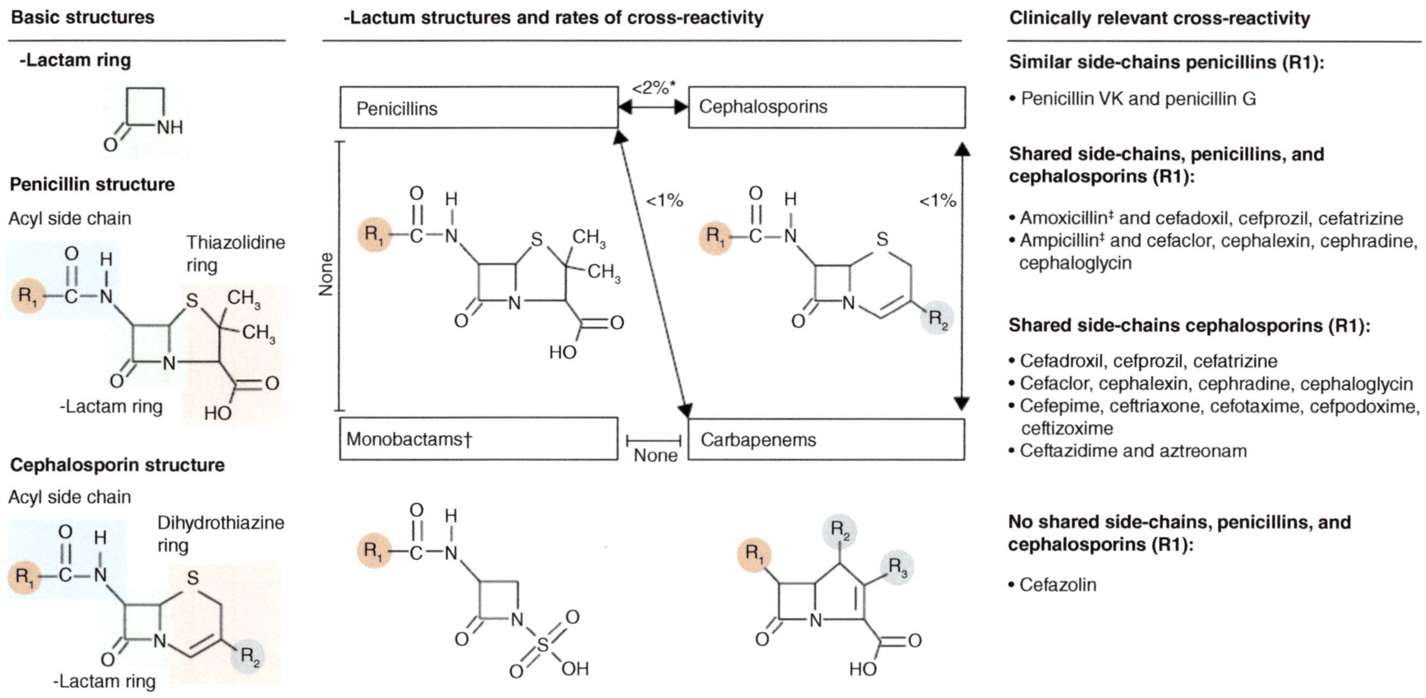

Fig. 16.1 Cross-reactivity between β-lactam antibiotics. Adapted from: Blumenthal. Antibiotic Allergy [34]

	Cephalosporin Parent Structure	Penicillin Parent Structure
	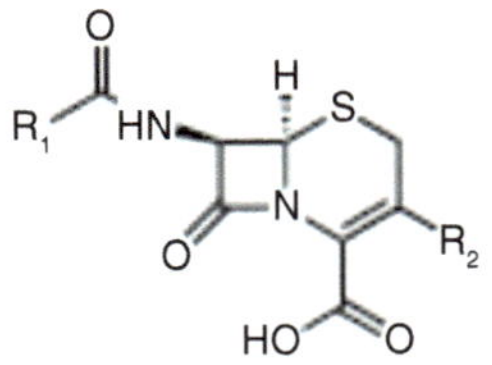	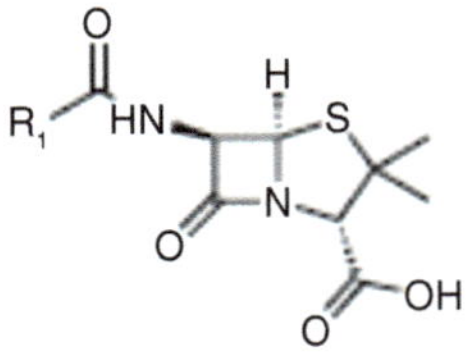
R1 Structure	Cephalosporins with denoted R1 moiety	Penicillins with denoted R1 moiety
Group 1 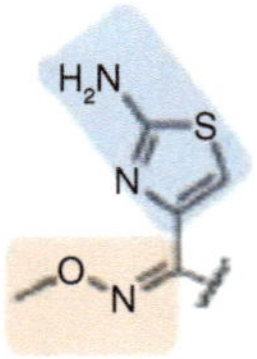	Ceftriaxone Cefotaxime Cefepime Cefpodoxime Cefditoren (may cross react with Group 2 & 3 Cephalosporins)	
Group 2 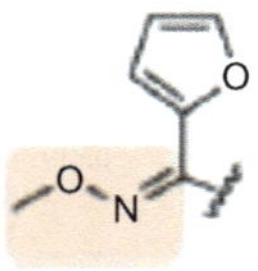	Cefuroxime (may cross react with Group 1 & 3 Cephalosporins)	
Group 3 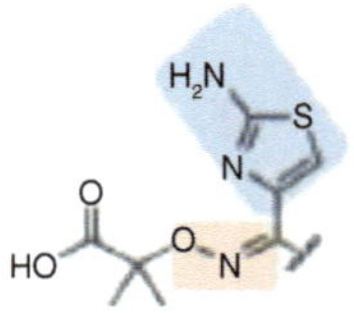	Ceftazidime (may cross react with Group 1 & Group 2 Cephalosporins)	Aztreonam

Fig. 16.2 Cephalosporins and penicillin antibiotics classified based on side chain similarity. Adapted from Khan. Drug Allergy: an updated practice parameter [31]

Group 4 A 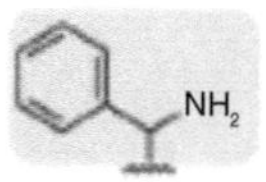	Cefaclor Cephalexin	Ampicillin
Group 4 B 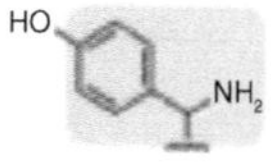	Cefadroxil Cefprozil	Amoxicillin
Group 5 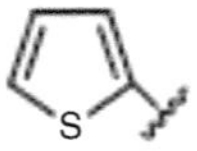	Cephalothin Cefoxitin	
Group 6 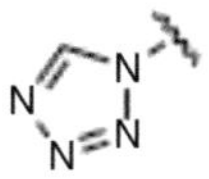	Cefazolin Ceftezole*	

Fig. 16.2 (continued)

proper time frame. Laboratory findings include reduction of serum C3 and C4, positive protein in urine analysis. C1q-binding assay and Raji cell radioimmunoassay are informative, but seldom used in clinical setting. The treatment of serum sickness-like reaction is supportive and anti-inflammatory. In mild cases, symptoms often resolve spontaneously in a few days after withdrawal of the culprit agent. In severe cases, non-steroidal anti-inflammatories and corticosteroids may be employed. Corticosteroids should be tapered over 2-week period [2, 36].

Cutaneous adverse drug reaction: Cutaneous adverse drug reaction (CADRs) are undesirable symptoms caused by a drug that affects skin and its adnexa (nails, hair, glands). CADRs can present with wide range of clinical symptoms from mild to moderate, self-limited cutaneous eruptions such as maculopapular exanthema to severe cutaneous adverse drug reactions (SCARs) such as Stevens-Johnson Syndrome (SJS)/Toxic Epidermal Necrolysis (TEN), Drug Reaction with Eosinophilia and Systemic Symptoms (DRESS), and Acute Generalized Exanthematous Pustulosis (AGEP). Antibiotics are the leading cause of SCARs, followed by anti-epileptic drugs, allopurinol, and NSAIDs (Fig. 16.3).

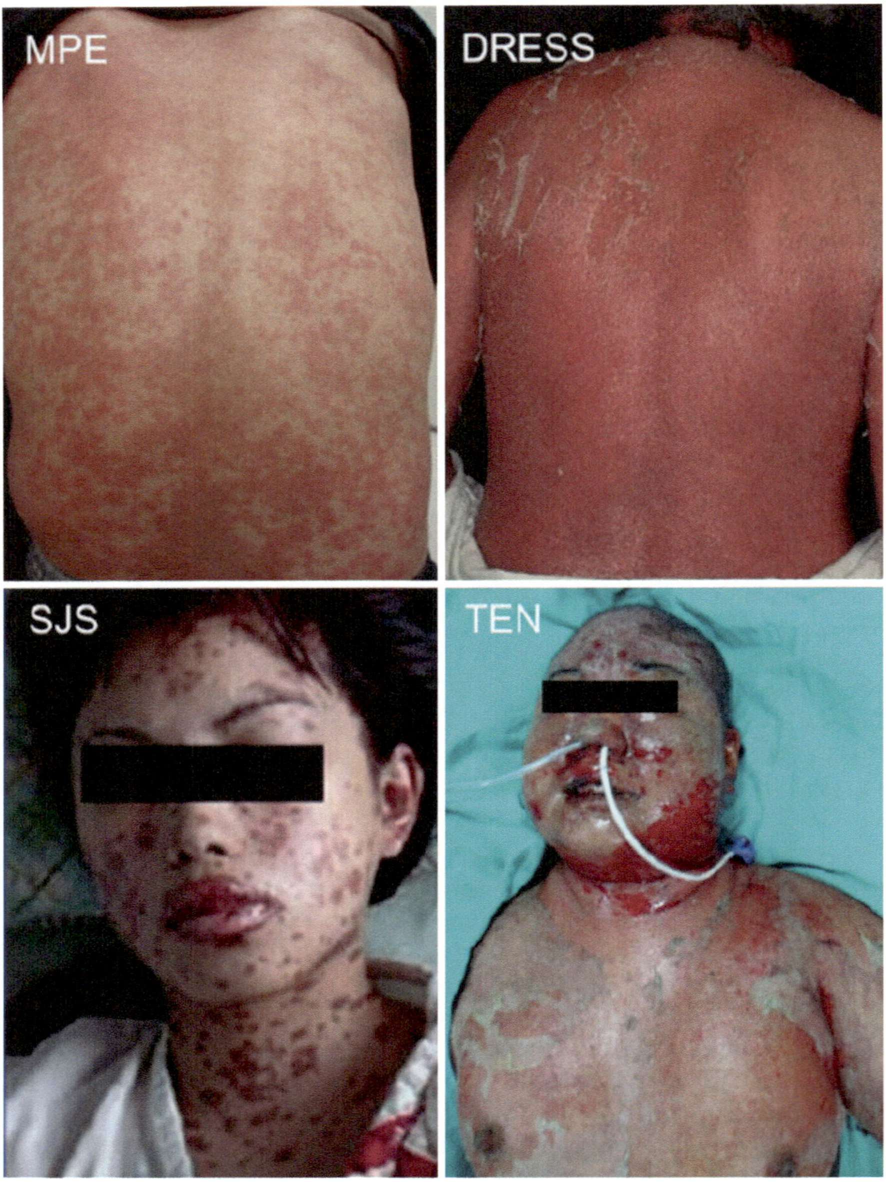

Fig. 16.3 Severe cutaneous adverse drug reactions. Adapted from Chung WH. J Dermatol [37]

Morbilliform or maculopapular drug reactions: Maculopapular exanthems are the most common presentation of CADRs. Rash usually begins 7–14 days after initiation of medication in non-sensitized patients. However, in previously sensitized patients, onset can be as soon as 6–12 h after drug intake. Maculopapular exanthems occur more frequently in patients with viral infections such as

Epstein-Barr virus (EBV) infections with incidence around 33% [38]. Clinically, patients present with diffuse, small, pink to red macules and papules start on trunk and progress to distal extremities with symmetrical distribution. The maculopapular exanthem is usually morbilliform and does not develop into blistering or sloughing of the skin. The rash usually resolves after 1–2 weeks with postinflammatory desquamation but without sequelae [39]. Most of such skin reactions are not severe or life-threatening. Treatment is symptomatic. If rash is mild and drug cannot be discontinued, it can continue with monitoring. Maculopapular drug reaction does not progress to severe SCADRs [40].

Stevens-Johnson Syndrome and Toxic Epidermal Necrolysis: Stevens-Johnson syndrome (SJS) was first described in 1922 by A.M. Stevens and F.C. Johnson. In 1956, A. Lyell coined the term "toxic epidermal necrolysis" (TEN). The current classification considers SJS and TEN as the same condition with different severity. SJS represents <10% of the body surface area (BSA) while TEN affects >30% of BSA. SJS/TEN overlap involves BSA between 10 and 30% [41]. SJS/TEN usually begins 4–28 days after the exposure to the drug. Initial manifestations include non-specific symptoms such as fever, malaise, headache, cough, and myalgias. These are followed by cutaneous lesions that start as erythematous, dark, purpuric macules in irregular shapes. Rash may evolve into two concentric rings with a necrotic center, as described as "target lesion." Pressing with a finger on erythematous area can result in skin detachment, a positive Nikolsky sign. More than 80% of patients will present with mucous membrane involvement. Lesions start with burning sensation of mucosal membranes (GI, GU, conjunctivae) followed by blisters that can rupture and become hemorrhagic erosions. In addition to cutaneous and mucosal membrane manifestations, patient often present with internal organ involvement such as liver, kidneys, bone marrow, lungs, and joints. Patients tend to develop secondary skin or systemic infections as a complication of SJS/TEN. The diagnosis of SJS is mainly based on history and classical mucocutaneous lesions. Skin biopsy will confirm the diagnosis. SJS/TEN is a serious systemic disease with high potential morbidity and mortality. A patient's risk of death can be assessed by using SCORTEN (TEN-specific severity of illness score) scale (Table 16.4).

Table 16.4 SCORTEN scoring system

Variable	Value
Age	>40 year
Malignancy	Present
Heart rate	>120/min
Body surface area involved at day 1	>10%
Serum BUN	>10 mg/dl
Serum bicarbonate	<20 mg/dl
Serum glucose	>14 mg/dl

Adapted from Guegan [42], one point is added for each positive variable. Mortality predicted as: 0–1 points = 3.2% mortality, 2 points = 12.1%, 3 points = 35.3%, 4–5 points = 83%, >5 points = 90%

Treatment of SJS/TEN is centered around intensive care similar to burn patients using multidisciplinary approach. The use of corticosteroid is controversial. However, other anti-inflammatory and immunomodulatory agents such as cyclosporine, cyclophosphamide, thalidomide, and IVIG have been employed to block the underlying immunological mechanism [43].

Drug reaction with eosinophilia and systemic syndrome (DRESS): DRESS is a rare, but serious hypersensitivity reaction with potential high mortality. The syndrome affects skin and internal organs such as liver, kidney, and heart. The pathogenesis is associated with patient's genetic makeup (HLA-B*1502, HLA-B*1508, HLA-B*5701, and HLA-B*5801), virus reactivation (HSV-6, HSV-7, CMV, and EBV), and characteristics of triggering medication [44, 45]. Antibiotics and antiepileptics are the most common drugs causing DRESS syndrome. Onset of symptoms usually is from 2 to 6 weeks after the initiation of treatment although a range between 3 and 105 days was reported [46]. The most common symptom is fever that usually is high grade (38–40 °C). The second most common feature is macular erythema rash that can progress to popular lesions. Lymphadenopathy is the third most common presentation. Leukocytosis and eosinophilia are common laboratory findings. Liver is the most common visceral organ involved in DRESS syndrome (about 50–60% of patients). It can present from mild elevation of LFT to severe fulminant hepatitis. Kidney is the second most common visceral organ involved in this syndrome with presentations from hematuria in mild case to nephritis in moderate form to acute renal failure in severe form [47]. Pulmonary involvement from mild cough to pneumonitis with acute respiratory distress syndrome has been reported. Muscle involvement can range from mild elevation of creatinine to myositis in moderate cases and rhabdomyolysis in severe cases. In severe cases, myocarditis and congestive heart failure can occur. Diagnosis is based on clinical presentations that involve multiple organs/systems. RegiSCAR is a simple and widely accepted scoring system to aid clinical decision-making. It is divided into definite (Score > 5), probable (Score 4–5), possible (Score 2–3), and not likely (Score < 2) for DRESS syndrome [48] (Table 16.5).

Treatment of DRESS is mainly supportive and symptom oriented. Antihistamine is used to treat pruritus. Systemic corticosteroid is recommended in patients with organ involvement such as liver, kidney, heart, and lungs. The course of steroid should be titrated until recovery of clinical symptoms and laboratory findings. For patients with severe hepatic damage, such as liver failure, liver transplant specialist needs to be consulted [49]. It has been reported that IVIG is beneficial in some patients with DRESS syndrome [50]. In patients with confirmed viral reactivation with severe symptoms, anti-viral agents (e.g., Ganciclovir) should be implemented in addition to IVIG. Cyclosporine can be considered in patient with organ involvement who fail to respond to a systemic corticosteroid.

Acute generalized exanthematous pustulosis (AGEP): AGEP that presents as generalized small nonfollicular sterile pustular skin rash with erythematous base with or without systemic symptoms, is one of the severe cutaneous adverse

Table 16.5 RegiSCAR system

Clinical manifestations	Scores					
	−1	0	1	2	Min.	Max.
General						
Fever ≥38.5° C	No/unknown	Yes	-	-	−1	0
Enlarged lymph nodes	-	No/unknown	Yes	-	0	1
Eosinophilia					0	2
Eosinophil count	-	No eosinophilia	0.7–1.49 x 10^9/L	≥1.5 x 10^9/L		
Eosinophil (%), if leukocyte count <4.0 × 10^9/L	-	-	10–19.9%	≥20%		
Atypical lymphocytes	-	No/unknown	Yes	-	0	1
Skin involvement					−2	2
Extent (% of body surface area)	-	No/unknown	>50%	-		
Skin rash suggesting DRESS	No	Unknown	Yes	-		
Skin biopsy suggesting DRESS	No	Yes/unknown	-	-		
Organ involvement (score 1: 1 organ involvement, score 2: ≥2 organs involvement)					0	2
Liver	-	No/unknown	Yes	-		
Kidney	-	No/unknown	Yes	-		
Lung	-	No/unknown	Yes	-		
Muscle/heart	-	No/unknown	Yes	-		
Pancreas	-	No/unknown	Yes	-		
Other organ	-	No/unknown	Yes	-		
Resolution ≥15 days	No/unknown	Yes	-	-	−1	0
Evaluation of other potential causes					0	1
(If none is positive and ≥3 of the following are negative)	-	-	Yes	-		
• Antinuclear antibody						
• Blood culture						
• Serology for hepatitis A/hepatitis B/hepatitis C						
• Chlamydia/mycoplasma						
Total score					**−4**	**9**

Max: maximum, min: minimum
Interpretation based on final score:
>5: definite, 4–5: probable, 2–3: possible, <2: no case

Adapted from Behera SK, Das S, Xavier AS, Selvarajan S. DRESS syndrome: a detailed insight [48]

reactions that was named by Beylot et al. in 1980. It is mediated by drug-specific T cells that induce apoptosis of keratinocytes, tissue destruction, and epidermal vesicle formation [51]. The onset of symptoms is usually within 48 h of drug intake. Patient may present with tens to hundreds of small, sterile, nonfollicular pustules on an erythematous base with no or minimal mucous membrane involvement. Fever and leukocytosis is common. It was reported 17% of the patients had organ involvement with liver, kidney, and lungs being the most common [52]. Hepatic involvement includes elevated liver enzymes, steatosis, and hepatomegaly. Pulmonary presentation includes pleural effusion and respiratory failure. Rarely, multiple organ dysfunction in AGEP may require ICU treatment [53]. Such multiple organ dysfunction is the cause of rare mortality in AGEP. After the causative drug is stopped, skin resolution typically occurs within a few days with desquamation over the affected area. Diagnosis of AGEP is mainly based on clinical presentation. Patch tests can be performed to confirm the culprit drug. A EuroSCAR scoring system was proposed in 2001. It is based on morphology of skin lesion, the presence of fever, the clinical course, and laboratory and histopathological findings [54] (Table 16.6).

The main treatment is discontinuation of the causative drug. Since most cases are benign with a self-limiting course, therapy is centered around supportive and symptomatic treatment. During the pustular phase, topical antiseptic solution could be used to prevent secondary infection. Topical steroid is used as anti-inflammatory therapy in prolonged cases. A short-term systemic steroid is used in some reports. However, it is considered as empirical as its effect in improving clinical course remains to be supported by randomized clinical studies [55].

Table 16.6 EuroSCAR scoring system

Morphology	
Pustules	
Typical[a]	+2
Compatible[b]	+1
Insufficient[c]	0
Erythema	
Typical	+2
Compatible	+1
Insufficient	0
Distribution/pattern	
Typical	+2
Compatible	+1
Insufficient	0
Postpustular desquamation	
Yes	+1
No/insufficient	+0
Course	
Mucosal involvement	
Yes	−2
No	0
Acute onset (≤10 d)	
Yes	0
No	−2
Resolution ≤15 days	
Yes	0
No	−4
Fever ≥38 °C	
Yes	+1
No	0
PNN ≥7000/mm^3	
Yes	+1
No	0
Histology	
Other disease	−10
Not representative/no histology	0
Exocytosis of PNN	+1
Subcorneal and/or intraepidermal *non* spongiform or NOS pustule(s) *with* papillary edema or subcorneal and/or intraepidermal *spongiform* or NOS pustule(s) *without* papillary edema (NOS=not otherwise specified)	+2
Spongiform subcorneal and/or intraepidermal pustule(s) *with* papillary edema	+3

Adapted from Sidoroff A. Acute generalized exanthematous pustulosis (AGEP) - A clinical reaction pattern [54]. Interpretation: 0: no AGEP, 1–4: possible, 5–7: probable, 8–12: definite

[a]Typical: typical morphology

[b]Compatible: not typical, but not strongly suggestive of other disease

[c]Insufficient: lesions can not be judged (mostly because of late stage of the disease or poor quality of pictures)

Answers and Discussion of Review Questions

1. A 60-year-old man presents with osteomyelitis. Infectious disease consultation recommends the use of Zosyn as treatment. Patient revealed that his mother told him that he developed rash after Amoxicillin treatment for ear infection when he was toddler. The characteristic of rash is not clear since his mother passed away 5 years ago. He has no received Penicillin or Amoxicillin because he was labeled as penicillin allergic. What is the best approach regarding antibiotic treatment for his osteomyelitis?

Amoxicillin often causes morbilliform kind of rash in pediatric population, particularly, when the patient has viral infection. This type of reaction is generally not allergic in nature. However, hives after penicillin family of antibiotics may indicate IgE-mediated drug allergy. Regarding Penicillin allergy, over time, patients tend to lose their sensitivity (about 10% per year). There, for low-risk patients like described in the question, it is reasonable to perform a single-dose challenge of the antibiotic under close monitoring. If tolerated, full course of treatment can follow.

2. A 30-year-old man developed wound infection after laceration on his right thumb. Urgent care facility placed him on Augmentin treatment. He previously tolerated Amoxicillin for bronchitis. The patient developed hives after 3 days of Augmentin treatment. Hives appeared first on face, then spread to trunk, arms, and legs within 12 h. By this time, wound culture grows Streptococcus. Sensitivity test shows sensitive to Ampicillin, Cephalexin, and Bactrim. His primary doctor stopped his Augmentin due to concern of Augmentin allergy. Patient reported that he developed skin rash after Bactrim when he was in college. In this case, can Cephalexin be used in this patient for wound treatment even if it is part of the β-lactam antibiotic category?

   Most allergic reaction to Penicillin is towards β-lactam core structure while allergy to cephalosporin is mainly mediated by side chain (R1 or R2). Therefore, in real practice, the cross-reactivity between Penicillin family and Cephalosporin antibiotics is very low (~1%). In general, it is safe to use cephalosporin in penicillin allergic patients.

3. A 45-year-old woman presents to the emergency department for fever, malaise, and a diffuse rash that almost completely covers her body. She reports that the symptoms started 4 weeks after she began to take Amoxicillin for strep throat. Your examination shows a diffuse, erythematous, maculopapular eruption, and facial swelling. There are no mucosal findings. Associated cervical lymphadenopathy and hepatomegaly are noted. Laboratory testing reveals peripheral eosinophilia. What is your diagnosis?

   The late onset, fever, skin rash, lymphadenopathy, and elevated eosinophilia are consistent with drug reaction with eosinophilia and systemic syndrome (DRESS). It is associated with viral reactivation (Typically HSV). Once diagnosed, the culprit medication should be promptly discontinued. Supportive and corticosteroid are cornerstones of treatment.

Summary

1. Penicillin allergy is a common claim in outpatient as well as inpatient settings. Most such patients can be delabeled through clinical evaluation including history, skin testing, and provocation of medication if necessary.
2. For true IgE-mediated β-Lactam allergic patients with clinical indication, desensitization can be performed.

3. Morbilliform type of rash is relatively common in patients with viral infection who receive Amoxicillin or Ampicillin treatment. If indicated, discontinuation of such antibiotics is not necessary.
4. Severe cutaneous drug reactions (SCADRs) to β-Lactam carry high morbidity and mortality. Early diagnosis and treatment is imperative. Reintroduction of β-Lactam antibiotics in such patients is contraindicated.

References

1. Castellani LR, Gold WL, MacFadden DR. A 25-year-old woman reporting an allergy to penicillin. CMAJ. 2015;187:1065–6.
2. Patterson-Fortin J, Harris CM, Niranjan-Azadi A, Melia M. Serum sickness-like reaction after the treatment of cellulitis with amoxicillin/clavulanate. BMJ Case Rep. 2016; https://doi.org/10.1136/bcr-2016-217608.
3. Song EK, Seon JK, Jeong MS. Delayed-type hypersensitivity reaction to piperacillin/tazobactam in a patient with an infected total knee replacement. J Bone Joint Surg Br. 2020;92:1596–9.
4. Lazarou J, Pomeranz BH, Corey PN. Incidence of adverse drug reactions in hospitalized patients: a meta-analysis of prospective studies. JAMA. 1998;279:1200–5.
5. Pichler WJ. Immune pathomechanism and classification of drug hypersensitivity. Allergy. 2019;74:1457–71.
6. Pichler WJ. Delayed drug hypersensitivity reactions. Ann Intern Med. 2003;139:683–93.
7. Bertram CM, Postelnick M, Mancini CM, Xiaoqing F, Zhang Y, Schulz LT, Bhowmick T, Lee F, Blumentha KG. Association of β-lactam allergy documentation and prophylactic antibiotic use in surgery: a National Cross-Sectional Study of hospitalized patients. Clin Infect Dis. 2021;72:e872–5.
8. VanderVelde KA, Suppes SL, Gibbs KA, Latz KH, Vanderpool AC, El Feghaly RE, Goldman JL. Increasing cefazolin use for surgical prophylaxis in penicillin-allergy-labeled patients. Antimicrob Steward Healthc Epidemiol. 2023;3:e11. https://doi.org/10.1017/ash.2022.360.
9. Stevoska S, Behm-Ferstl V, Zott S, Stadler C, Schieder S, Luger M, Gotterbarm T, Klasan A. The impact of patient-reported penicillin or cephalosporin allergy on the occurrence of the Periprosthetic joint infection in primary knee and hip arthroplasty. Antibiotics (Basel). 2022;11:1345.
10. Bahoravitch TJ, Jami M, Nayar SK, Agarwal A, Kreulen RT, Best MJ, Srikumaran U. Total shoulder arthroplasty: antibiotic allergies increase risk of postoperative complications. J Am Acad Orthop Surg. 2022;30(19):e1249–59. https://doi.org/10.5435/JAAOS-D-21-01167. Epub 2022 May 17
11. Blumenthal KG, Ryan EE, Li Y, Lee H, Kuhlen JL, Shenoy ES. The impact of a reported penicillin allergy on surgical site infection risk. Clin Infect Dis. 2018;66(3):329–36. https://doi.org/10.1093/cid/cix794. PMID: 29361015; PMCID: PMC5850334
12. Niu T, Zhang Y, Li Z, Bian Y, Zhang J, Wang Y. The association between penicillin allergy and surgical site infection after orthopedic surgeries: a retrospective cohort study. Front Cell Infect Microbiol. 2023;21(13):1182778. https://doi.org/10.3389/fcimb.2023.1182778. PMID: 37153141; PMCID: PMC10160653
13. Sogn DD, Evans R 3rd, Shepherd GM, Casale TB, Condemi J, Greenberger PA, Kohler PF, Saxon A, Summers RJ, VanArsdel PP Jr, et al. Results of the National Institute of Allergy and Infectious Diseases Collaborative Clinical Trial to test the predictive value of skin testing with major and minor penicillin derivatives in hospitalized adults. Arch Intern Med. 1992;152(5):1025–32.

14. Bull AL, Worth LJ, Richards MJ. Impact of vancomycin surgical antibiotic prophylaxis on the development of methicillin-sensitive staphylococcus aureus surgical site infections: report from Australian Surveillance Data (VICNISS). Ann Surg. 2012;256(6):1089–92. https://doi.org/10.1097/SLA.0b013e31825fa398.
15. Berríos-Torres SI, Yi SH, Bratzler DW, Ma A, Mu Y, Zhu L, Jernigan JA. Activity of commonly used antimicrobial prophylaxis regimens against pathogens causing coronary artery bypass graft and arthroplasty surgical site infections in the United States, 2006–2009. Infect Control Hosp Epidemiol. 2014;35(3):231–9. https://doi.org/10.1086/675289. Epub 2014 Jan 29
16. Yee J, Dixon CM, McLean AP, Meakins JL. Clostridium difficile disease in a department of surgery. The significance of prophylactic antibiotics. Arch Surg. 1991;126(2):241–6. https://doi.org/10.1001/archsurg.1991.01410260131019.
17. Castells M, Khan DA, Phillips EJ. Penicillin allergy. Reply. N Engl J Med. 2020;382(14):1380. https://doi.org/10.1056/NEJMc2000115.
18. Banerji A, Solensky R, Phillips EJ, Khan DA. Drug allergy practice parameter updates to incorporate into your clinical practice. J Allergy Clin Immunol Pract. 2023;11(2):356–368.e5. https://doi.org/10.1016/j.jaip.2022.12.002. Epub 2022 Dec 20
19. Wang Z, Shaker M, Hsu BK. Pearls for practice from the 2022 joint task force drug allergy practice parameter. Curr Opin Pediatr. 2023;35(3):368–79. https://doi.org/10.1097/MOP.0000000000001240. Epub 2023 Mar 17
20. Sousa-Pinto B, Tarrio I, Blumenthal KG, Araújo L, Azevedo LF, Delgado L, Fonseca JA. Accuracy of penicillin allergy diagnostic tests: a systematic review and meta-analysis. J Allergy Clin Immunol. 2021;147(1):296–308. https://doi.org/10.1016/j.jaci.2020.04.058. Epub 2020 May 21. PMID: 32446963; PMCID: PMC8019189
21. Solensky R, Jacobs J, Lester M, Lieberman P, McCafferty F, Nilsson T, Park M, Schwarz G, Soong W, Wagelie-Steffen A, Wedner HJ, Weiss M, Windom H, Tonascia J, Yates KP, Mendelson LM, Wolfe J, Adkinson NF. Penicillin allergy evaluation: a prospective, multi-center, open-label evaluation of a comprehensive penicillin skin test kit. J Allergy Clin Immunol Pract. 2019;7(6):1876–1885.e3. https://doi.org/10.1016/j.jaip.2019.02.040. Epub 2019 Mar 13
22. Adkinson NF Jr, Thompson WL, Maddrey WC, Lichtenstein LM. Routine use of penicillin skin testing on an inpatient service. N Engl J Med. 1971;285(1):22–4. https://doi.org/10.1056/NEJM197107012850104.
23. Patterson RA, Stankewicz HA. Penicillin allergy (2022 Jun 23). In: StatPearls [Internet]. Treasure Island (FL): StatPearls Publishing; 2023.
24. Yates AB. Management of patients with a history of allergy to beta-lactam antibiotics. Am J Med. 2008;121(7):572–6. https://doi.org/10.1016/j.amjmed.2007.12.005.
25. Phillips EJ, Bigliardi P, Bircher AJ, Broyles A, Chang YS, Chung WH, Lehloenya R, Mockenhaupt M, Peter J, Pirmohamed M, Roujeau JC, Shear NH, Tanno LK, Trubiano J, Valluzzi R, Barbaud A. Controversies in drug allergy: testing for delayed reactions. J Allergy Clin Immunol. 2019;143(1):66–73. https://doi.org/10.1016/j.jaci.2018.10.030. Epub 2018 Dec 17. PMID: 30573342; PMCID: PMC6429556
26. Dash CH. Penicillin allergy and the cephalosporins. J Antimicrob Chemother. 1975;1(3 Suppl):107–18. https://doi.org/10.1093/jac/1.suppl_3.107.
27. Petz LD. Immunologic reactions of humans to cephalosporins. Postgrad Med J. 1971;47(Suppl):64–9.
28. Bratzler DW, Dellinger EP, Olsen KM, Perl TM, Auwaerter PG, Bolon MK, Fish DN, Napolitano LM, Sawyer RG, Slain D, Steinberg JP, Weinstein RA, American Society of Health-System Pharmacists; Infectious Disease Society of America; Surgical Infection Society; Society for Healthcare Epidemiology of America. Clinical practice guidelines for antimicrobial prophylaxis in surgery. Am J Health Syst Pharm. 2013;70(3):195–283. https://doi.org/10.2146/ajhp120568.

29. Stone CA Jr, Trubiano J, Coleman DT, Rukasin CRF, Phillips EJ. The challenge of de-labeling penicillin allergy. Allergy. 2020;75(2):273–88. https://doi.org/10.1111/all.13848. Epub 2019 May 26. PMID: 31049971; PMCID: PMC6824919
30. Khan DA, Banerji A, Bernstein JA, Bilgicer B, Blumenthal K, Castells M, Ein D, Lang DM, Phillips E. Cephalosporin allergy: current understanding and future challenges. J Allergy Clin Immunol Pract. 2019;7(7):2105–14. https://doi.org/10.1016/j.jaip.2019.06.001. PMID: 31495420; PMCID: PMC6955146
31. Joint Task Force on Practice Parameters; American Academy of Allergy, Asthma and Immunology; American College of Allergy, Asthma and Immunology; Joint Council of Allergy, Asthma and Immunology. Drug allergy: an updated practice parameter. Ann Allergy Asthma Immunol. 2010;105(4):259–73. https://doi.org/10.1016/j.anai.2010.08.002.
32. Kurcz BP, Allan DG, Nestler AJ, Lister EL, Yarnell WC, Delfino KR, Thuppal S, Horberg JV. Documented penicillin allergies should not preclude use of preoperative cefazolin in hip and knee arthroplasty. J Am Acad Orthop Surg. 2023;31(2):e107–17. https://doi.org/10.5435/JAAOS-D-22-00122.
33. Bhathal S, Joseph E, Nailor MD, Goodlet KJ. Adherence and outcomes of a surgical prophylaxis guideline promoting cephalosporin use among patients with penicillin allergy. Surgery. 2022;172(6):1598–603. https://doi.org/10.1016/j.surg.2022.01.020. Epub 2022 Feb 17
34. Blumenthal KG, Peter JG, Trubiano JA, Phillips EJ. Antibiotic allergy. Lancet. 2019;393(10167):183–98. https://doi.org/10.1016/S0140-6736(18)32218-9. Epub 2018 Dec 14. PMID: 30558872; PMCID: PMC6563335
35. von Pirquet CE. Allergy. Arch Intern Med. 1911;7:383–436.
36. Tatum AJ, Ditto AM, Patterson R. Severe serum sickness-like reaction to oral penicillin drugs: three case reports. Ann Allergy Asthma Immunol. 2001;86(3):330–4. https://doi.org/10.1016/S1081-1206(10)63308-X.
37. Chung WH, Wang CW, Dao RL. Severe cutaneous adverse drug reactions. J Dermatol. 2016;43(7):758–66. https://doi.org/10.1111/1346-8138.13430. Epub 2016 May 6
38. Chovel-Sella A, Ben Tov A, Lahav E, Mor O, Rudich H, Paret G, Reif S. Incidence of rash after amoxicillin treatment in children with infectious mononucleosis. Pediatrics. 2013;131(5):e1424–7. https://doi.org/10.1542/peds.2012-1575. Epub 2013 Apr 15
39. Bircher AJ. Uncomplicated drug-induced disseminated exanthemas. Chem Immunol Allergy. 2012;97:79–97. https://doi.org/10.1159/000335617. Epub 2012 May 3
40. Noguera-Morel L, Hernández-Martín Á, Torrelo A. Cutaneous drug reactions in the pediatric population. Pediatr Clin N Am. 2014;61(2):403–26. https://doi.org/10.1016/j.pcl.2013.12.001. Epub 2014 Jan 28
41. Bastuji-Garin S, Rzany B, Stern RS, Shear NH, Naldi L, Roujeau JC. Clinical classification of cases of toxic epidermal necrolysis, Stevens-Johnson syndrome, and erythema multiforme. Arch Dermatol. 1993;129(1):92–6.
42. Guégan S, Bastuji-Garin S, Poszepczynska-Guigné E, Roujeau JC, Revuz J. Performance of the SCORTEN during the first five days of hospitalization to predict the prognosis of epidermal necrolysis. J Invest Dermatol. 2006;126(2):272–6. https://doi.org/10.1038/sj.jid.5700068.
43. Viard I, Wehrli P, Bullani R, Schneider P, Holler N, Salomon D, Hunziker T, Saurat JH, Tschopp J, French LE. Inhibition of toxic epidermal necrolysis by blockade of CD95 with human intravenous immunoglobulin. Science. 1998;282(5388):490–3. https://doi.org/10.1126/science.282.5388.490.
44. Hung SI, Chung WH, Jee SH, Chen WC, Chang YT, Lee WR, Hu SL, Wu MT, Chen GS, Wong TW, Hsiao PF, Chen WH, Shih HY, Fang WH, Wei CY, Lou YH, Huang YL, Lin JJ, Chen YT. Genetic susceptibility to carbamazepine-induced cutaneous adverse drug reactions. Pharmacogenet Genomics. 2006;16(4):297–306. https://doi.org/10.1097/01.fpc.0000199500.46842.4a.
45. Tohyama M, Hashimoto K, Yasukawa M, Kimura H, Horikawa T, Nakajima K, Urano Y, Matsumoto K, Iijima M, Shear NH. Association of human herpesvirus 6 reactivation

with the flaring and severity of drug-induced hypersensitivity syndrome. Br J Dermatol. 2007;157(5):934–40. https://doi.org/10.1111/j.1365-2133.2007.08167.x. Epub 2007 Sep 13
46. Um SJ, Lee SK, Kim YH, Kim KH, Son CH, Roh MS, Lee MK. Clinical features of drug-induced hypersensitivity syndrome in 38 patients. J Investig Allergol Clin Immunol. 2010;20(7):556–62.
47. Kumari R, Timshina DK, Thappa DM. Drug hypersensitivity syndrome. Indian J Dermatol Venereol Leprol. 2011;77(1):7–15. https://doi.org/10.4103/0378-6323.74964.
48. Behera SK, Das S, Xavier AS, Selvarajan S. DRESS syndrome: a detailed insight. Hosp Pract (1995). 2018;46(3):152–62. https://doi.org/10.1080/21548331.2018.1451205. Epub 2018 Mar 15
49. Descamps V, Ben Saïd B, Sassolas B, Truchetet F, Avenel-Audran M, Girardin P, Guinnepain MT, Mathelier-Fusade P, Assier H, Milpied B, Modiano P, Lebrun-Vignes B, Barbaud A, groupe Toxidermies de la Société française de dermatologie. Prise en charge du drug reaction with eosinophilia and systemic symptoms (DRESS) [Management of drug reaction with eosinophilia and systemic symptoms (DRESS)]. Ann Dermatol Venereol. 2010;137(11):703–8. https://doi.org/10.1016/j.annder.2010.04.024. French, Epub 2010 Aug 5
50. Singer EM, Wanat KA, Rosenbach MA. A case of recalcitrant DRESS syndrome with multiple autoimmune sequelae treated with intravenous immunoglobulins. JAMA Dermatol. 2013;149(4):494–5. https://doi.org/10.1001/jamadermatol.2013.1949.
51. Schmid S, Kuechler PC, Britschgi M, Steiner UC, Yawalkar N, Limat A, Baltensperger K, Braathen L, Pichler WJ. Acute generalized exanthematous pustulosis: role of cytotoxic T cells in pustule formation. Am J Pathol. 2002;161(6):2079–86. https://doi.org/10.1016/S0002-9440(10)64486-0. PMID: 12466124; PMCID: PMC1850901
52. Hotz C, Valeyrie-Allanore L, Haddad C, Bouvresse S, Ortonne N, Duong TA, Ingen-Housz-Oro S, Roujeau JC, Wolkenstein P, Chosidow O. Systemic involvement of acute generalized exanthematous pustulosis: a retrospective study on 58 patients. Br J Dermatol. 2013;169(6):1223–32. https://doi.org/10.1111/bjd.12502.
53. Mohyuddin GR, Al Asad M, Scratchko L, Khaleeq G. Acute generalized exanthematous pustulosis with multiple organ dysfunction syndrome. Am J Crit Care. 2013;22(3):270–3. https://doi.org/10.4037/ajcc2013987.
54. Sidoroff A, Halevy S, Bavinck JN, Vaillant L, Roujeau JC. Acute generalized exanthematous pustulosis (AGEP)--a clinical reaction pattern. J Cutan Pathol. 2001;28(3):113–9. https://doi.org/10.1034/j.1600-0560.2001.028003113.x.
55. Buettiker U, Keller M, Pichler WJ, Braathen LR, Yawalkar N. Oral prednisolone induced acute generalized exanthematous pustulosis due to corticosteroids of group a confirmed by epicutaneous testing and lymphocyte transformation tests. Dermatology. 2006;213(1):40–3. https://doi.org/10.1159/000092837.

Index

W. A. Zuelzer, S. Metikala (eds.), *Unusual Conditions That Every Orthopaedic Surgeon Should Know*, https://doi.org/10.1007/978-3-031-58946-1

GPSR Compliance

The European Union's (EU) General Product Safety Regulation (GPSR) is a set of rules that requires consumer products to be safe and our obligations to ensure this.

If you have any concerns about our products, you can contact us on ProductSafety@springernature.com

In case Publisher is established outside the EU, the EU authorized representative is:

Springer Nature Customer Service Center GmbH
Europaplatz 3
69115 Heidelberg, Germany

Batch number: 09336662

Printed by Printforce, the Netherlands